T0188435

Haematology

Haematology

From the Image to the Diagnosis

Mike Leach MB ChB, FRCP, FRCPath
Consultant Haematologist and Honorary Senior Lecturer
Haematology Laboratories and West of Scotland Cancer Centre
Gartnavel General Hospital, Glasgow, UK

Barbara J. Bain MB BS, FRACP, FRCPath
Professor of Diagnostic Haematology
St Mary's Hospital Campus, Imperial College London
and Honorary Consultant Haematologist
St Mary's Hospital, London, UK

There is always more to learn – the study of haematology is a constant journey, not a destination

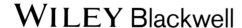

Registered Offices
John Wiley & Sons, Inc., 111 River Street, Hoboken, NJ 07030, USA
John Wiley & Sons Ltd, The Atrium, Southern Gate, Chichester, West Sussex, PO19 8SQ, UK

Editorial Office
9600 Garsington Road, Oxford, OX4 2DQ, UK

For details of our global editorial offices, customer services, and more information about Wiley products visit us at www.wiley.com.

Wiley also publishes its books in a variety of electronic formats and by print-on-demand. Some content that appears in standard print versions of this book may not be available in other formats.

Library of Congress Cataloging-in-Publication Data

Names: Leach, Richard M. (Haematologist), author. | Bain, Barbara J.,
    author.
Title: Haematology : from the image to the diagnosis / Mike Leach, Barbara
    J. Bain.
Description: Hoboken, NJ : Wiley-Blackwell, 2022. | Includes
    bibliographical references and index.
Identifiers: LCCN 2021010953 (print) | LCCN 2021010954 (ebook) | ISBN
    9781119777502 (hardback) | ISBN 9781119777519 (adobe pdf) | ISBN
    9781119777526 (epub)
Subjects: MESH: Hematologic Diseases–diagnosis | Blood Physiological
    Phenomena | Examination Questions | Case Reports
Classification: LCC RC636 (print) | LCC RC636 (ebook) | NLM WH 18.2 |
    DDC 616.1/5–dc23
LC record available at https://lccn.loc.gov/2021010953
LC ebook record available at https://lccn.loc.gov/2021010954

Cover Design: Wiley
Cover Image: © Mike Leach

Set in 9.5/12.5pt STIXTwoText by Straive, Pondicherry, India

Printed in Singapore
M114550_180621

Contents

Preface

Despite the tremendous advances that have occurred in diagnostic haematopathology in recent decades, haematology remains firmly based on a clinical assessment of the patient, on basic laboratory tests and on a critical assessment of peripheral blood and bone marrow films. In this book we seek to show how an appreciation of blood and bone marrow morphology, assessed with knowledge of the clinical context, can lead to a provisional or, sometimes, a definitive diagnosis that guides further investigation and management. Each of the 101 themes is followed by a related multiple choice question with the preferred answers and further discussion being found in the second part of the book. The multiple choice questions can have more than one true answer. The themes are sometimes single cases and sometimes a composite of related cases. The book is directed at consultants and trainees in haematology and haematopathology and at clinical and biomedical scientists in these disciplines. We hope that readers will share our enjoyment of the constant sense of discovery that accompanies haematological morphology.

All magnifications are stated in terms of the objective used. Common abbreviations that may be used without definition are given on page xi. Other abbreviations are defined on first use in a theme. All images are of films stained with a May–Grünwald–Giemsa stain unless stated otherwise. The cases are not arranged thematically, since a more random arrangement better approximates to real life.

We wish to thank our clinical and laboratory colleagues with whom we have collaborated over many years.

Mike Leach and Barbara Bain, January 2021

Abbreviations

Full blood count (FBC) components

WBC	white blood cell count
RBC	red blood cell count
Hb	haemoglobin concentration
Hct	haematocrit
MCV	mean cell volume
MCH	mean cell haemoglobin
MCHC	mean cell haemoglobin concentration

Others

AA	aplastic anaemia
AL	acute leukaemia
ALK	anaplastic lymphoma kinase
ALL	acute lymphoblastic leukaemia
ALP	alkaline phosphatase
ALT	alanine transaminase
AML	acute myeloid leukaemia
ANA	antinuclear antibody
APL	acute promyelocytic leukaemia
APTT	activated partial thromboplastin time
AST	aspartate transaminase
ATLL	adult T-cell leukaemia/lymphoma
BL	Burkitt lymphoma
c	cytoplasmic
CD	cluster of differentiation
CHOP	cyclophosphamide, doxorubicin, vincristine and prednisolone
CLL	chronic lymphocytic leukaemia
CML	chronic myeloid leukaemia
CMML	chronic myelomonocytic leukaemia
CNS	central nervous system
CRP	C-reactive protein
CSF	cerebrospinal fluid
CT	computed tomography

DIC	disseminated intravascular coagulation
DLBCL	diffuse large B-cell lymphoma
DNA	deoxyribonucleic acid
EBV	Epstein–Barr virus
ESR	erythrocyte sedimentation rate
ET	essential thrombocythaemia
FISH	fluorescence *in situ* hybridisation
FDG	fluorodeoxyglucose
FL	follicular lymphoma
GP	general practitioner
H&E	haematoxylin and eosin (stain)
HCL	hairy cell leukaemia
HL	Hodgkin lymphoma
HLA-DR	human leukocyte antigen DR
HTLV-1	human T-cell lymphotropic virus type 1
Ig	immunoglobulin
IgA	immunoglobulin A
IgG	immunoglobulin G
IgM	immunoglobulin M
iu	international unit
LBL	lymphoblastic lymphoma
LDH	lactate dehydrogenase
LGL	large granular lymphocyte
LPD	lymphoproliferative disorder
MCL	mantle cell lymphoma
MDS	myelodysplastic syndrome
MDS/MPN	myelodysplastic/myeloproliferative neoplasm
M:E	myeloid:erythroid
MGG	May–Grünwald–Giemsa (stain)
MPN	myeloproliferative neoplasm
MPO	myeloperoxidase
MRI	magnetic resonance imaging
NLPHL	nodular lymphocyte predominant Hodgkin lymphoma
NR	normal range
NRBC	nucleated red blood cells
PET	positron emission tomography
PCR	polymerase chain reaction
PRCA	pure red cell aplasia
PT	prothrombin time
R-CHOP	rituximab, cyclophosphamide, doxorubicin, vincristine and prednisolone
RNA	ribonucleic acid
RS	Reed–Sternberg
SLE	systemic lupus erythematosus
T-ALL	T-lymphoblastic leukaemia
TdT	terminal deoxynucleotidyl transferase
T-LBL	T-lymphoblastic lymphoma
TT	thrombin time
u	unit
WM	Waldenström macroglobulinaemia

Normal ranges for commonly used tests (for adults)

FBC and differential count

	Males	Females
WBC ($\times 10^9$/l)	3.7–9.5	3.9–11.1
RBC ($\times 10^{12}$/l)	4.32–5.66	3.88–4.99
Hb (g/l)	133–167	118–148
MCV (fl)	82–98	
MCH (pg)	27.3–32.6	
MCHC (g/l)	316–349	
Neutrophils ($\times 10^9$/l)	1.7–6.1	1.7–7.5
Lymphocytes ($\times 10^9$/l)	1.0–3.2	
Monocytes ($\times 10^9$/l)	0.2–0.6	
Eosinophils ($\times 10^9$/l)	0.03–0.46	
Basophils ($\times 10^9$/l)	0.2–0.29	
Platelets ($\times 10^9$/l)	143–332	169–358

From Bain BJ (2017) *A Beginner's Guide to Blood Cells*, 3rd Edn. Wiley Blackwell, Oxford.

Coagulation tests

Prothrombin time	9–13 s
Activated partial thromboplastin time	27–38 s
Thrombin time	11–15 s
Fibrinogen	2–4.5 g/l
D dimer	<230 ng/ml

Other tests

Albumin	35–50 g/l
Ferritin	15–300 µg/l (males); 14–200 µg/l (females)
Bilirubin	1–20 µmol/l
Alanine transaminase	0–50 u/l
Aspartate transaminase	0–40 u/l
Alkaline phosphatase	30–130 u/l
C-reactive protein	<5 mg/l
Erythrocyte sedimentation rate	<10 mm in 1 h (males); <20 mm in 1 h (females)

Haematology

From the Image to the Diagnosis

1 Anaplastic large cell lymphoma with haemophagocytic syndrome

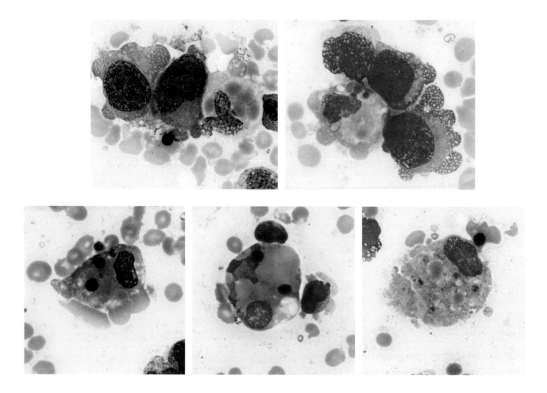

A 50-year-old man from another health board was transferred to a local hospital for a surgical biopsy of a mediastinal lymph node. He had presented 6 weeks previously with fever, sweats and weight loss. No infective or neoplastic aetiology had been identified. He had progressive pancytopenia and hyperferritinaemia and a diagnosis of idiopathic haemophagocytic syndrome had been considered. He had already been treated at the base hospital with corticosteroids and etoposide. CT imaging, however, had shown abnormal mediastinal lymph nodes, which would not have been accessible by percutaneous needle biopsy.

On arrival at the local cardiothoracic unit he was clearly unwell. The full blood count showed Hb 90 g/l, WBC 2.5 × 10^9/l, neutrophils 1.5 × 10^9/l and platelets 25 × 10^9/l. The coagulation screen showed PT 18 s, APTT 45 s, TT 18 s, fibrinogen 1.4 g/l and D dimer 5500 ng/ml (NR <230). Serum ferritin was >10 000 μg/l. The anaesthetic team phoned to ask for advice regarding management of the coagulopathy prior to surgery. The blood film showed rouleaux and was leucoerythroblastic with a few toxic granulated neutrophils but no neoplastic cell population was evident. We decided to cancel the surgery, review the imaging and perform a bone marrow aspirate and trephine biopsy. A CT scan showed definitely pathological mediastinal lymph nodes. The bone marrow aspirate showed a population of very large lymphoid cells with round or ovoid nuclei, indistinct nucleoli and partially condensed nuclear chromatin without cytoplasmic granules (top images). The cytoplasm of these cells showed prominent vacuolation, often concentrated in apparent pseudopodia (top images). In addition, there was a substantial population of macrophages showing haemophagocytosis, particularly of red cells and their precursors (all images above ×100 objective).

Haematology: From the Image to the Diagnosis, First Edition. Mike Leach and Barbara J. Bain.
© 2022 John Wiley & Sons Ltd. Published 2022 by John Wiley & Sons Ltd.

The clinical, laboratory and morphological findings were in keeping with a haemophagocytic syndrome. Flow cytometry on the large cell population in the marrow aspirate showed these cells to express CD45, CD2, CD3, CD4 and CD30. No myeloid or B-lineage antigens were expressed. The bone marrow trephine biopsy sections were also abnormal, showing prominent macrophages displaying haemophagocytosis on H&E staining (below, left image) and CD68R (below, centre image, immunoperoxidase), whilst the large neoplastic cells were highlighted using CD30 (below, right, immunoperoxidase) (all images below ×50). Immunohistochemistry showed the large cells to be ALK negative. The diagnosis was now confirmed as ALK-negative anaplastic large cell lymphoma. The patient was transferred back to his local hospital with a view to commencing CHOP chemotherapy but after one cycle of treatment he deteriorated further and sadly died.

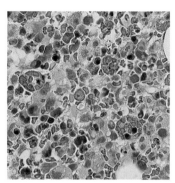 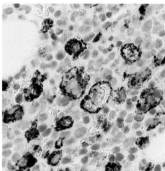 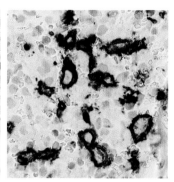

Haemophagocytic syndrome is a rare constellation of clinicopathological features including fever, weight loss, sweats and organomegaly, together with laboratory abnormalities including cytopenias, hyperferritinaemia, hypertriglyceridaemia, coagulopathy and bone marrow haemophagocytosis. Interestingly, according to strict diagnostic criteria, and despite the name, demonstration of the latter is not absolutely essential. In adults the typical triggers for a confirmed haemophagocytic syndrome are infective or neoplastic. In adult patients a neoplastic cause is very likely and high-grade T-cell and NK-cell neoplasms are the usual culprits. In paediatric practice there are a number of inherited immunodeficiency syndromes that strongly predispose to a haemophagocytic syndrome, but neoplastic and infective triggers similar to the above have also to be considered. It is absolutely essential to consider a neoplastic cause in adult patients; this focuses attention on looking for an underlying neoplasm with subsequent targeted treatment, in which case the haemophagocytic syndrome will gradually resolve.

MCQ

ALK-negative anaplastic large cell lymphoma:

1 Generally occurs at an older age than ALK-positive cases
2 Has a better prognosis than ALK-positive anaplastic large cell lymphoma
3 Has similar histological and immunophenotypic features to breast implant-associated anaplastic large cell lymphoma
4 Is usually associated with t(2;5)(p23.2-23.1;q35.1)
5 Usually presents with localised disease

For answers and discussion, see page 206.

2   Bone marrow AL amyloidosis

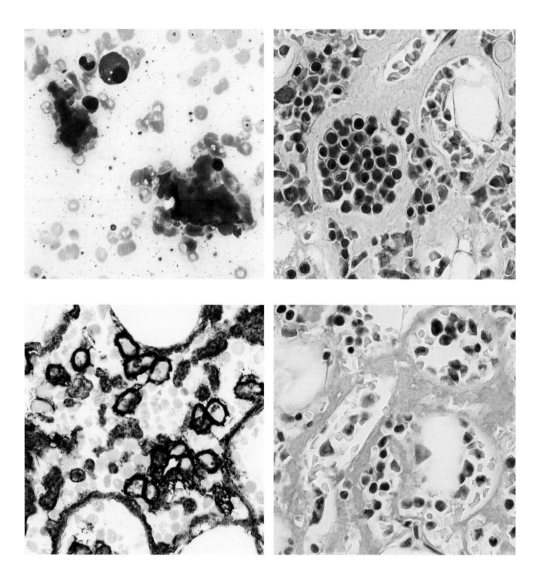

A 47-year-old man presented with peripheral oedema due to nephrotic syndrome and a kidney biopsy was planned. Full blood count showed Hb 154 g/l, WBC 7.8×10^9/l and platelets 355×10^9/l. Serum creatinine was 136 µmol/l, estimated glomerular filtration rate (eGFR) 49 ml/min/1.73 m^2, albumin 17 g/l and urine protein 5.4 g/l. A serum IgA lambda paraprotein (9 g/l) and excess serum free lambda light chains at 103.5 mg/l (NR 5.7–26.3) were identified.

A bone marrow aspirate identified deposits of amorphous, purple-staining material suggestive of amyloid protein (top left image) (all images ×50 objective). The trephine biopsy sections showed diffuse eosinophilic amorphous material (top right, H&E) in keeping with amyloid deposited around fat cells, around erythroid islands, in the walls of small vessels and throughout the interstitium. Immunohistochemistry for CD138 revealed 7% plasma cells with non-specific binding to the amyloid deposits (bottom left, immunoperoxidase) the latter deposits staining also with Sirius red (bottom right). These findings are indicative of extensive bone marrow amyloid deposition due to primary AL amyloidosis. In view of these findings the renal biopsy was now not deemed necessary.

This case illustrates the striking morphological abnormalities encountered in amyloidosis; accurate recognition of these features is important in bringing together a unified clinical diagnosis.

A second patient presented with back pain and vertebral collapse. MRI suggested a marrow infiltrative disease such as myeloma. Indeed, he was shown to have raised serum free lambda light chains (367 mg/l) but no paraprotein was detected. The bone marrow aspirate, however, was hypocellular and showed low level (<1%) involvement by plasma cells so the diagnosis was questioned. The trephine biopsy sections showed heavy involvement by AL amyloidosis (all images below, H&E, left ×10, centre and right ×50) occupying well over 80% of the marrow space, with notable involvement of vessel walls. In the cellular areas well over 90% of cells were neoplastic plasma cells. Elsewhere small pockets of malignant plasma cells were identified (below centre). Extensive bone marrow amyloidosis can influence accurate assessment of plasma cell populations and can delay accurate diagnosis.

 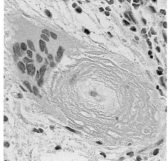 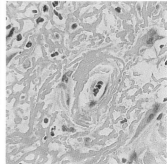

MCQ

Amyloid in tissue sections can be identified by positive staining with:

1 Congo red
2 Martius scarlet blue
3 Methenamine silver
4 Prussian blue
5 Sirius red

For answers and discussion, see page 206.

3 Cup-like blast morphology in acute myeloid leukaemia

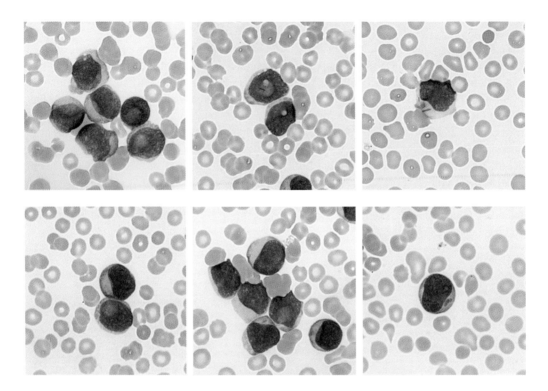

A 54-year-old woman attended Accident and Emergency with fever, progressive facial pain and bleeding following a tooth extraction 1 week previously. On examination she was systemically unwell and febrile with features of a deep perimandibular soft tissue/tooth socket infection. She had prominent widespread bruising. The full blood count showed Hb 106 g/l, WBC 291 × 10⁹/l, neutrophils 0.7 × 10⁹/l and platelets 49 × 10⁹/l. A coagulation screen showed PT 13 s, APTT 30 s, thrombin time 12.4 s, fibrinogen 1.0 g/l and D dimer 14 059 ng/ml (NR <230). The blood film showed a large population of myeloid blasts. Many of them displayed deep nuclear invaginations (cup-like morphology) as shown centrally (top left and centre, bottom left and centre) or indenting one side of the nucleus (top left, bottom left and centre) (all images ×100 objective). Some blasts showed small but well-defined nucleoli (top left, top right and bottom right). There was fine cytoplasmic granulation in some cells and some had Auer rods (top centre and right) whilst a small proportion had pseudo-Chédiak–Higashi granules (top right, bottom right). The blasts had a CD34−, HLA-DR−, CD117+, CD13+, CD33+, CD15−, CD14−, CD64+ and MPO+ immunophenotype resembling that often seen in acute promyelocytic leukaemia (APL), but the morphological features were not consistent with this diagnosis. T- and B-lineage markers were not expressed. The karyotype was normal but both *NPM1* and *FLT3* were mutated with *FLT3* showing an internal tandem duplication (*FLT3*-ITD).

The clinical presentation here of an acute myeloid leukaemia with bleeding, bruising and coagulopathy together with a CD34−, HLA-DR−, pan-myeloid+, CD64+ immunophenotype should lead to consideration of APL as management of this entity clearly differs from that of other AML subtypes. However, a thoughtful examination of the blood film suggests an alternative diagnosis.

Haematology: From the Image to the Diagnosis, First Edition. Mike Leach and Barbara J. Bain.
© 2022 John Wiley & Sons Ltd. Published 2022 by John Wiley & Sons Ltd.

MCQ

Acute myeloid leukaemia with mutated *NPM1* is typically associated with:

1 An abnormal karyotype
2 Cup-shaped nuclei
3 Cytoplasmic expression of NPM1
4 Expression of CD34
5 Poor prognosis

For answers and discussion, see page 206.

4 Neutrophil morphology

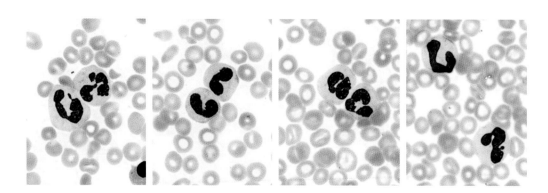

The neutrophil has been a focus of attention for haematologists for many decades and this remains true today for many reasons. These phagocytic and bactericidal cells are a key player in innate immunity but have many other roles in systemic inflammation, cytokine signalling and tissue remodelling and repair. Quantitative and qualitative disorders of neutrophils can have serious consequences for the patient and, importantly, recognising the nature and existence of these abnormalities can be instrumental in diagnosis. Furthermore, we generate iatrogenic neutropenia when treating many haematological diseases, so a full appreciation of the importance of the neutrophil lies at the core of haematology practice. The patient history and examination will provide the foundation for clinical assessment but careful focused supporting laboratory examination is always key to generating a specific diagnosis. We are all familiar with the characteristics of the normal neutrophil but defining clear morphological abnormalities can be more challenging due to the nuances of normality, clinical circumstances and coexisting disease and its treatment. Neutrophil morphology can be informative in many different clinical situations. The blood film images above, from a woman with a myelodysplastic syndrome, show neutrophils displaying profound hypogranularity (all images ×100 objective); in addition, some cells show abnormal nuclear segmentation (extreme left, centre right). Furthermore, one cell (extreme right) shows an unusual location of the drumstick, which preferentially arises from the distal half of a terminal segment (extreme left) (Karni *et al.* 2001).

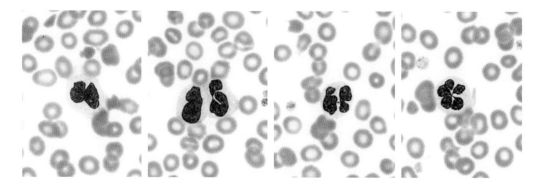

The images above show more examples of abnormal nuclear segmentation in MDS; in simplistic terms the neutrophil nucleus should show a 'string of sausages' type orientation of nuclear

Haematology: From the Image to the Diagnosis, First Edition. Mike Leach and Barbara J. Bain.
© 2022 John Wiley & Sons Ltd. Published 2022 by John Wiley & Sons Ltd.

segments. Though not 100% specific, we would encourage you to use this idea as a basis of defining normality. Note the variety of abnormal segmentation in each image above and the particularly odd orientation of nuclear lobes in the image extreme right.

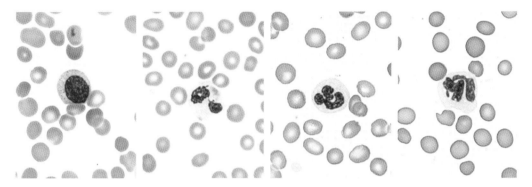

Further examples are illustrated above; note the mature but non-lobated nucleus in the neutrophil extreme left. Attention to the abnormal nuclear morphology might be lost when the eye is drawn to the cytoplasmic hypogranularity but the nuclear features shown here are significant.

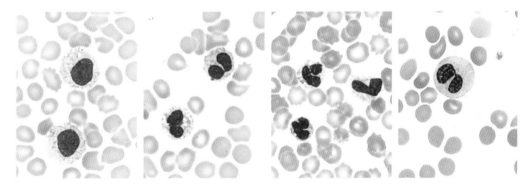

Importantly, changes in neutrophil morphology can be reactive in nature so the clinical circumstances should be accounted for at the time of the blood film report, if the latter is to be fully informative. The images above are all from the peripheral blood of a patient with overwhelming bacterial sepsis; note the neutrophil hyposegmentation, including non-lobated neutrophils and pseudo-Pelger forms, together with cytoplasmic vacuolation and toxic granulation. Compare the above with the inherited condition Pelger–Huët anomaly (see Theme 38).

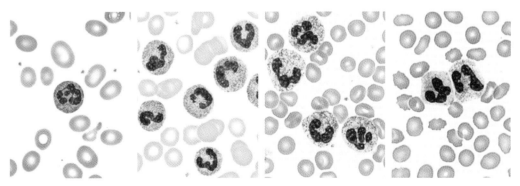

Neutrophil hypersegmentation can also be a feature of dysplasia but more frequently is seen in vitamin B12 or folic acid deficiency (above left). Reactive neutrophilia is common in inflammatory, infective and neoplastic conditions. The left centre image above is from a patient with a reactive neutrophilia as a response to corticosteroid therapy for small cell lung carcinoma. The image right centre shows a toxic type neutrophilia resulting from granulocyte colony-stimulating factor (G-CSF) therapy and the image extreme right is from a patient with septicaemia with neutrophils demonstrating Döhle bodies. Furthermore, and relevant to other cases in this text, neutrophil morphology can inform the diagnosis of inherited disease (see Theme 90).

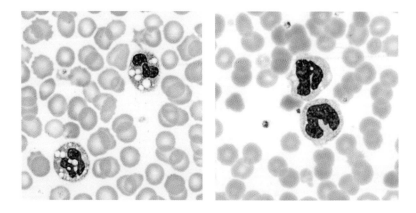

The left image (above) shows prominent neutrophil cytoplasmic vacuolation due to lipid accumulation in a patient with neutral lipid storage disease, a finding known as Jordans anomaly. The right image is from a patient with recurrent serious bacterial infections due to neutrophil-specific granule deficiency (previously known as lactoferrin deficiency). The automated analyser misinterpreted these cells as monocytes as they have very similar light scatter characteristics.

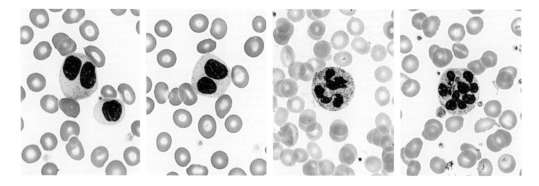

Other neutrophil abnormalities that can be found in MDS include binucleated macropolycytes (above images, extreme left and centre left, both with marked hypogranularity) and other tetraploid cells (segmented macropolycytes, above centre right and extreme right).

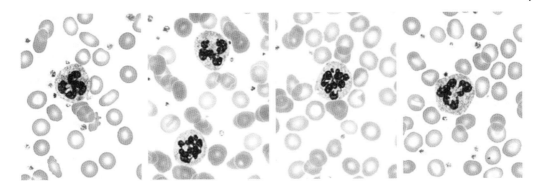

Other features of MDS include detached nuclear fragments, ring nuclei and nuclei with irregular projections (all images above) and with chromatin condensed into dense blocks (all images above) (Bain 2015). The spectrum of neutrophil morphological abnormalities that are informative in the diagnosis of MDS and AML are well summarised by the International Working Group on Morphology of MDS (IWGM-MDS) (Goasguen *et al.* 2013).

References

Bain BJ (2015) *Blood Cells*, 5th Edn. Wiley-Blackwell, Oxford, pp. 99–107.

Goasguen JE, Bennett JM, Bain BJ, Brunning R, Vallespie MT, Tomonaga M *et al.*; International Working Group on Morphology of MDS (IWGM-MDS) (2013) Proposal for refining the definition of dysgranulopoiesis in acute myeloid leukemia and myelodysplastic syndromes. *Leuk Res*, **38**, 447–453.

Karni RJ, Wangh LJ and Sanchez JA (2001) Nonrandom location and orientation of the inactive X chromosome in human neutrophil nuclei. *Chromosoma*, **110**, 267–274.

MCQ

A botryoid ('grape-like') nucleus in a neutrophil can be a feature of:

1 Burns
2 Granulocyte colony-stimulating factor (G-CSF) therapy
3 Hyperthermia
4 Myelodysplastic syndrome
5 Sepsis

For answers and discussion, see page 206.

5 Primary myelofibrosis

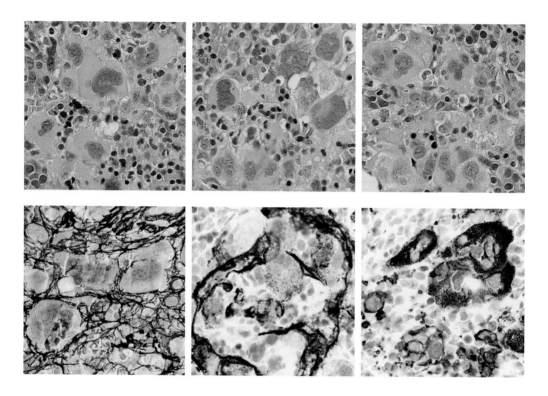

A 40-year-old man underwent allogeneic stem cell transplantation for *JAK2*-mutated primary myelofibrosis. His disease has recurred, and now 7 years later, he has been enrolled into a phase 1 clinical trial. He has massive splenomegaly which causes abdominal discomfort and early satiety but his blood counts are reasonably well preserved: Hb 126 g/l, WBC 5.3 × 10^9/l, neutrophils 4.1 × 10^9/l and platelets 348 × 10^9/l. A bone marrow trephine biopsy was taken as a baseline at enrolment and the sections are illustrated above. On H&E staining the marrow showed marked hypercellularity, approaching 100%, largely due to a marked increase in large pleomorphic mega-karyocytes (top images ×50 objective). These showed inevitable gross clustering. There was a marked increase in stainable reticulin to grade 3/3 with the reticulin fibres often laid down circum-ferentially around the megakaryocytes (bottom left). There was a marked increase in marrow sinu-soids (note the CD34 expression by the endothelial cells) and the megakaryocytes showed aberrant CD34 expression (CD34, bottom centre, immunoperoxidase). The variation in megakaryocyte size is also illustrated here with giant forms being common, though much smaller forms are also evi-dent (CD42b, bottom right, immunoperoxidase).

Primary myelofibrosis is a myeloproliferative neoplasm characterised by megakaryocyte prolif-eration, associated progressive bone marrow fibrosis/osteosclerosis and a propensity to evolve to acute myeloid leukaemia. Due to compromise of the bone marrow compartment, extramedullary haemopoiesis follows with involvement of the liver and particularly the spleen. Progressive bone marrow fibrosis causes bone marrow failure which is further compounded by hypersplenism.

Haematology: From the Image to the Diagnosis, First Edition. Mike Leach and Barbara J. Bain.
© 2022 John Wiley & Sons Ltd. Published 2022 by John Wiley & Sons Ltd.

Patients develop abdominal pain and early satiety due to splenomegaly together with night sweats, fatigue and weight loss from the catabolic effect of the disease. Treatments such as ruxolitinib, a JAK-STAT pathway inhibitor, are useful for splenic symptoms and sweats. Ruxolitinib prolongs survival in myelofibrosis but the only potential curative treatment is allogeneic bone marrow transplantation. There is an unmet need for effective treatment of myelofibrosis.

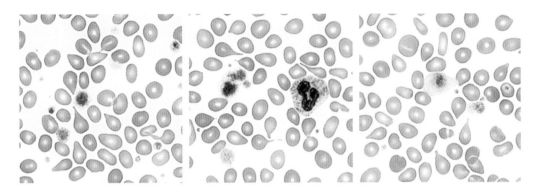

The blood film can show important features (images above ×100), but these are not specific for the diagnosis which is based on bone marrow assessment. Note the teardrop poikilocytes and the macrothrombocytes with abnormal granulation. Platelet morphology is consistently abnormal in myelofibrosis. Myelofibrosis can also develop as a secondary phenomenon in other myeloproliferative neoplasms and the clinical consequences are similar to those described above, often with a loss of proliferative behaviour of the disorder with progressive splenomegaly and cytopenias.

MCQ

Molecular mechanisms underlying primary myelofibrosis include:

1 *BCR-ABL1*
2 *CALR* mutation
3 *JAK2* V617F
4 *JAK2* exon 12 mutation
5 *MPL* mutation

For answers and discussion, see page 206.

6 Sarcoidosis

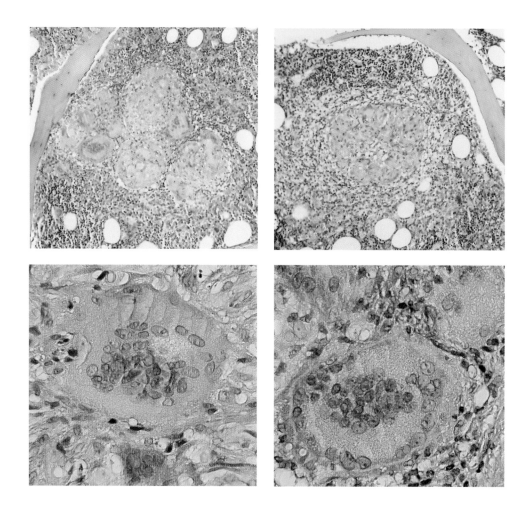

A 50-year-old man was referred for investigation of low-volume lymphadenopathy and mild splenomegaly noted on a CT scan performed as part of the investigation of loin pain. Renal stones had
been suspected. He had no specific respiratory symptoms but did describe occasional night sweats.
Widespread small-volume lymphadenopathy involving cervical, axillary, mediastinal and mesenteric nodes had been identified. The spleen measured 15 cm in long axis. Notably the lung imaging
showed some non-specific lower zone inflammatory/infective changes. His full blood count
showed Hb 127 g/l, WBC 4.3×10^9/l, neutrophils 2.5×10^9/l, lymphocytes 0.6×10^9/l and platelets
206×10^9/l. Serum angiotensin-converting enzyme (ACE) and LDH were both normal. He underwent a bone marrow aspirate and trephine biopsy. The aspirate was initially reported as showing
reactive changes but no specific pathology. The trephine biopsy sections were abnormal, showing
very well demarcated non-caseating granulomas (top images, H&E ×10 objective). There were very
prominent multinucleated giant cells present within the granulomas (bottom images, H&E ×50
objective). There was no evidence of a low-grade or high-grade lymphoma. The working diagnosis,

Haematology: From the Image to the Diagnosis, First Edition. Mike Leach and Barbara J. Bain.
© 2022 John Wiley & Sons Ltd. Published 2022 by John Wiley & Sons Ltd.

despite the normal serum ACE level, was sarcoidosis. A lymph node core biopsy also showed non-caseating granulomas. The patient was referred to the Respiratory team who performed a trans-bronchial lung biopsy which showed features of intra-alveolar inflammation and a small granuloma. A Ziehl–Neelsen stain and mycobacterial cultures were negative.

Sarcoidosis is an intriguing condition where there are many pathological features of a cell-mediated reaction to an unknown stimulus. It is typically a pulmonary disease (suggesting a primary pulmonary pathogen) but can evolve into a systemic disorder with potentially serious consequences (neurosarcoidosis and myocardial sarcoidosis). The diagnosis is one of exclusion as no single investigation carries high specificity and the serum ACE level, classically described as being elevated, can be normal. Hodgkin lymphoma enters into the differential diagnosis since sarcoidosis can cause weight loss, night sweats and fatigue with hilar and mediastinal lymphadenopathy.

On reviewing the bone marrow aspirate a number of disrupted granulomas were evident (images below ×50). This presents a good example as to how co-reporting of the aspirate and trephine biopsy specimen can yield a unified diagnosis. Many haematologists reporting and identifying these aspirate abnormalities in isolation would likely fail to appreciate their significance.

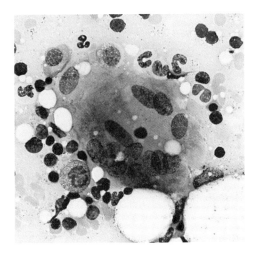 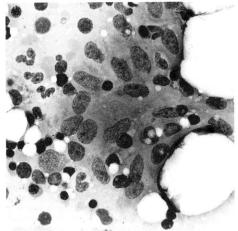

MCQ

Caseating granulomas can be a feature of:

1 Fungal infection
2 Granulomatous response to follicular lymphoma
3 Granulomatous response to multiple myeloma
4 Sarcoidosis
5 Tuberculosis

For answers and discussion, see page 206.

7 Visceral leishmaniasis

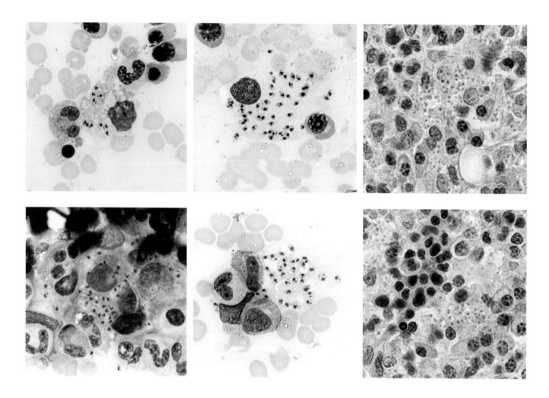

A 5-year-old boy was referred for investigation of anorexia, abdominal bloating and intermittent fever. On examination he appeared pale and underweight and had palpable splenomegaly. His full blood count showed Hb 100 g/l, WBC 4×10^9/l, neutrophils 2×10^9/l and platelets 247×10^9/l. The blood film showed no specific features. He had a polyclonal increase in immunoglobulins, low serum albumin at 26 g/l and a direct Coombs test that was positive for IgG. CT imaging confirmed splenomegaly but no lymphadenopathy was apparent. A lymphoma was suspected, but in the absence of a suitable biopsy target, bone marrow aspiration and trephine biopsy were performed.

The aspirate was particulate with cellular trails. There was no lymphomatous infiltrate. There were, however, increased numbers of macrophages containing *Leishmania* promastigotes (left and centre images ×100 objective). Note that the macrophage cytoplasm was disrupted in some cells with the parasites appearing free in the film (centre images). Note that each parasite has a nucleus and a smaller rod-shaped kinetoplast. Microscopy alone is sufficient to make a diagnosis but serology and molecular studies can be used for confirmation and determining species, respectively. The bone marrow trephine biopsy sections showed maximal cellularity with large numbers of macrophages harbouring parasites being visible (right images ×50). On further questioning regarding the travel history, it was learned that the family had visited Malta on a 2-week holiday some months previously. The patient was treated with intravenous liposomal amphotericin and made a full recovery.

The term leishmaniasis encompasses multiple clinical syndromes resulting from *Phlebotomus* sand fly transmission of a variety of *Leishmania* species; cutaneous, mucocutaneous and visceral

Haematology: From the Image to the Diagnosis, First Edition. Mike Leach and Barbara J. Bain.
© 2022 John Wiley & Sons Ltd. Published 2022 by John Wiley & Sons Ltd.

forms (the case described above) of the disease result, sometimes many months or years after primary infection. It is present in the tropics, subtropics and southern Europe including the Mediterranean area. It is endemic in dogs in Malta with the implicated organism being *Leishmania infantum*. Visceral leishmaniasis is a serious infection which should never be overlooked and bone marrow biopsy material should be carefully scrutinised whenever this diagnosis is possible. In this case, the marrow biopsy was taken looking for involvement by lymphoma and the condition was encountered almost by accident. This was also the case for another patient who presented with a perianal ulcer. The biopsy showed granulomatous inflammation and a diagnosis of Crohn's disease was assumed. He was commenced on azathioprine therapy but developed progressive pancytopenia. A bone marrow aspirate and trephine biopsy were taken, assuming the cause to be drug toxicity but *Leishmania* parasites were seen and accurately identified in the aspirate films. Review of the skin biopsy showed the granulomatous skin ulcer to be due to cutaneous *Leishmania* infection.

In tropical and subtropical countries where the infection is endemic, a rapid field hospital method of making a diagnosis is microscopy of a splenic aspirate, taken under local anaesthetic. The images below (×100) are of an MGG-stained splenic aspirate showing visceral leishmaniasis.

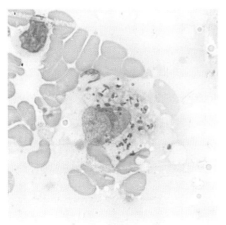 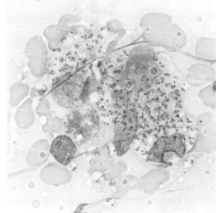

MCQ

Leishmaniasis involving the bone marrow:

1 Can be complicated by a haemophagocytic syndrome
2 Can cause granuloma formation
3 Can lead to significant dyserythropoiesis
4 Is easily detected with Grocott's methenamine silver stain
5 Is often associated with increased plasma cells

For answers and discussion, see page 206.

8   Gelatinous transformation of the bone marrow

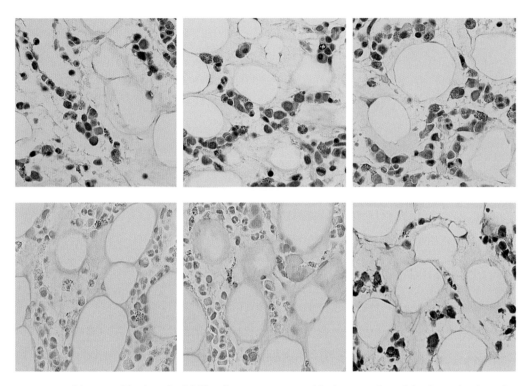

A 60-year-old man with chronic debility due to neurosarcoidosis was referred for investigation of a normocytic anaemia with Hb 100 g/l and normal leucocyte and platelet counts. The blood film was not informative. He underwent bone marrow aspiration. The aspirate was hypocellular but did not show any definitive diagnostic features. The bone marrow trephine biopsy specimen was abnormal, showing hypocellularity with reduction of haemopoietic activity around the marrow fat spaces (top images, H&E) (all images ×50 objective). The hypocellular areas show preserved architecture and an amorphous myxoid (mucoid) interstitium. Subsequent staining with Alcian blue (bottom left and centre) and periodic acid–Schiff (bottom right) confirmed the diagnosis of gelatinous transformation, also known as myxoid degeneration.

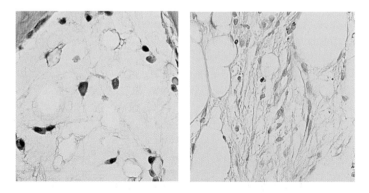

Haematology: From the Image to the Diagnosis, First Edition. Mike Leach and Barbara J. Bain.
© 2022 John Wiley & Sons Ltd. Published 2022 by John Wiley & Sons Ltd.

Typically, this condition involves the marrow diffusely (above left, H&E and right, Alcian blue ×50), resulting in peripheral blood cytopenias with neutropenia and anaemia being most frequent. Gelatinous transformation of the bone marrow is an important condition to recognise and should not be mistaken for marrow aplasia or marrow necrosis. It is typically seen as part of the catabolic response to chronic debilitating disease (malignant or non-malignant) and/or malnutrition. The condition will regress on treating the underlying cause.

MCQ

Myxoid degeneration (gelatinous transformation) can be a feature of:

1 Acquired immune deficiency syndrome
2 Anorexia nervosa
3 Extreme exercise
4 Metastatic carcinoma
5 Morbid obesity

For answers and discussion, see page 206.

9 Acanthocytic red cell disorders

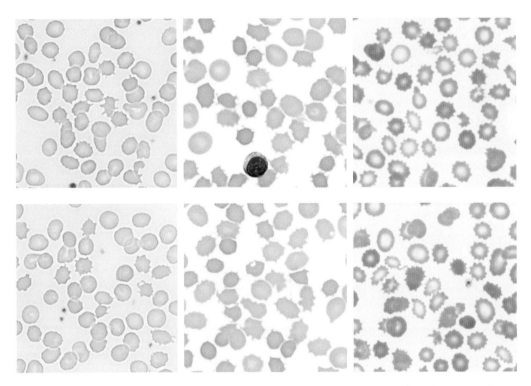

A 50-year-old man with a progressive myopathy and cardiomyopathy was referred to a neurologist because of early cognitive decline and tic-like involuntary movements. His full blood count was normal but a blood film was requested. This showed prominent acanthocytes; these are dense cells with prominent cytoplasmic projections (spicules), which are irregular in length and shape (*acanthus* is Greek for 'thorny') (left images ×100 objective). Routine renal and liver biochemistry and serum lipids were normal. A diagnosis of McLeod syndrome was considered and confirmed when a mutation in the *XK* gene at Xp21.1 was identified. McLeod syndrome is an X-linked multisystem disorder, being one of a number of the rare neuroacanthocytic disorders. The condition is characterised by acanthocytosis, mild compensated haemolysis, weak expression of Kell blood group antigens, myopathy, cardiomyopathy and progressive neurological decline with cognitive impairment, involuntary movements, seizures and peripheral neuropathy. Peripheral blood morphology may provide a useful pointer to the diagnosis, as in this case.

A second patient, a 15-year-old boy was referred to ophthalmology with a progressive decline in visual acuity. He was found to have retinitis pigmentosa. He had a very low total cholesterol level, and low-density and very low-density lipoproteins (LDL and VLDL) were absent. His full blood count was normal but the requested blood film showed acanthocytes (centre images ×100). A diagnosis of abetalipoproteinaemia was considered and confirmed when biallelic mutation of the microsomal triglyceride transfer protein gene (*MTTP*) was identified. Abetalipoproteinaemia is a rare autosomal recessively inherited condition of lipid metabolism in which LDL and VLDL are severely reduced. The condition is characterised by fat malabsorption, spinocerebellar

Haematology: From the Image to the Diagnosis, First Edition. Mike Leach and Barbara J. Bain.
© 2022 John Wiley & Sons Ltd. Published 2022 by John Wiley & Sons Ltd.

degeneration, acanthocytosis and retinitis pigmentosa. The MTTP protein influences intracellular lipid transport in the small bowel and liver. Symptoms usually first appear in infants and children, and when the condition is identified disease progression can be slowed using dietary vitamin E and medium chain fatty acid supplementation.

A third patient, a 32-year-old man with malnutrition from severe exocrine pancreatic insufficiency of unknown aetiology was hospitalised with a respiratory infection. He was poorly compliant with pancreatic enzyme supplements and appeared ill, grossly malnourished and wasted. His full blood count showed Hb 109 g/l, MCV 86.5 fl, MCH 26.3 pg, WBC 6.2×10^9/l and platelets 218×10^9/l. Serum ferritin was low at 9 µg/l and a blood film was requested. This showed significant hypochromia, consistent with iron deficiency, but also marked acanthocytosis with some of these cells appearing very dense (right images ×100). His lipid profile was abnormal, showing total cholesterol 2.2 mmol/l (optimal <5.2), triglycerides 0.8 mmol/l (NR 0.2–2.3), high-density lipoprotein 0.6 mmol/l (optimal >1), LDL 1.2 mmol/l (optimal <2.59) and VLDL 0.4 mmol/l (NR 0.1–1.7). Serum apolipoprotein B levels were 0.6 g/l (NR 0.6–1.3) and screening for mutation in *MTTP* was negative. A diagnosis of acquired acanthocytosis, with iron deficiency secondary to severe lipid malabsorption from pancreatic exocrine failure was made.

MCQ

Acanthocytes in a blood film can be the result of:

1 Anorexia nervosa
2 Liver failure
3 Splenectomy
4 Storage artefact
5 Transfusion of blood at the end of its shelf life

For answers and discussion, see page 206.

10 T-cell large granular lymphocytic leukaemia

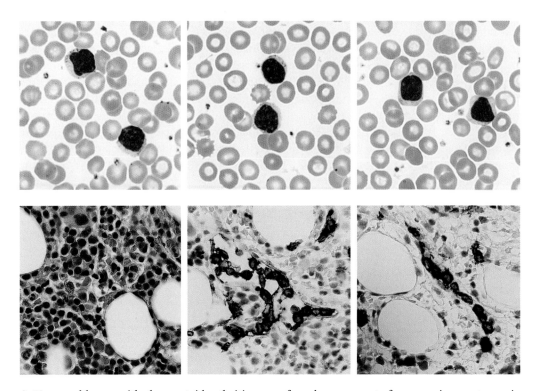

A 53-year-old man with rheumatoid arthritis was referred on account of progressive neutropenia whilst on weekly methotrexate therapy. Importantly, the methotrexate was withheld but the neutropenia continued and in fact worsened. At the time of referral the full blood count showed Hb 159 g/l, WBC 6.5×10^9/l, neutrophils 0.6×10^9/l, lymphocytes 5.1×10^9/l and platelets 133×10^9/l. The lymphocytosis had actually evolved during the period when methotrexate was suspended. The blood film showed prominent large granular lymphocytes (top images ×100 objective) and on immunophenotyping these expressed CD8, weak CD5, CD2, CD3 and CD57, whilst expression of CD7 and CD26 was lost, suggesting a clonal T-cell disorder. The bone marrow trephine biopsy sections showed a cellular marrow with a subtle interstitial (bottom left, H&E ×50) and intrasinusoidal (CD3, bottom centre and right, immunoperoxidase ×50) T-cell infiltrate. T-cell receptor gene rearrangement studies showed a clonal population, and sequencing of *STAT3* and *STAT5B* genes showed a gain of function mutation in *STAT3*, Y640F, which has been associated with a therapeutic response to methotrexate. The clinical advice was therefore to restart methotrexate treatment. This resulted in improvement in rheumatic symptoms but also in resolution of lymphocytosis and neutropenia: Hb 160 g/l, WBC 5.0×10^9/l, neutrophils 2.1×10^9/l, lymphocytes 2.9×10^9/l and platelets 162×10^9/l.

Large granular lymphocytic leukaemia is a condition which should always be at the forefront of the mind of haematologists when investigating patients with cytopenias, particularly in the context of a known connective tissue disorder. Although a lymphocytosis is often apparent, the condition should also be considered when the count sits within the normal range. It is then important to

Haematology: From the Image to the Diagnosis, First Edition. Mike Leach and Barbara J. Bain.
© 2022 John Wiley & Sons Ltd. Published 2022 by John Wiley & Sons Ltd.

scrutinise the blood film for granular lymphocytes and consider using flow cytometry to identify a possible aberrant T-cell population.

MCQ

T-cell large granular lymphocytic leukaemia:

1 Can lead to anaemia due to pure red cell aplasia or autoimmune haemolytic anaemia
2 Has specific diagnostic features on trephine biopsy
3 Shows an association with Felty syndrome
4 Shows an association with thymoma
5 Typically shows expression of CD3, CD8 and CD57

For answers and discussion, see page 206.

11 Pure erythroid leukaemia

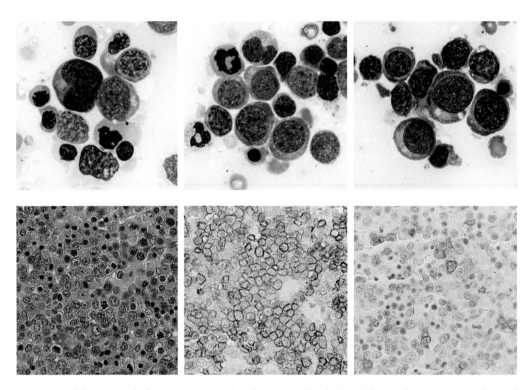

A 40-year-old, previously fit man presented with progressive fatigue. Physical examination showed pallor and mild icterus. His full blood count showed Hb 87 g/l, WBC 1.7 × 10^9/l, neutrophils 0.8 × 10^9/l and platelets 26 × 10^9/l. His blood film showed no specific features but, importantly, red cell fragments, spherocytes and blast cells were not seen. Serum bilirubin and LDH were both mildly elevated. A direct Coombs test was negative and no auto- or allo-antibodies were identified. He had a significantly raised haemoglobin F at 10.9%. The bone marrow aspirate and trephine biopsy sections were reviewed by the haematologists at the source hospital and a working diagnosis of myelodysplastic syndrome with haemolysis was proposed. Flow cytometric studies on the marrow aspirate, gating on the largest cells based on the forward scatter/side scatter (FSC/SSC) profile, identified CD34+ cells at 2% of events, whilst CD117+ cells were increased at 12% of events. The karyotype was normal. The patient was discussed at the regional multidisciplinary team meeting where the diagnosis was questioned and a central haematopathology review was recommended.

On review of the very cellular bone marrow aspirate, marked erythroid hyperplasia was evident (M:E ratio 1:10) with a notable left shift in erythroid precursors, prominent proerythroblasts, relatively mild erythroid dysplasia and karyorrhectic forms (top images ×100 objective). There was no excess of myeloblasts but dysplastic neutrophils were present (top centre). Importantly, the marrow was not megaloblastic. The trephine biopsy sections showed 100% cellularity with marked erythroid hyperplasia with left shift (bottom left, H&E and bottom centre, glycophorin C, immunoperoxidase ×50). A proportion of proerythroblasts also showed expression of CD117 (bottom right, immunoperoxidase ×50). There was no excess of CD34+ cells. A diagnosis of pure erythroid

Haematology: From the Image to the Diagnosis, First Edition. Mike Leach and Barbara J. Bain.
© 2022 John Wiley & Sons Ltd. Published 2022 by John Wiley & Sons Ltd.

leukaemia was made. Subsequent myeloid next generation sequencing identified an *NRAS* mutation (c.35G>A) and two mutations in *WT1* (c.758A>G and c.759C>A).

Pure erythroid leukaemia is a rare neoplastic bone marrow disorder characterised by a proliferation of immature erythroid cells (>80% of bone marrow cells with at least 30% proerythroblasts) and no significant myeloblast component. Patients typically present with pancytopenia and the condition can appear *de novo*, can evolve from a myelodysplastic syndrome or can be therapy-related. It is important that the erythroid hyperplasia is not attributed to haemolysis (the evidence in this patient was not convincing) or to a myelodysplastic syndrome. In the latter, erythroid hyperplasia and dysplasia is common but the marked left shift with predominance of proerythroblasts and myeloid hypoplasia is not seen. Furthermore, *de novo* pure erythroid leukaemia, as in this 40-year-old patient, has a more acute presentation rather than the more gradual onset of cytopenias typically associated with MDS. A reversion to primitive erythropoiesis with increased haemoglobin F levels can occur in erythroleukaemia. There is no specific cytogenetic abnormality associated with pure erythroid leukaemia; complex karyotypes with loss of chromosomes 5 and 7, 5q– and 7q– are common, whilst favourable cytogenetics is very rare. The prognosis is poor when the condition evolves from MDS or is therapy-related (these cases being categorised differently), but may be more favourable and similar to other subtypes of AML if it arises as a primary condition (Santos *et al.* 2009).

Reference

Santos FPS, Faderl S, Garcia-Manero G, Koller C, Beran M, O'Brien S *et al.* (2009) Adult acute erythroid leukaemia: an analysis of 91 patients treated at a single institution. *Leukemia*, **23**, 2275–2280.

MCQ

Proerythroblasts in pure erythroid leukaemia often express:

1 CD34
2 CD61
3 CD117
4 E-cadherin (CD234)
5 Glycophorin A (CD235a)

For answers and discussion, see page 206.

12 Reactive mesothelial cells

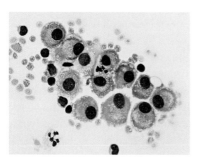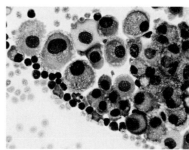

A 53-year-old woman presented with chest pain and dyspnoea. On CT imaging a large mediastinal mass was identified associated with bilateral pleural effusions. On biopsy the mass was shown to be a myeloid sarcoma. There was an associated t(10;11)(p12;q14.2); (*PICALM-MLLT10*). The full blood count was normal and a bone marrow aspirate showed no evidence of acute leukaemia. The patient was treated with two cycles of acute myeloid leukaemia induction chemotherapy with marked regression of the mass, but a left pleural effusion, though improved, persisted. A pleural fluid sample was aspirated due to concerns regarding persisting disease. A cytospin preparation is shown above (×50 objective). Note the population of large cells with vacuolated blue cytoplasm and an eccentric nucleus. These features are typical of pleural mesothelial cells; they do not represent a neoplastic population but might be interpreted as such by the inexperienced. In addition, note the small compact lymphoid cells, which are reactive T lymphocytes that are prevalent in reactive effusions (the diagonal line of cells, image right). Morphological and flow cytometry assessment of the fluid specimen identified no precursor myeloid cells. The patient completed a further two cycles of treatment and the effusion fully resolved. She remains well and disease free on follow-up.

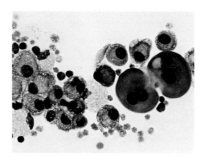

Mesothelial cells are often seen in pleural and ascitic taps. They are shed into the fluid environment when other disease processes cause pleural irritation or interfere with pleural lymphatic drainage. These cells have characteristic morphology as illustrated here, but do not express CD45 or haemopoietic lineage markers. They can on occasion be binucleated (image above ×50) and show significant size variation. They should not be mistaken for carcinoma or other

Haematology: From the Image to the Diagnosis, First Edition. Mike Leach and Barbara J. Bain.
© 2022 John Wiley & Sons Ltd. Published 2022 by John Wiley & Sons Ltd.

non-haemopoietic neoplasms. This is another good example of where a careful morphological assessment is necessary and careful correlation with other important points in the history is absolutely essential.

PICALM-MLLT10 is most often found in T-acute lymphoblastic leukaemia but also occurs in acute myeloid leukaemia and mixed phenotype acute leukaemia.

MCQ

Myeloid sarcoma:

1 Can be the first sign of relapse of acute myeloid leukaemia
2 Can have a green colour
3 Can be associated with t(8;21)(q22;q22.1)
4 Is common in acute promyelocytic leukaemia
5 Occurs only at a single site

For answers and discussion, see page 206.

13   Plasmablastic myeloma

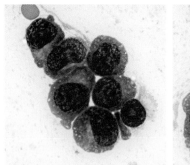 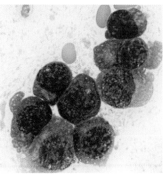 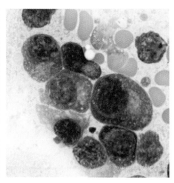

A 76-year-old woman treated with multiple lines of therapy for multiple myeloma presented to clinic with generalised debility and recent heavy nose bleeds. Her paraprotein levels had been noted to be on the rise despite lenalidomide and dexamethasone therapy. The full blood count showed Hb 95 g/l, WBC 3.5×10^9/l, neutrophils 1.5×10^9/l and platelets 18×10^9/l. An IgG para-protein quantitation was 69 g/l. It was clear that the disease was becoming refractory to therapy but a bone marrow aspirate was taken in view of the problematic thrombocytopenia and bleeding. The aspirate was markedly hypercellular and well over 90% of cells were large pleomorphic plasma cells, some showing prominent nucleoli (images above ×100 objective). Normal haemopoiesis was markedly reduced and megakaryocytes in particular were scarce.

The malignant plasma cells of multiple myeloma are usually easy to recognise allowing accurate quantitation using a manual differential count. The morphology of plasma cells in refractory myeloma, however, often changes with increasing pleomorphism, increasing cell size and multi-nuclearity. The cells can sometimes resemble those of a high-grade lymphoma. In addition many of these patients start to shed plasma cells into the peripheral blood (also noted in this case, not shown). Despite their morphological abnormality, the lineage is indicated in this patient by the strongly basophilic cytoplasm and the paler paranuclear Golgi zone. These features are important in helping recognise plasma cells when the nuclear morphology is atypical (images below ×100). Note the variation in nuclear morphology with bilobed and even binucleated forms but the Golgi zone and intense blue cytoplasm are prominent; all of these cells are plasma cells. As an adjunct, note the cytoplasmic fragments and particles due to the intense fragility of plasma cells on handling.

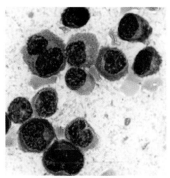 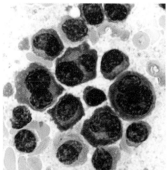 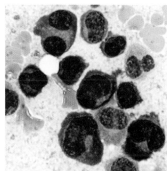

Haematology: From the Image to the Diagnosis, First Edition. Mike Leach and Barbara J. Bain.
© 2022 John Wiley & Sons Ltd. Published 2022 by John Wiley & Sons Ltd.

It may be worth reassessing the marrow in patients developing severe cytopenias since, in addition to the above features, some patients sadly develop a treatment-related myelodysplastic syndrome or acute leukaemia.

MCQ

Plasmablastic myeloma:

1 Can represent disease evolution
2 Has a high proliferation index on Ki-67 staining
3 Has a worse prognosis than other cases of myeloma
4 Is associated with worse renal function than other cases of myeloma
5 Is associated with a higher serum calcium than other cases of myeloma

For answers and discussion, see page 206.

14 Septicaemia

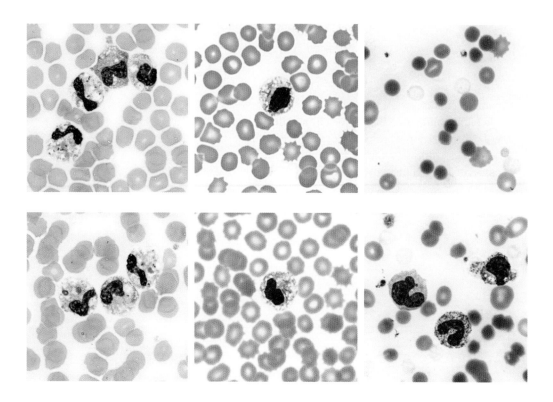

A 5-year-old girl was admitted as an emergency after a collapse following a fever at home. On assessment she was acutely unwell and hypotensive and had generalised petechiae. The clinical picture was of severe sepsis and after blood cultures had been taken she was commenced on broad-spectrum antibiotics. The full blood count showed Hb 120 g/l, WBC 20 × 10⁹/l, neutrophils 17 × 10⁹/l and platelets 32 × 10⁹/l. The coagulation profile was indicative of disseminated intravascular coagulation (DIC). The blood film (left images ×100 objective) showed neutrophilia with left shift; in particular there was prominent neutrophil vacuolation and there were cytoplasmic inclusions consistent with the appearance of diplococci. Note also the prominent Döhle bodies in the neutrophils (bottom left). Meningococcal septicaemia now seemed likely and was confirmed on blood cultures and PCR studies.

A second patient, a 62-year-old man, was admitted following a collapse after a 2-day prodrome of feeling non-specifically unwell. He had been bitten on the hand by a dog some days previously. He was febrile and hypotensive and had widespread petechiae. His condition deteriorated and he required intubation, ventilation and inotropic support. His full blood count showed Hb 137 g/l, WBC 24.2 × 10⁹/l, neutrophils 22.7 × 10⁹/l and platelets 9 × 10⁹/l. The coagulation screen was again indicative of DIC (PT 25 s, APTT 92 s, TT 17 s, fibrinogen 1.5 g/l and D dimer 88 726 ng/ml). The blood film showed neutrophilia with left shift and some neutrophils had rod-shaped bacterial inclusions (centre images). Blood cultures grew the Gram-negative bacillus, *Capnocytophaga canimorsus*, which is a serious human pathogen that often forms part of normal canine and feline flora.

Haematology: From the Image to the Diagnosis, First Edition. Mike Leach and Barbara J. Bain.
© 2022 John Wiley & Sons Ltd. Published 2022 by John Wiley & Sons Ltd.

A third patient, a 66-year-old woman was in hospital with obstructive jaundice due to liver metastases from ovarian carcinoma and had external biliary stents *in situ*. She was receiving weekly paclitaxel chemotherapy. She became acutely unwell, developing hypotension and jaundice. The full blood count showed Hb 57 g/l, WBC 7.3×10^9/l and platelets 177×10^9/l. As in the previous cases, the blood film was informative; it showed profound red cell spherocytosis (right images) with red cell ghosts (top right image) and toxic granulation of neutrophils (bottom right image) but no bacterial inclusions were seen. Despite resuscitation efforts the patient died shortly afterwards. Blood cultures subsequently grew *Clostridium perfringens*. This bacterium can be a commensal of the normal hepatobiliary and gastrointestinal tracts but becomes a serious and life-threatening pathogen when it gains access to the blood, most likely in this case in relation to the stent. It produces an alpha lecithinase enzyme which directly lyses the red cell membrane, inducing an acute haemolytic anaemia that further compounds the septicaemia. The blood film features are typical of this condition; the spherocytes are due to membrane perforation, as are the ghost cells where all red cell haemoglobin has been leaked. By the time the blood film has been assessed, most affected patients have succumbed to this form of septicaemia but in some cases the morphological features may indicate the need for rapid active management and save a life.

MCQ

Neutrophil vacuolation can be a feature of:

1 Bacterial infection
2 Chédiak–Higashi syndrome
3 Ethanol toxicity
4 Neonatal necrotising enterocolitis
5 Neutral lipid storage disease

For answers and discussion, see page 206.

15   An unstable haemoglobin and a myeloproliferative neoplasm

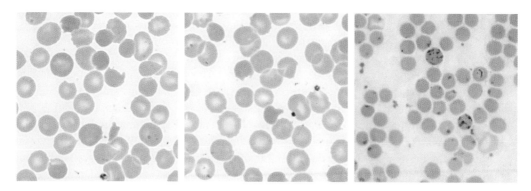

A 26-year-old man was well known to the Haematology clinic and had a chronic compensated haemo-lytic anaemia due to the unstable haemoglobin, haemoglobin Köln. He suffered exacerbations of hae-molysis with intercurrent infection but his condition would settle thereafter. A typical full blood count showed Hb 114 g/l, WBC 4.7×10^9/l, neutrophils 2.4×10^9/l and platelets 154×10^9/l. His blood film is illustrated above; bite cells and irregularly contracted cells are evident (left and centre ×100 objective) and Heinz bodies were prominent (right, methyl violet ×100). Somewhat unexpectedly, he developed progressive and ultimately massive splenomegaly though his haemolytic disorder appeared clinically unchanged. CT scanning showed a 25 cm spleen with no focal abnormality; there was no evidence of chronic liver disease or portal hypertension and no lymphadenopathy was apparent. His full blood count now showed Hb 125 g/l, WBC 12.7×10^9/l, neutrophils 8.9×10^9/l and platelets 1830×10^9/l. He underwent a splenectomy in view of progressive splenic symptoms. The spleen weighed 2700 g (normal 200 g). Histological examination showed massive expansion of the red pulp with congested sinuses and extramedullary haemopoiesis. There was no evidence of lymphoma.

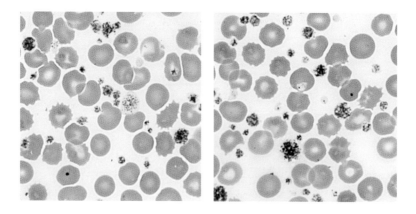

The post-operative blood film is shown above (×100). There is a marked thrombocytosis with profound platelet anisocytosis and hyposplenic features but bite cells are not now obvious. An unrelated myeloproliferative neoplasm was now considered likely and a bone marrow trephine biopsy was taken. The sections showed a hypercellular marrow with expansion of all lineages

Haematology: From the Image to the Diagnosis, First Edition. Mike Leach and Barbara J. Bain.
© 2022 John Wiley & Sons Ltd. Published 2022 by John Wiley & Sons Ltd.

(below left, H&E) (all images below ×50), increased reticulin staining (grade 2–3/3, below centre) and megakaryocyte clustering (below right, immunoperoxidase for CD42b).

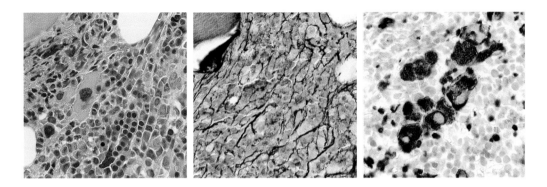

The features here support a diagnosis of a myeloproliferative neoplasm and molecular studies showed a pathogenic intragenic *CALR* deletion. In the circumstances it is difficult to accurately classify this myeloproliferative neoplasm but the diagnosis is likely to be primary myelofibrosis. This patient has two unrelated disorders which had caused understandable diagnostic difficulty. It is important to link any new development to a known disorder but it is also advisable that the clinician keeps an open mind, and considers all potential options when patients show an unexpected clinical evolution.

MCQ

Unstable haemoglobins:

1 Affect only the α or β globin chain
2 Can be associated with the presence of two variant haemoglobins as well as haemoglobin A
3 Can be detected by instability on heating or exposure to isopropanol
4 Have normal oxygen affinity
5 When clinically manifest, usually indicate homozygosity

For answers and discussion, see page 206.

16 Sickle cell anaemia in crisis

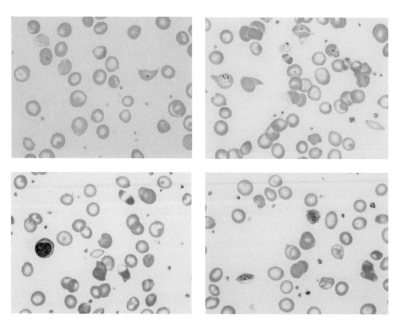

A 33-year-old woman with known sickle cell anaemia, newly arrived in the United Kingdom, presented to Accident and Emergency with a painful crisis. She was breathless, febrile and faintly jaundiced. Her FBC showed Hb 51 g/l, RBC 1.72×10^{12}/l, Hct 0.165, MCV 95.8 fl, MCH 29.8 pg, MCHC 311 g/l, WBC 13.8×10^9/l and platelet count 445×10^9/l. Bilirubin was increased to 141 µmol/l and ALT was mildly increased to 55 u/l. CRP was markedly increased to 137 mg/l. Examination of the blood film (all images ×100 objective) showed boat-shaped cells (top) but surprisingly infrequent sickle cells. There were some nucleated red blood cells and polychromasia was present. The changes of hyposplenism were present, specifically Howell–Jolly bodies (top), rare acanthocytes (top right), target cells (bottom left), giant platelets (bottom right) and thrombocytosis. An unusual feature was the presence of cells with haemoglobin condensed at the two poles of the cell and of irregularly contracted cells including hemighosts (top right and bottom left). An even more unusual feature was the presence of *Plasmodium falciparum* gametocytes (bottom right) and trophozoites (top). HPLC showed absent haemoglobin A, haemoglobin S 86.5% and haemoglobin F 5.1%.

Sickle cell trait protects from falciparum malaria but the converse is true of sickle cell anaemia, in which malaria can be life-threatening. Opportunistic detection of malaria parasites in a patient in whom the diagnosis has not been suspected clinically can be life-saving. Another warning sign in this patient is the presence of irregularly contracted cells and hemighosts. This observation correlates with the presence of hypoxia (Siow *et al.* 2017).

Haematology: From the Image to the Diagnosis, First Edition. Mike Leach and Barbara J. Bain.
© 2022 John Wiley & Sons Ltd. Published 2022 by John Wiley & Sons Ltd.

Reference

Siow W, Matthey F and Bain BJ (2017) The significance of irregularly contracted cells and hemighosts in sickle cell disease. *Am J Hematol*, **92**, 966–967.

MCQ

Causes of worsening anaemia that would be likely in a 30-year-old African or Afro-Caribbean woman with sickle cell anaemia include:

1 Folic acid deficiency
2 Haemolytic crisis
3 Parvovirus B19 infection
4 Splenic infarction
5 Splenic sequestration

For answers and discussion, see page 206.

17   Acute myeloid leukaemia with t(8;21)(q22;q22.1)

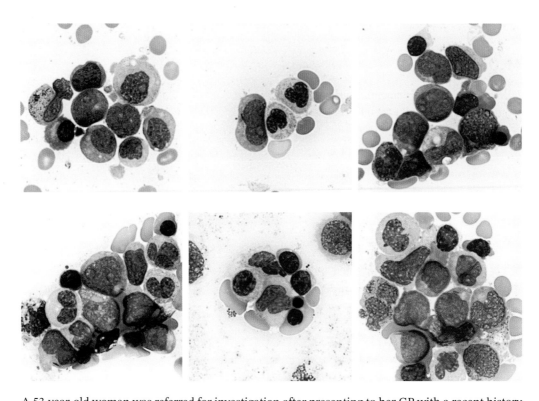

A 53-year-old woman was referred for investigation after presenting to her GP with a recent history of lethargy, myalgia, fever and headache. Her FBC showed Hb 100 g/l, WBC 3.4×10^9/l, neutrophils 0.5×10^9/l and platelets 39×10^9/l. The blood film showed small numbers of myeloblasts with some containing Auer rods. The bone marrow aspirate showed a prominent myeloblast population (approximately 40% of nucleated cells) with cytoplasmic granules (all images ×100 objective) with some showing Auer rods (top centre, top right, bottom left, bottom right). There was myeloid maturation to neutrophils with some cells showing hypogranularity (myelocytes, top left and neutrophils, bottom left, bottom right) but significantly, the nuclear morphology of maturing cells was also abnormal. Note the abnormal neutrophil segmentation (top centre, bottom right) and pseudo-Pelger–Huët anomaly (bottom left) including complete failure of segmentation resulting in a round nucleus (bottom centre). This subtype of AML can often be predicted on the basis of the marked granulocyte dysplasia, particularly the abnormalities in nuclear morphology in the maturing myeloid cells.

The blast cells had a CD34+, CD117+, MPO+, CD13+, CD33+, CD15+, CD19+ immunophenotype. Cytoplasmic CD3 and CD79a were not expressed. Note the CD117/CD15 co-expression; this indicates a myeloid maturation defect as CD15 is normally only acquired by maturing myeloid cells (neutrophil or monocyte lineage) when CD117 is lost. This feature can be useful in tracking minimal (or measurable) residual disease using flow cytometry as it is not seen in normal marrow cells. The karyotype was 46,XX,t(8;21)(q22;q22.1),del(9)(q13q22) indicating a *RUNX1-RUNX1T1* rearrangement and a favourable prognosis. Additional chromosomal changes, especially deletion

Haematology: From the Image to the Diagnosis, First Edition. Mike Leach and Barbara J. Bain.
© 2022 John Wiley & Sons Ltd. Published 2022 by John Wiley & Sons Ltd.

of the long arm of chromosome 9, are common in this entity and this does not influence prognosis. The morphological features described here are typical of AML with this recurrent cytogenetic abnormality. The patient was treated with four cycles of chemotherapy and remains in remission 5 years later.

MCQ

Acute myeloid leukaemia with t(8;21)(q22;q22.1); *RUNX1-RUNX1T1*:

1 Can be diagnosed despite blast cells being less than 20% in blood and bone marrow
2 May have an increase in bone marrow eosinophils and precursors
3 Often shows trilineage dysplasia
4 Should be classified as mixed phenotype acute leukaemia when there is expression of CD19, CD79a and PAX5
5 Shows an association with systemic mastocytosis with a *KIT* D816V mutation

For answers and discussion, see page 206.

18 Chronic neutrophilic leukaemia

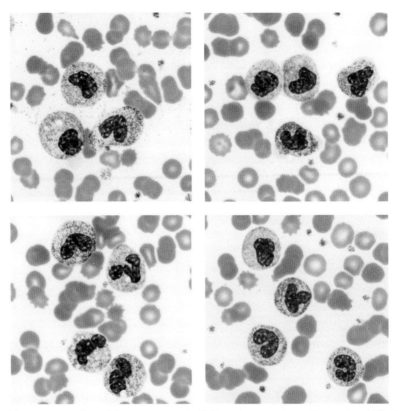

A 72-year-old man was referred for assessment of chronic asymptomatic neutrophilia. The initial blood tests had been triggered by a clinical diagnosis of gout. He had shown a chronic unexplained persistent neutrophilia and the most recent full blood count showed Hb 130 g/l, WBC 115 × 10^9/l, neutrophils 92 × 10^9/l and platelets 132 × 10^9/l. The blood film showed neutrophilia with minimal dysplasia, minimal left shift and no excess of blast cells. The neutrophils showed normal or increased granulation and some were vacuolated (all images ×100 objective). A bone marrow aspirate showed myeloid hyperplasia with no excess of blasts, eosinophils or basophils. Molecular analysis did not show *BCR-ABL1*. Two mutations in *CSF3R* were identified: T618I in exon 12 and E778X in exon 17. These findings are in keeping with a diagnosis of chronic neutrophilic leukaemia (CNL).

Chronic neutrophilic leukaemia is a rare myeloid disorder characterised by a chronic neutrophilia with mature neutrophils, often splenomegaly and the absence of a reactive trigger. Serum LDH and vitamin B12 levels are typically high and G-CSF levels are low. The diagnosis was largely one of exclusion until a strong association with mutations in the *CSF3R* gene was demonstrated. This is important in that mutations in *CSF3R* identify this as a clonal rather than reactive disorder and this is a defining feature in the 2016 WHO classification (Bain *et al.* 2017). In addition, there should be peripheral blood leucocytosis ≥25 × 10^9/l with at least 80% being mature neutrophils or band cells

Haematology: From the Image to the Diagnosis, First Edition. Mike Leach and Barbara J. Bain.
© 2022 John Wiley & Sons Ltd. Published 2022 by John Wiley & Sons Ltd.

and <10% being neutrophil precursors with no monocytosis. The type of *CSF3R* mutation appears to influence prognosis, being worse in the majority of patients who have this mutation (Szuber *et al.* 2018). Mutations in *CSF3R* are not essential for diagnosis but when absent the situation should be carefully reviewed and a leukaemoid reaction should be considered. In addition to *CSF3R*, mutations in *ASXL1*, *SETBP1*, *SRSF2* and rarely *JAK2* have been reported. Traditionally, CNL has been treated with chemotherapy, interferon or hypomethylating agents but responses have often been partial and not sustained. Without effective disease control many patients ultimately progress to blast crisis. More recently, the use of the JAK inhibitor ruxolitinib has been explored as CNL shows aberrant activation of the *JAK/STAT* pathway (Szuber *et al.* 2020).

References

Bain BJ, Brunning RD, Orazi A and Thiele J (2017) Chronic neutrophilic leukaemia. *In* Swerdlow SH, Campo E, Harris NL, Jaffe ES, Pileri S, Stein H and Thiele J (Eds) *WHO Classification of Tumours of Haematopoietic and Lymphoid Tissues,* revised 4th Edn. IARC Press, Lyon, pp. 37–38.

Szuber N, Finke CM, Lasho TL, Elliott MA. Hanson CA, Pardanani A and Tefferi A (2018) *CSF3R*-mutated chronic neutrophilic leukemia: long-term outcome in 19 consecutive patients and risk model for survival. *Blood Cancer J*, **8**, 21.

Szuber N, Elliott M and Tefferi A (2020) Chronic neutrophilic leukaemia: 2020 update on diagnosis, molecular genetics, prognosis and management. *Am J Haematol*, **95**, 212–224.

MCQ

Increased neutrophil granulation ('toxic' granulation) is a usual feature of:

1 Chronic myeloid leukaemia, *BCR-ABL1*-positive
2 Chronic neutrophilic leukaemia
3 G-CSF (filgrastim) therapy
4 Leukaemoid reaction to multiple myeloma
5 Sepsis

For answers and discussion, see page 206.

19   Essential thrombocythaemia

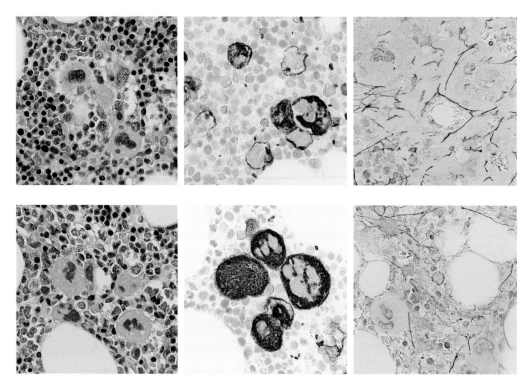

A 40-year-old man was referred on account of a persisting thrombocytosis. He was a smoker but gave no other past medical history of note and physical examination was unremarkable. The full blood count showed Hb 144 g/l, WBC 6.7×10^9/l, neutrophils 3.5×10^9/l and platelets 621×10^9/l. Serum ferritin was 120 µg/l. He had normal serum biochemistry and the ESR and CRP were normal. The blood film showed mild platelet anisocytosis but no other abnormality. The working diagnosis was essential thrombocythaemia (ET) but mutations in *JAK2* and *MPL* genes and deletions in *CALR* gene were not identified. The bone marrow trephine biopsy sections were mildly hypercellular (60%) and showed increased numbers of megakaryocytes forming clusters (left images, H&E, centre images, immunoperoxidase for CD42b) (all images ×50 objective). The megakaryocyte morphology was largely normal but some larger forms were recognised (lower centre image). There was some mild focal increase in reticulin staining (grade 1 of 3, right images). Erythroid and myeloid activity were normal and no abnormal infiltrate was noted. A diagnosis of ET was made.

Essential thrombocythaemia is a myeloproliferative neoplasm characterised by persistent thrombocytosis in the absence of anaemia or polycythaemia. Around 85% of cases will show abnormalities in *JAK2, CALR* or *MPL* but so called 'triple-negative' cases do exist (Cazzola and Kralovics 2014). In such circumstances the diagnosis is one of exclusion when persistence of thrombocytosis is shown, reactive causes are excluded and the bone marrow morphology supports the diagnosis and excludes other myeloproliferative neoplasms (polycythaemia vera, primary myelofibrosis and chronic myeloid leukaemia). Bone marrow trephine biopsy sections typically show only mild hypercellularity, an increase in medium to large megakaryocytes with focal aggregations or 'clustering' with only a minimal, if any, increase in reticulin staining. A cluster requires three or more megakaryocytes to be adjacent to, or touching, each other. Cases that are suspicious for ET, but without sufficient features for a definitive diagnosis, are not uncommon. A proportion of these triple-negative cases show either a low allele burden, an alternative mutation site in *JAK2* or *MPL* or a mutation only identified by examining platelet RNA (Angona *et al.* 2016), but evidence of clonality is currently not demonstrable in all cases that appear to be true ET.

References

Angona A, Fernández-Rodríguez C, Alvarez-Larrán A, Camacho L, Longarón R, Torres E *et al.* (2016) Molecular characterisation of triple negative essential thrombocythaemia patients by platelet analysis and targeted sequencing. *Blood Cancer J*, **6**, e463.

Cazzola M and Kralovics R (2014) From Janus kinase 2 to calreticulin: the clinically relevant genomic landscape of myeloproliferative neoplasms. *Blood*, **123**, 3714–3719.

MCQ

Essential thrombocythaemia:

1 Causes itch in a minority of patients
2 Is associated with *JAK2* V617F in more than half of patients
3 Is most often an incidental diagnosis in an asymptomatic patient
4 Is Ph+, *BCR-ABL1*+ in only a minority of patients
5 Typically has small platelets

For answers and discussion, see page 206.

20   Hairy cell leukaemia

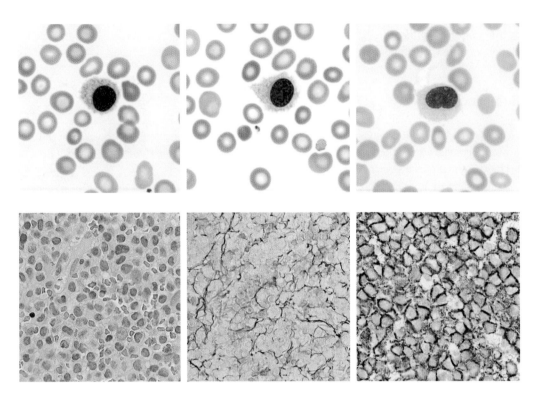

A 43-year-old man presented with fatigue and early satiety. His automated full blood count showed Hb 75 g/l, WBC 15.3×10^9/l, lymphocytes 3.62×10^9/l, neutrophils 0.6×10^9/l, monocytes 11.1×10^9/l and platelets 32×10^9/l. He had an easily palpable spleen without lymphadenopathy. The blood film showed plentiful hairy cells with a typical round or ovoid nucleus, absent nucleoli and pale blue fluffy irregular cytoplasm (top images ×100 objective): some cells showed an indented peanut-shaped nucleus (top right). The marrow trephine biopsy sections (×50) showed a diffuse infiltrate of lymphoid cells with voluminous cytoplasm (bottom left, H&E), generating grade 1–2/3 fibrosis (bottom centre, reticulin stain) with strong uniform CD20 positivity (bottom right, immunoperoxidase). Flow cytometric studies on the peripheral blood lymphoid cells indicated a CD19+, CD20+, CD79b+, CD22+, FMC7+, HLA-DR+, CD10+, CD11c+, CD25+, CD103+, CD123+ and lambda-restricted immunophenotype. The diagnosis is hairy cell leukaemia (HCL), a rare mature B-cell neoplasm typically causing splenomegaly and cytopenias, most notably neutropenia and monocytopenia (note that the automated analyser has miscounted the hairy cells as monocytes). The disease typically infiltrates the bone marrow in a diffuse pattern with associated fibrosis. Bone marrow aspirates are typically 'dry' so a careful assessment of the blood film is frequently useful in anticipating this condition.

The images on the facing page are of peripheral blood from a patient with splenic marginal zone lymphoma (SMZL). There are some morphological similarities to HCL but the cells here are a little smaller and have less voluminous cytoplasm showing fronds and tufts (×100). The cytoplasmic

Haematology: From the Image to the Diagnosis, First Edition. Mike Leach and Barbara J. Bain.
© 2022 John Wiley & Sons Ltd. Published 2022 by John Wiley & Sons Ltd.

border is somewhat easier to define. The cells here showed a mature pan-B phenotype with CD11c positivity whilst CD25, CD103 and CD123 were not expressed.

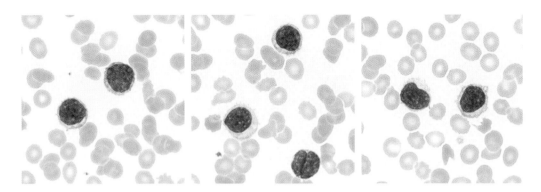

The pattern of bone marrow infiltration also differs in SMZL. This condition can show a degree of interstitial infiltration but it more typically demonstrates focal nodular, paratrabecular and intrasinusoidal disease.

Hairy cell leukaemia variant, in which the neoplastic cells have prominent nucleoli, must also be distinguished from HCL. Despite the name, this condition has no close relationship to hairy cell leukaemia.

MCQ

Hairy cell leukaemia:

1 Can be distinguished from chronic lymphocytic leukaemia on the basis of CD200 expression
2 Is associated with a *BRAF* V600E mutation in the majority of patients
3 Is best distinguished from hairy cell leukaemia variant by expression of CD25, CD123 and CD200
4 Requires assessment of tartrate-resistant acid phosphatase (TRAP) activity for a firm diagnosis
5 Usually has collagen fibrosis

For answers and discussion, see page 206.

21   Mantle cell lymphoma in leukaemic phase

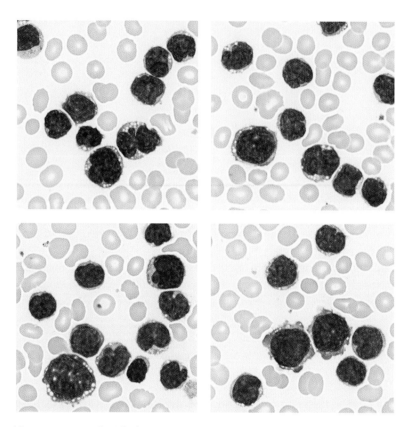

A 66-year-old man presented with dizziness, headaches and difficulty walking. On assessment he was globally confused but had no specific neurological deficit. His full blood count showed Hb 79 g/l, WBC 602×10^9/l and platelets 70×10^9/l. He had splenomegaly but no significant lymphadenopathy. His blood film showed pleomorphic lymphoid cells varying in size from small to large, with condensed nuclear chromatin and prominent nuclear clefts and convolutions, with many of the larger cells showing cytoplasmic vacuoles (all images ×100 objective). Immunophenotyping studies identified a mature CD5−, kappa-restricted, B-cell lymphoproliferative disorder expressing CD19, CD20, CD79b, FMC7 and CD38. Immunohistochemistry on the marrow trephine biopsy sections showed the cells to express nuclear cyclin D1 and on karyotypic analysis a t(11;14)(q13;q32) trans-location was identified with, in addition, loss of the short arm of chromosome 17 in 60% of cells. The features here are most consistent with leukaemic non-nodal mantle cell lymphoma.

   In view of the presentation, in keeping with cerebral leucostasis, he was treated by leucapheresis and emergency chemotherapy incorporating high-dose corticosteroids, cyclophosphamide and vincristine. This was followed by six courses of high-dose cytarabine and rituximab with an incom-plete clinical response with persisting splenomegaly on CT imaging. The splenic anatomy remained abnormal with focal hypodense lesions and a splenectomy was performed. This showed extramed-ullary haemopoiesis but no evidence of residual lymphoma. This patient remains well and in remission 12 years later.

Haematology: From the Image to the Diagnosis, First Edition. Mike Leach and Barbara J. Bain.
© 2022 John Wiley & Sons Ltd. Published 2022 by John Wiley & Sons Ltd.

Mantle cell lymphoma constitutes between 3 and 10% of non-Hodgkin lymphomas. Typically, it involves lymph nodes, but the spleen and bone marrow are also often infiltrated. The disease also has an affinity for the gastrointestinal tract but this may not necessarily be symptomatic. A subset of patients, as in the case presented here, show a leukaemic presentation with splenomegaly but without lymphadenopathy. Leukaemic non-nodal mantle cell lymphoma is biologically different and paradoxically, despite the leukaemic manifestation, usually has a more indolent course and an appreciably better prognosis (Nadeu *et al.* 2020). More aggressive forms of the disease can show mutations in *TP53, MYC* and *CDKN2A*. The latter is an important tumour suppressor gene encoding proteins which in turn inhibit MDM2 (a physiological inhibitor of the TP53 pathway). Loss or mutation of either *CDKN2A* or *TP53* leads to chemotherapy resistance and *MYC* mutation is typically associated with proliferative disease. Note the CD5 negativity here; approximately 5% of mantle cell lymphomas are CD5 negative so morphological assessment alongside genetic and immunohistochemical studies are still required in achieving the correct diagnosis.

Reference

Nadeu F, Martin-Garcia D, Clot G, Díaz-Navarro A, Duran-Ferrer M, Navarro A *et al.* (2020) Genomic and epigenomic insights into the origin, pathogenesis, and clinical behavior of mantle cell lymphoma subtypes. *Blood*, **136**, 1419–1432.

MCQ

Mantle cell lymphoma:

1 Can result from translocations involving *CCND1, CCND2* or *CCND3*
2 Is derived from marginal zone lymphocytes
3 Is the most common pathology underlying multiple lymphomatous polyposis
4 May show SOX11 expression on immunohistochemistry
5 Usually expresses CD200

For answers and discussion, see page 206.

22 Infantile osteopetrosis

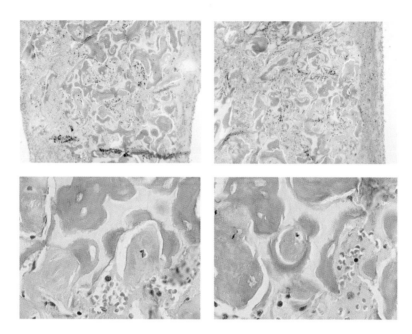

A 6-month-old boy, born to consanguineous parents, presented with failure to thrive, developmental delay and pancytopenia. He was found to have significant hearing impairment. His full blood count showed Hb 80 g/l, WBC 2×10^9/l, neutrophils 0.8×10^9/l and platelets 50×10^9/l. The blood film was leucoerythroblastic but abnormal cells were not identified. The bone marrow aspirate was markedly hypocellular. The bone marrow trephine biopsy sections were highly abnormal, showing prominent disorganised trabecular structure and whorls with a significant encroachment on, and reduction in activity of, normal haemopoietic marrow (top images ×10 objective, bottom images ×50). The normal haemopoietic marrow space appears overrun by abnormal disorganised marrow trabeculae. The clinical presentation and marrow findings are indicative of inherited infantile osteopetrosis.

Infantile osteopetrosis is a serious autosomal recessively inherited disorder of osteoclast malfunction. It presents in infancy with progressive pancytopenia and cranial nerve compromise due to uncontrolled bony overgrowth resulting from an osteoclast-based remodelling failure. The most serious early consequences are progressive hearing and visual loss due to compression of the auditory and optical nerves, respectively. The condition needs to be recognised and treated early since, as osteoclasts are derived from bone marrow stem cells, the only effective therapy is allogeneic bone marrow transplantation.

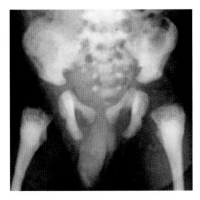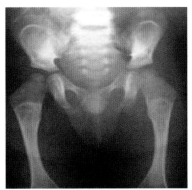

The images above are plain X-rays of the pelvis in a child with osteopetrosis before (left) and after (right) allogeneic stem cell transplantation.[1] Note the marked improvement in bone density due to the donor-derived stem cells and subsequent osteoclast-related bone resorption and remodelling. The transplant also helps re-establish the haemopoietic marrow space and thus blood count recovery.

Note

1 Images courtesy of Professor Rob Wynn and Cambridge University Press.

MCQ

Infantile osteopetrosis can be associated with:

1 Autosomal recessive or dominant inheritance
2 Decreased osteoclasts
3 Fragile bones
4 Responsiveness to vitamin D that renders transplantation unnecessary
5 Increased osteoclasts

For answers and discussion, see page 206.

23 Reactive eosinophilia

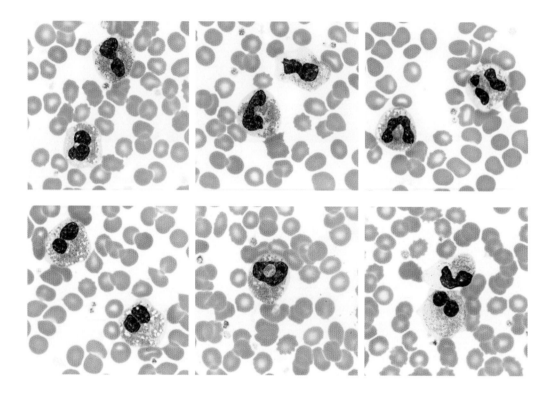

A 79-year-old man with a 60-year smoking history presented with the recent onset of anorexia and weight loss with rapidly appearing skin nodules. He had no new respiratory symptoms though he had a longstanding cough attributed to chronic obstructive pulmonary disease. His full blood count showed Hb 133 g/l, WBC 58 × 10^9/l, eosinophils 35 × 10^9/l and platelets 500 × 10^9/l. The blood film confirmed a marked eosinophilia with a number of abnormalities of eosinophil morphology. Hypogranular eosinophils are prominent (all images ×100 objective) with some cells showing 50% loss of cytoplasmic granules (top left). There is also eosinophil cytoplasmic vacuolation (bottom left) and some basophilic granulation (top centre and bottom right). Finally, there are cells with nuclear abnormalities with some showing separation of nuclear components (top right) and even a ring nucleus (bottom centre). It might be assumed that such dramatic morphological abnormalities indicate a primary haematological disorder but this is not the case. A CT scan of chest, abdomen and pelvis showed a solid pulmonary lesion with irregular margins, mediastinal lymphadenopathy and bilateral adrenal masses. A skin biopsy showed a poorly differentiated carcinoma of possible primary lung origin.

Eosinophil morphology has intrigued experienced morphologists for decades. In contrast to neutrophils, dysplastic features are actually very common in reactive eosinophilias and morphological features are not reliable in predicting when eosinophilia might be a component of a myeloid neoplasm (Goasguen *et al.* 2020). It is important therefore to interpret all available investigative data and to consider reactive eosinophilia even when morphological abnormalities are apparent

Haematology: From the Image to the Diagnosis, First Edition. Mike Leach and Barbara J. Bain.

© 2022 John Wiley & Sons Ltd. Published 2022 by John Wiley & Sons Ltd.

(Leach 2020). The fruitless pursuit of a primary haematological disorder could divert from the actual diagnosis. It did not delay diagnosis in the patient described as easily accessible skin tissue was available but in other patients this might not necessarily be the case.

References

Goasguen JE, Bennett JM, Bain BJ, Brunning R, Zini G, Vallespi M-T *et al.*; International Working Group on Morphology of MDS (2020) The role of eosinophil morphology in distinguishing between reactive eosinophilia and eosinophilia as a feature of a myeloid neoplasm. *Br J Haematol*, **191**, 497–504.
Leach M (2020) The diagnostic utility of eosinophil morphology. *Br J Haematol*, **191**, 325.

MCQ

Reactive eosinophilia can occur in:

1 Acute lymphoblastic leukaemia
2 Acute myeloid leukaemia associated with inv(16)
3 Babesiosis
4 Filariasis
5 Strongyloidiasis

For answers and discussion, see page 206.

24 Stomatocytic red cell disorders

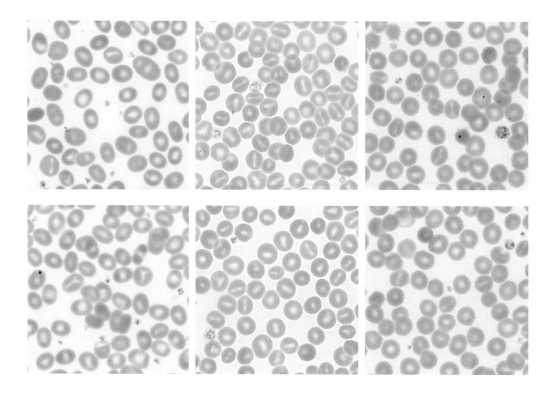

A 30-year-old woman, born in the Philippines, presented at the booking clinic with a pregnancy of 12 weeks' duration. She gave no prior history of anaemia or blood disorder. Her full blood count showed Hb 130 g/l, WBC 9×10^9/l and platelets 247×10^9/l. The blood film showed prominent ovalocytes, many of which were also macrocytic and stomatocytic. Notably, there were double, transverse and longitudinal stomas (left images ×100 objective) and some cells had Y-shaped stomas (bottom left). The morphological features here, in particular the macro-ovalocytes with double stomas (knizocytes, image top left) together with the ethnic origin of the patient, are indicative of a diagnosis of Southeast Asian ovalocytosis. This condition results from mutations in the *SLC4A1* gene resulting in a variant band 3 protein which increases membrane stiffness. In the resting state there is normally minimal or absent haemolysis but this can be significant in the perinatal period. Carriers of this polymorphism have a survival advantage against all forms of malaria.

A second patient, a 37-year-old man, was referred for investigation of mild chronic thrombocytopenia; the full blood count showed Hb 140 g/l, WBC 5×10^9/l and platelets 80×10^9/l. There was no personal or family bleeding history and clinical examination was normal. The blood film showed prominent stomatocytes and macrothrombocytopenia but no neutrophil inclusions were present (centre images ×100). Routine biochemistry and serum lipid levels were normal. Serum phytosterol levels, however, were grossly elevated at up to 20 times the upper limit of normal. He was a compound heterozygote for mutations in the *ABCG5* gene and these findings are in keeping with a diagnosis of hereditary phytosterolaemia, also known as sitosterolaemia. This is an under-recognised disorder of plant lipid (phytosterol) absorption and excretion characterised by red cell stomatocytosis, macrothrombocytopenia and sometimes a mild haemolytic anaemia with splenomegaly. It is an important condition to be aware of as it can lead to abnormal lipid deposition in tissues (xanthelasma and xanthomas) and in blood vessels, leading to accelerated atherosclerosis. Patients may benefit from treatment with ezetimibe, which blocks absorption of phytosterols and may protect patients from the aforementioned complications.

A third patient, a 60-year-old man with a historical diagnosis of hereditary spherocytosis treated with splenectomy at 18 years of age after an episode of parvovirus-induced red cell aplasia, was referred for reassessment after developing life-threatening pulmonary embolism following a long-haul flight. His full blood count showed Hb 140 g/l, WBC $13 \times 10^9/l$ and platelets $507 \times 10^9/l$. There was no personal or family history of thrombosis and physical examination was normal. There was no laboratory evidence of an inherited thrombophilia and no molecular evidence of a myeloproliferative neoplasm. His blood film showed well-haemoglobinised red cells with prominent stomatocytes in addition to hyposplenic features (right images ×100). His historical pre-splenectomy osmotic fragility test was traced and found to be normal as were red cell eosin-5-maleimide (EMA) binding studies by flow cytometry. Red cell membrane polyacrylamide gel electrophoresis showed no abnormality. The features here are in keeping with a diagnosis of overhydrated hereditary stomatocytosis, a mild, often well-compensated haemolytic anaemia most often caused by mutations in the *RHAG* gene that result in loss of membrane stomatin, causing abnormal sodium and potassium homeostasis and increased intracellular water. Splenectomy significantly increases the risk of venous thrombosis; the patient is now on life-long anticoagulation with rivaroxaban.

MCQ

Stomatocytosis can be a feature of:

1 Alcoholic excess and alcoholic liver disease
2 Hereditary xerocytosis
3 Hydroxycarbamide therapy
4 Triose phosphate isomerase deficiency
5 Zieve syndrome

For answers and discussion, see page 206.

25   Reactive lymphocytosis due to viral infection

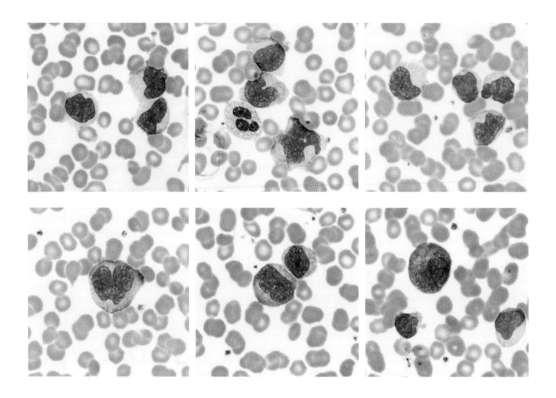

An 18-year-old 'fresher' medical student was referred to the university medical service with a fever, sore throat and cervical lymphadenopathy. His full blood count showed Hb 144 g/l, WBC 74×10^9/l, neutrophils 7.4×10^9/l, lymphocytes 66×10^9/l and platelets 203×10^9/l. The liver enzyme profile showed increased transaminases (AST 300 u/l, ALT 279 u/l) and a Monospot® test (which later became available) was positive. Epstein–Barr virus (EBV) was subsequently detected in his blood at 5606 copies/ml. The blood film caused some initial concern amongst the trainees due to the magnitude of lymphocytosis, but further careful morphological review from more senior members of the department was reassuring. Notably, the blood film shows a population of medium to large pleomorphic lymphocytes (all images ×100 objective), with some showing fine cytoplasmic granules. The cells have voluminous cytoplasm and tend to be indented by adjacent red cells (top images). Importantly, some cells have blastoid morphology, being larger with a prominent nucleolus and having more pronounced cytoplasmic basophilia. Flow cytometry identified a large population of CD8+, CD5+, CD2+, HLA-DR+, CD7+/− cells which were not expressing precursor antigens, CD30 or CD25. The morphological diagnosis is a reactive lymphocytosis due to viral infection, in this case EBV infection. The flow cytometric studies are in keeping with this as expression of HLA-DR is an activation marker of T cells and such cells frequently show some loss of CD7 expression. The activated cells are cytotoxic CD8+ T lymphocytes even though EBV targets the B-lymphoid population.

Haematology: From the Image to the Diagnosis, First Edition. Mike Leach and Barbara J. Bain.
© 2022 John Wiley & Sons Ltd. Published 2022 by John Wiley & Sons Ltd.

Reactive lymphocytosis is relatively common in clinical practice and the morphological features described above are typical. Neoplastic disorders tend to have more monomorphic appearances, but of course a careful assessment of the clinical circumstances is always necessary. T-cell neoplasms are remarkably variable in their presentation but the clinical history, morphology, laboratory investigations and flow cytometric findings were all consistent with a reactive process. Importantly, a wide range of viruses and other organisms can induce such a reaction; these include EBV, cytomegalovirus, human immunodeficiency virus (HIV), toxoplasma and pertussis. Most often the responsible organism is benign but if HIV is implicated it is important that this is identified. A positive test for a heterophile antibody is a pointer to EBV infection but not all cases are positive. Immunophenotyping is not generally indicated but was performed in this case because of initial concern about the possibility of a lymphoma.

MCQ

Infectious mononucleosis due to the Epstein–Barr virus:

1 Can be associated with pure red cell aplasia
2 Can be complicated by haemophagocytic lymphohistiocytosis
3 Can be followed by aplastic anaemia
4 Is associated with a subsequent increased incidence of Hodgkin lymphoma
5 Predisposes to B-lineage acute lymphoblastic leukaemia

For answers and discussion, see page 206.

26 Therapy-related acute myeloid leukaemia with eosinophilia

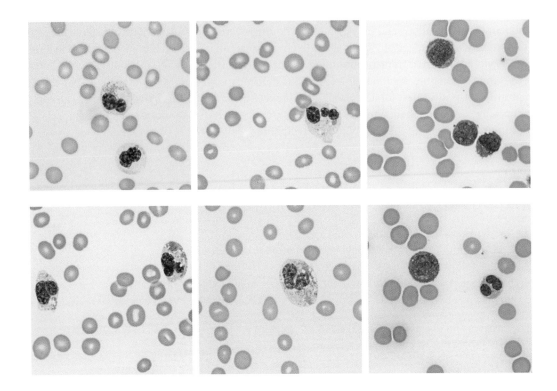

A 70-year-old man developed therapy-related acute myeloid leukaemia (t-AML) some years after starting chlorambucil therapy for chronic lymphocytic leukaemia. His FBC showed Hb 63 g/l, WBC 48.9 × 10^9/l, neutrophils 1.0 × 10^9/l, lymphocytes 5.5 × 10^9/l, eosinophils 19.6 × 10^9/l, monocytes 1.4 × 10^9/l, myelocytes 0.4 × 10^9/l, blast cells 21 × 10^9/l and platelet count 11 × 10^9/l. There were two nucleated red blood cells per 100 leucocytes. Many of the eosinophils were cytologically abnormal: 25% were hypogranular, 46% were vacuolated and 17% were both hypogranular and vacuolated (all images ×100 objective). Occasional eosinophils had fine basophilic granules (bottom centre) or non-lobated nuclei. Neutrophils were cytologically normal. The myeloblasts were small and compact with little cytoplasm and prominent nucleoli (right images).

Clonal eosinophils in myeloid neoplasms tend to have more marked cytological abnormalities than those in reactive eosinophilia but there is considerable overlap. It is therefore essential for cytological abnormalities to be assessed together with other disease features. When there is an increase in blast cells, as in the current patient, or when there are clearly dysplastic features in other lineages, such as hypogranular neutrophils, the diagnosis is straightforward. However, if an increase in cytologically abnormal eosinophils occurs without other morphological clues, cytogenetic and molecular analysis may well be needed to confirm the diagnosis of a myeloid neoplasm.

Haematology: From the Image to the Diagnosis, First Edition. Mike Leach and Barbara J. Bain.
© 2022 John Wiley & Sons Ltd. Published 2022 by John Wiley & Sons Ltd.

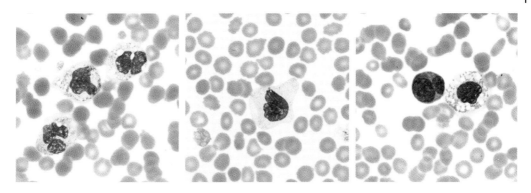

The images above (×100 objective) show hypogranular and vacuolated eosinophils; the cell in the centre image is virtually agranular. Note also the dysplastic platelet (centre) and the megakaryoblast (right); these latter two features together with the eosinophil morphology suggest a clonal haemopoietic disorder, in this case primary myelofibrosis.

Therapy-related AML is an unfortunate consequence of bone marrow exposure to chemotherapy or radiotherapy used as treatment for neoplastic disease in haematology and oncology practice. As more of these conditions are cured with modern therapy, often using a combination of surgery, chemotherapy and radiotherapy, in breast cancer for example, more patients are surviving to develop therapy-related myeloid neoplasms. It is not uncommon within haematology to see therapy-related AML resulting from treatment of another haematological disease, as in the patient described here. We have seen such cases as a result of previous successful treatment for Hodgkin lymphoma, diffuse large B-cell lymphoma, blastic plasmacytoid dendritic cell neoplasm and acute promyelocytic leukaemia. To be cured of a good-prognosis leukaemia and develop a poor-prognosis leukaemia as a consequence is particularly difficult to face.

MCQ

Therapy-related acute leukaemia:

1 Can be associated with 5q−, monosomy 5, 7q− and monosomy 7
2 Can be lymphoblastic or myeloid
3 Has an equally poor prognosis, regardless of the causative agent, the blast percentage or any cytogenetic abnormalities present
4 Has identical characteristics whether it follows alkylating agents or topoisomerase II inhibitors
5 Increases in incidence with the age of exposure to the causative agent

For answers and discussion, see page 206.

27 Red cell fragmentation syndromes

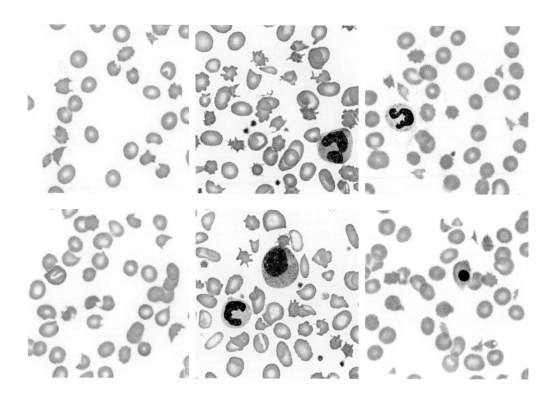

A 40-year-old man undergoing allogeneic stem cell transplantation for chronic myeloid leukaemia developed a worsening anaemia, renal dysfunction and jaundice on day 30 of the procedure. His full blood count showed Hb 90 g/l, WBC 1.0×10^9/l, neutrophils 0.3×10^9/l and platelets 10×10^9/l. The blood film showed prominent red cell fragmentation but with minimal polychromasia (left images ×100 objective). The reticulocyte count was 20×10^9/l. A diagnosis of ciclosporin-induced microangiopathic haemolytic anaemia seemed likely and the patient's clinical condition and laboratory parameters improved when the drug was withheld.

A second patient, a 70-year-old man known to the Oncology department with a diagnosis of a mucinous gastric carcinoma, was admitted with weight loss, pallor and jaundice. His full blood count showed Hb 73 g/l, WBC 27×10^9/l, neutrophils 18×10^9/l and platelets 399×10^9/l. The blood film showed red cell fragmentation, contracted poikilocytes and acanthocytes with neutrophilia and left shift to myelocytes (centre images ×100). CT scanning showed widespread dissemination of disease with involvement of perigastric nodes, peritoneum and liver. The coagulation profile was in keeping with disseminated intravascular coagulation (DIC). A diagnosis of metastatic carcinoma with associated DIC and secondary microangiopathic haemolytic anaemia was made.

A third patient, a 50-year-old woman with a serious inherited cardiomyopathy, awaiting cardiac transplantation, was admitted for management of severe cardiac failure. A ventricular assist device was implanted to augment cardiac output whilst a potential donor was sourced but the increasing

Haematology: From the Image to the Diagnosis, First Edition. Mike Leach and Barbara J. Bain.
© 2022 John Wiley & Sons Ltd. Published 2022 by John Wiley & Sons Ltd.

drive on the device generated a worsening anaemia, rising LDH and jaundice. The full blood count showed Hb 85 g/l, WBC 40×10^9/l, neutrophils 32×10^9/l and platelets 19×10^9/l. The blood film showed red cell fragmentation, with nucleated red cells (right images ×100), indicating significant bone marrow stress. On the basis of these findings the mechanical ventricular assist treatment was moderated and the red cell fragmentation syndrome improved. She survived through to the cardiac transplant procedure.

MCQ

Microangiopathic haemolytic anaemia can result from:

1 A defective prosthetic cardiac valve
2 Haemolytic uraemic syndrome following *Escherichia coli* O157:H7 infection
3 Pregnancy-associated HELLP syndrome
4 Severe aortic or mitral valve disease
5 Thrombotic thrombocytopenic purpura

For answers and discussion, see page 206.

28   NK/T-cell lymphoma in leukaemic phase

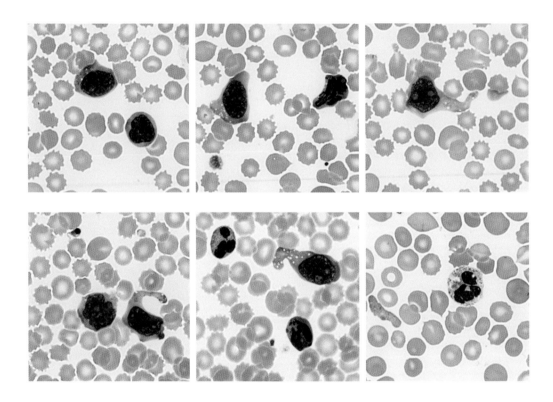

A 70-year-old woman had been non-specifically unwell for 6 weeks with anorexia and weight loss. She came to the attention of the Haematology department on account of her blood count, which showed Hb 107 g/l, WBC 21.2×10^9/l, neutrophils 4.7×10^9/l and platelets 56×10^9/l. The blood film showed a significant population of large pleomorphic lymphoid cells with an ovoid clefted nucleus, prominent nucleoli and basophilic vacuolated cytoplasm with prominent projections and fine granules (all top images, bottom left and centre) (all images ×100 objective). There were prominent cytoplasmic fragments in the film (top centre and right; bottom left and right) and even neutrophils showing phagocytosis of cytoplasmic debris (bottom right). Note the karyorrhexis of a malignant cell (bottom centre). A high-grade neoplasm was suspected. Flow cytometric studies gating on a blast gate identified a CD45+, HLA-DR+, CD7+, CD56+, cCD3+ neoplasm. An NK/T-cell lymphoma in leukaemic phase was suspected.

Haematology: From the Image to the Diagnosis, First Edition. Mike Leach and Barbara J. Bain.
© 2022 John Wiley & Sons Ltd. Published 2022 by John Wiley & Sons Ltd.

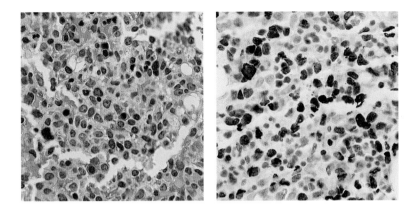

The bone marrow trephine biopsy sections showed an infiltrate of similar cells with a CD3+, CD7+, CD30-weak, CD56+, Epstein–Barr virus (EBV) early RNA (EBER)+ phenotype. An H&E-stained section of the trephine biopsy specimen is shown above (left image ×50) and EBV *in situ* hybridisation shows positivity in the neoplastic cells (right image ×50).

The diagnosis here is leukaemic phase of extranodal NK/T-cell lymphoma, nasal type. This is a rare neoplasm with aggressive behaviour and extranodal presentation (typically nasal, testis, gut, bone marrow, spleen or liver). A leukaemic presentation is very rare and carries a particularly poor prognosis.

MCQ

Extranodal NK/T-cell lymphoma, nasal type:

1 Does not involve lymph nodes
2 Is angiocentric
3 Is strongly associated with EBV
4 Is usually cCD3 negative on flow cytometry
5 Occurs only in Chinese and other Asian populations

For answers and discussion, see page 206.

29 Myelodysplastic syndrome with del(5q)

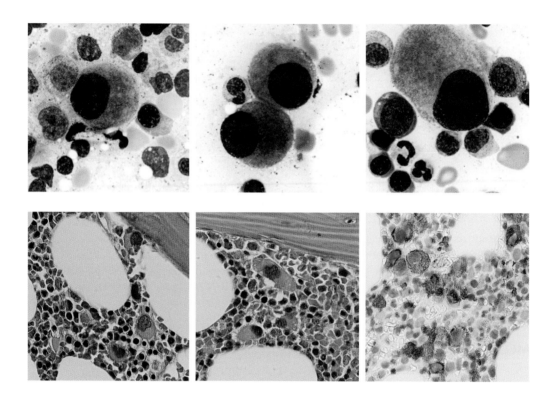

A 70-year-old man was referred for investigation of a mild macrocytic anaemia and thrombocytopenia. His full blood count showed Hb 90 g/l, MCV 103 fl, WBC 6×10^9/l, neutrophils 3×10^9/l and platelets 123×10^9/l. The blood film showed mild macrocytosis and anisopoikilocytosis, the leucocytes appeared normal and the platelet count was genuine. Haematinic assays were normal and the reticulocyte count was 45×10^9/l. Urea and electrolytes, liver enzyme profile, bone biochemistry and thyroid function tests were all normal. The bone marrow aspirate notably showed small and non-lobated megakaryocytes (top images ×100 objective) and this was a remarkably consistent feature. There was mild dyserythropoiesis and normal granulopoiesis. The trephine biopsy specimen showed the same non-lobated megakaryocytes, some of which were abnormally located adjacent to bony trabeculae (bottom left and centre ×50), further highlighted by CD42b staining (bottom right, immunoperoxidase ×50). Metaphase cytogenetic studies showed an isolated 5q chromosomal deletion.

Myelodysplastic syndrome with chromosome 5q deletion, sometimes referred to as the 5q− syndrome, is a subtype of MDS typically presenting with a mild anaemia. When this chromosomal abnormality is identified in isolation the condition normally carries a good prognosis and frequently responds well to directed treatment as long as there is not a coexistent *TP53* mutation. The morphological abnormalities of megakaryocytes shown here are typical, so much so that the cytogenetic counterpart can often be predicted. Non-lobated megakaryocytes can be seen in a multitude of other myeloid disorders, including other MDS subtypes, myeloproliferative and

Haematology: From the Image to the Diagnosis, First Edition. Mike Leach and Barbara J. Bain.
© 2022 John Wiley & Sons Ltd. Published 2022 by John Wiley & Sons Ltd.

myelodysplastic/myeloproliferative neoplasms and AML, but they are normally one feature amongst a myriad of other megakaryocyte abnormalities. The megakaryocyte morphology in MDS with 5q– is remarkably consistent.

MCQ

The WHO category of myelodysplastic syndrome with isolated del(5q):

1 By definition, cannot have any other cytogenetic abnormality
2 By definition, can have thrombocytopenia but not thrombocytosis
3 Can benefit from lenalidomide therapy
4 Has a poor prognosis
5 Is more common in females

For answers and discussion, see page 206.

30 Classical Hodgkin lymphoma

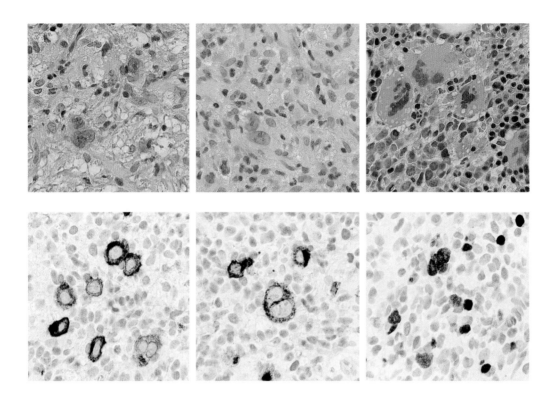

A previously fit 35-year-old man presented with progressive fatigue and night sweats with the latter occurring every night. Physical examination revealed pathological lymph nodes in the left groin. A CT scan showed widespread lymphadenopathy including involvement of the mediastinum and in addition a PET/CT scan suggested pathological fluorodeoxyglucose uptake in multiple bone foci including the right superior posterior iliac crest. Bone marrow trephine biopsy sections were markedly abnormal, showing an abnormal nodular infiltrate of large cells with complex bilobed nuclei and prominent nucleoli surrounded by histiocytes, lymphocytes and plasma cells (top left and centre, H&E, all images ×50 objective). These large cells have typical characteristics of Reed–Sternberg and Hodgkin cells. Other areas showed reactive features including hypercellularity with increased megakaryocytes, lymphocytes, plasma cells and eosinophils (top right).

Immunohistochemical studies showed the large cells to express CD30 (bottom left), CD15 (bottom centre) and weak nuclear PAX5 (bottom right); note also the strong expression of PAX5 in the smaller normal mature B cells. No other T-cell or B-cell specific antigens were expressed and CD45 expression in the large cells was absent. The features here are indicative of a diagnosis of classical Hodgkin lymphoma. The patient had a Hasenclever score of 4 and was therefore treated with escalated BEACOPP therapy. An interim PET/CT showed no pathological nodal uptake and a full six cycles of therapy were subsequently delivered. He is currently well and in remission 12 months after completing treatment.

Haematology: From the Image to the Diagnosis, First Edition. Mike Leach and Barbara J. Bain.
© 2022 John Wiley & Sons Ltd. Published 2022 by John Wiley & Sons Ltd.

MCQ

Classical Hodgkin lymphoma:

1 Has the Epstein–Barr virus (EBV) as an aetiological factor in a significant proportion of cases
2 Is a neoplasm of uncertain lineage
3 Is increased in frequency in patients carrying the human immunodeficiency virus (HIV)
4 Is more common in children and adolescents in developing countries than in developed countries
5 When the bone marrow is infiltrated, can usually be diagnosed by the presence of Reed–Sternberg cells and mononuclear Hodgkin cells in a bone marrow aspirate

For answers and discussion, see page 206.

31 Cryoglobulinaemia

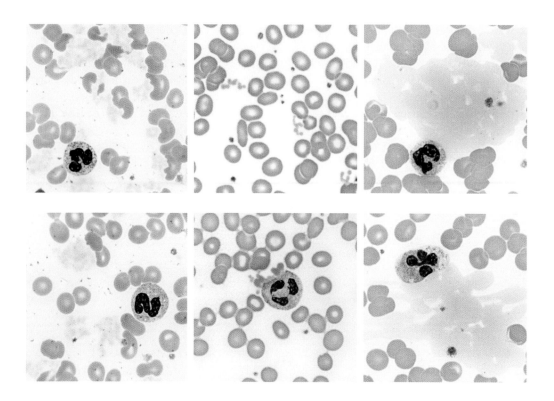

A 59-year-old man with a known diagnosis of lymphoplasmacytic lymphoma had a full blood count performed, this showing Hb 110 g/l, WBC 5.1×10^9/l and platelets 2300×10^9/l. The apparent high platelet count required a blood film to be examined. This revealed severe distortion of red cell morphology by an amorphous pale blue precipitate (left images ×100 objective), which had formed on cooling of the sample. A type I cryoglobulin, derived from an IgM paraprotein, was detected. The apparent thrombocytosis and red cell changes were spurious. A repeat FBC performed on a fresh warmed specimen showed a normal platelet count.

A second patient, a 70-year-old woman with a known diagnosis of multiple myeloma had a full blood count performed, this showing Hb 110 g/l, WBC 8×10^9/l and platelets 353×10^9/l. The blood film in this case shows small globules and strings of pink precipitate, whilst the red cell morphology was preserved (centre images ×100). A type I cryoglobulin derived from an IgG paraprotein was detected.

A third patient, a 65-year-old woman with a history of rheumatoid arthritis, presented with joint pains, mottled skin and ischaemic ears and toes. Her FBC showed Hb 65 g/l, WBC 9.4×10^9/l and platelets 433×10^9/l. The blood film showed large aggregates of a blue precipitate forming in zones within the film and displacing red cells (right images ×100). A type III cryoglobulin derived from polyclonal IgM and IgG was identified and a diagnosis of mixed cryoglobulinaemia with associated vasculitis was made.

Haematology: From the Image to the Diagnosis, First Edition. Mike Leach and Barbara J. Bain.
© 2022 John Wiley & Sons Ltd. Published 2022 by John Wiley & Sons Ltd.

Cryoglobulins are monoclonal or polyclonal immunoglobulins that precipitate on cooling below 37°C. They can often be seen as precipitates in blood films and their identification is important. They can cause clinical abnormalities, misquantitation of paraproteins and spurious blood counts, typically with false elevations of the platelet count when the cryoglobulin particles have impedance characteristics and size similar to platelets. In some cases the cryoglobulin actually binds to platelets (images below ×100), causing spurious thrombocytopenia. Cryoglobulin can also be ingested by neutrophils and monocytes or appear as crystalline deposits in blood films. Careful examination of the blood film is crucial in all of these scenarios.

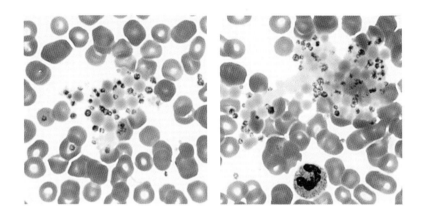

MCQ

Type II cryoglobulinaemia:

1 Can be a feature of hepatitis C infection
2 Can occur in Sjögren syndrome
3 Has no monoclonal component
4 Is occasionally a feature of a lymphoproliferative disorder
5 Is typically found in multiple myeloma

For answers and discussion, see page 206.

32   Congenital dyserythropoietic anaemia

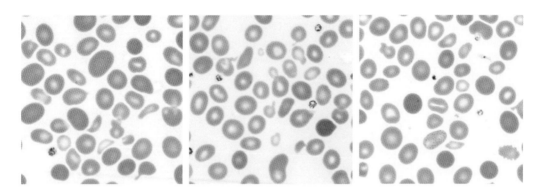

A 22-year-old woman was referred for investigation of a macrocytic anaemia whilst her brother (similarly affected) was simultaneously referred to another Haematology team. The GP referral letter suggested that her mother had a diagnosis of hereditary spherocytosis but this was not confirmed on subsequent investigation; the mother's blood film, haemolytic indices and eosin-5-maleimide (EMA) binding studies were all normal. The patient's full blood count showed Hb 110 g/l, MCV 115 fl, WBC 6×10^9/l and platelets 257×10^9/l. Serum vitamin B12 and folate assays were normal but serum ferritin was elevated at 550 μg/l. She had a chronically elevated serum bilirubin and LDH, and haptoglobin was absent but the reticulocyte count was normal. The direct Coombs test was negative and there was no clinical or serological evidence of a connective tissue disorder. She had a history of orthopaedic procedures for multiple bone exostoses. Her blood film was strikingly abnormal (images above ×100 objective) showing marked anisopoikilocytosis, oval macrocytes, micropoikilocytes, a few spherocytes, teardrop forms and basophilic stippling. There was marked variation in the degree of haemoglobinisation between cells. These features are not suggestive of any inherited disorder of the red cell membrane, red cell enzymes or haemoglobin. Neither parent was known to have a red cell disorder so an autosomal recessively inherited condition was certainly possible.

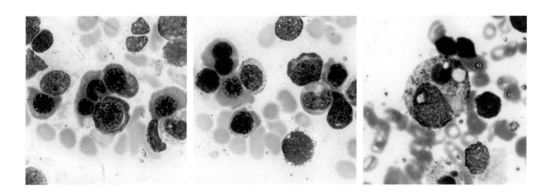

Haematology: From the Image to the Diagnosis, First Edition. Mike Leach and Barbara J. Bain.
© 2022 John Wiley & Sons Ltd. Published 2022 by John Wiley & Sons Ltd.

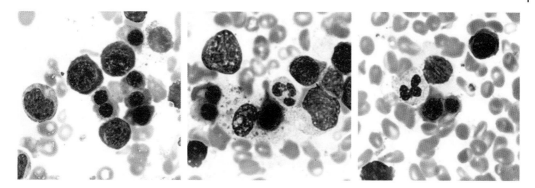

The bone marrow aspirate was cellular and highly informative (images above and on facing page ×100). There was erythroid hyperplasia with frequent dysplasia, including abnormal nuclear maturation, nuclear irregularity, binuclearity, poor haemoglobinisation and cytoplasmic stippling. The image lower right (above) shows internuclear chromatin bridging. Importantly, there was no dysplasia of the myeloid and megakaryocyte series and no excess of blasts. Ring sideroblasts were not present on Perls staining. There was evidence of excess erythroid cell karyorrhexis and active haemophagocytosis (bottom right, facing page). The intramedullary cell death due to failure of maturation accounts for the apparent haemolytic laboratory indices. These findings, together with the family history, suggested a possible diagnosis of congenital dyserythropoietic anaemia (CDA). Bone marrow analysis of the index case showed compound heterozygosity for mutations in the codanin (*CDAN1*) gene, c.2015C>T and c.3338T>C, confirming this diagnosis. Her brother showed an identical genotype.

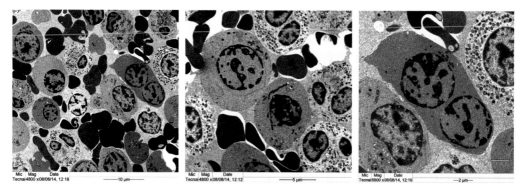

Electron microscopy studies of the patient's bone marrow showed the erythroid precursors to have abnormal nuclear chromatin morphology with an open 'Swiss cheese' type appearance, characteristically seen in CDA type I (images above, magnification shown).

MCQ

Congenital dyserythropoietic anaemia type I is characterised by:

1 A positive acid lysis test
2 Frequent splenomegaly and gallstones
3 Giant erythroblasts with multiple nuclei
4 Internuclear chromatin bridges
5 Responsiveness to interferon

For answers and discussion, see page 206.

33 Acute monoblastic leukaemia with t(9;11)(p21.3;q23.3)

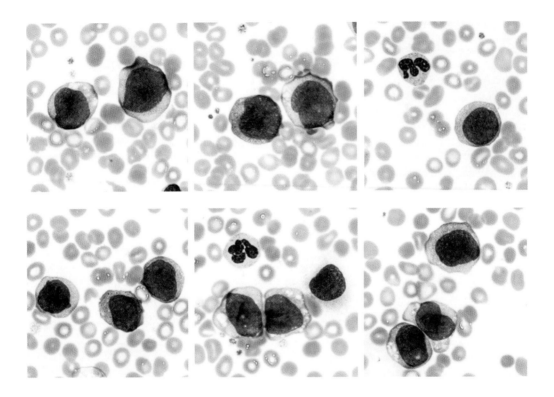

A 49-year-old woman presented with fatigue and swollen painful gingivae. Her FBC showed Hb 80 g/l, WBC 20 × 10⁹/l, neutrophils 0.7 × 10⁹/l and platelets 59 × 10⁹/l. The blood film showed a population of large blasts with ovoid or round nuclei, prominent nucleoli and copious pale blue, finely granulated and sometimes vacuolated cytoplasm (all images ×100 objective). Other similar cells had indented or lobated nuclei. Note the dysplastic neutrophils showing abnormal segmentation (top right) and hypogranularity (bottom centre). The images here show the typical morphology of monoblastic leukaemia. This was confirmed with flow cytometry showing these cells to have a CD34−, CD45+, CD15+, CD13+, CD33+, CD11c+, CD14−, CD64+, MPO−, HLA-DR+ immunophenotype. T- and B-lineage antigens were not expressed. The karyotype was 47,XX,+8,t(9;11)(p21.3;q23.3), which results in a *KMT2A-MLLT3* fusion gene. This karyotype, which is often associated with monocytic or monoblastic leukaemia, carries an intermediate prognosis. *NPM1* mutation and *FLT3* internal tandem duplication were excluded.

The patient achieved remission with induction chemotherapy and this was consolidated with a further three cycles. The gum swelling fully resolved within 2 weeks of starting treatment. One year later the patient developed a generalised persistent headache, worse on coughing. She was noted to have papilloedema but the FBC remained normal. A CSF specimen was obtained and the cytospin is shown below.

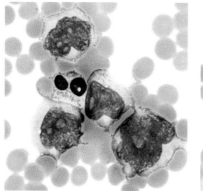 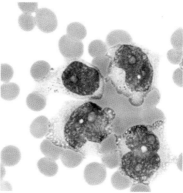

Again, note the large nucleolated blast cells and promonocytes in a blood-stained CSF with morphology very similar to those seen in blood at diagnosis. The immunophenotype of these cells was also identical to that seen previously, confirming CNS relapse of monoblastic leukaemia.

MCQ

Acute monoblastic/monocytic leukaemia associated with t(9;11)(p21.3;q23.3):

1 Can occur following therapy with topoisomerase II-interactive drugs
2 Is more likely than acute myeloblastic leukaemia to have infiltration of gums, skin and other extramedullary sites
3 Not infrequently expresses CD4, CD11b, CD14, CD64 and strong HLA-DR
4 Often has blast cells that do not express CD34 or myeloperoxidase
5 Should be confirmed by non-specific esterase staining

For answers and discussion, see page 206.

34 Chronic myeloid leukaemia presenting with myeloid sarcoma

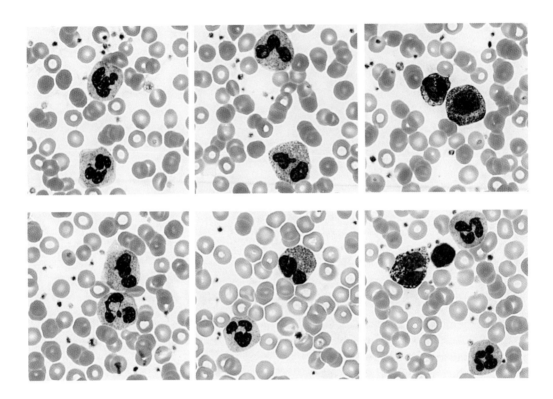

An 8-year-old boy presented with pain and swelling over the distal left femur. Physical examination revealed no other abnormality. His FBC showed Hb 118 g/l, WBC 14.9×10^9/l, (neutrophils 10.1×10^9/l, lymphocytes 3.1×10^9/l, monocytes 0.3×10^9/l, eosinophils 0.69×10^9/l, basophils 0.8×10^9/l) and platelet count 1060×10^9/l. The blood film showed mature neutrophils and an occasional band cell. Notably there was a mild eosinophilia (centre images) and prominent basophils (right images) including basophil myelocytes (top right) (all images ×100 objective). No blasts were identified. The marked thrombocytosis was confirmed and the platelets were generally small. Despite the absence of a prominent leucocytosis these features are highly suggestive of a diagnosis of chronic myeloid leukaemia (CML) and an e14a2 (p210) *BCR-ABL1* fusion transcript was identified indicating the presence of t(9;22)(q34.1;q11.2). The bone marrow aspirate and trephine biopsy sections showed 20% myeloblasts with a CD34+, CD117+, MPO+, CD13+, CD33+, CD7+ immunophenotype indicating blast crisis of CML. MRI of both femurs showed a large focal soft tissue mass in the distal left femur with cortical destruction (image below).

Haematology: From the Image to the Diagnosis, First Edition. Mike Leach and Barbara J. Bain.
© 2022 John Wiley & Sons Ltd. Published 2022 by John Wiley & Sons Ltd.

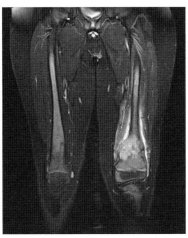

A needle biopsy of the lesion showed a myeloid tumour with up to 40% blast cells in some areas; the phenotype of these cells was identical to that identified in the marrow biopsy and analysis of touch preparations of the lesion showed a *BCR-ABL1* fusion in 64% of nuclei, confirming a myeloid sarcoma derived from CML. The patient was treated using a combination of mitoxantrone, cytarabine and dasatinib followed by an unrelated donor stem cell transplant. He remains in remission 2 years later with no measurable residual disease.

Chronic myeloid leukaemia typically presents with marked neutrophilia, eosinophilia and basophilia with a myeloid left shift to blast cells. Thrombocytosis may or may not be present. A subset of patients present with extreme thrombocytosis (between 1000 and 4000 × 10^9/l) with mild or absent neutrophilia but, importantly, eosinophilia and basophilia are usually evident in these cases. If recognised and treated appropriately, these cases appear to have a favourable prognosis (Sora *et al*. 2018). It is therefore essential to analyse the blood film carefully in all patients presenting with thrombocytosis so that these cases are not misclassified as essential thrombocythaemia (ET). Of course, CML will always show a *BCR-ABL1* fusion gene and this should be sought in all patients presenting as described. Erroneous diagnosis of molecularly negative ET in such circumstances could have disastrous therapeutic consequences for the patient.

Reference

Sora F, Iurlo A, Sica S, Latagliata R, Annunziata M, Galimberti S *et al*. (2018) Chronic myeloid leukaemia with extreme thrombocytosis at presentation: incidence, clinical findings and outcome. *Br J Haematol*, **181**, 267–270.

MCQ

The peripheral blood in *BCR-ABL1*-positive chronic myeloid leukaemia (CML):

1 Can show occasional nucleated red blood cells and megakaryocyte nuclei
2 Characteristically shows a double peak of myelocytes and neutrophils
3 Has monocytes increased in proportion to the increase in neutrophils
4 Often shows hypogranular neutrophils
5 Rarely shows thrombocytosis without leucocytosis

For answers and discussion, see page 206.

35 Glucose-6-phosphate dehydrogenase deficiency

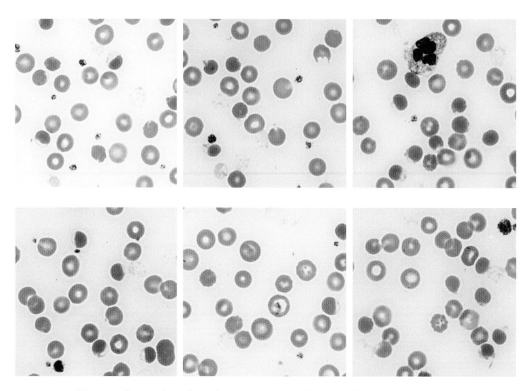

A 59-year-old man of French-Italian descent, visiting the United Kingdom, and with no prior medical history, was admitted to hospital with fever, lethargy, jaundice and abdominal pain. His full blood count showed Hb 74 g/l, WBC 12.9×10^9/l, neutrophils 9.1×10^9/l and platelets 171×10^9/l. Serum bilirubin was markedly elevated at 248 μmol/l with AST 110 u/l, ALT 25 u/l and LDH 1624 iu/l whilst haptoglobin was absent. CT imaging showed right lower lobe subsegmental pulmonary embolism but no other abnormality was seen. He therefore had a presentation in keeping with an acute-onset haemolytic anaemia but the mechanism was initially not clear. His blood film was key to making a diagnosis. This showed marked red cell abnormalities with blister cells (all images ×100 objective), ghost cells (all images), hemighosts (top left), bite cells (top centre), irregularly contracted cells, basophilic stippling (bottom right) and Pappenheimer bodies (bottom centre). Note the neutrophil showing toxic granulation and vacuolation (top right) and the plasma colour tint due to free haemoglobin. These morphological features are typical of an acute haemolytic episode associated with glucose-6-phosphate dehydrogenase (G6PD) deficiency. The medical team, in the light of this finding, went back to question the patient and he reported having eaten a significant volume of fava beans (broad beans) in the days preceding this event. On recovery, a red cell G6PD assay showed levels less than 2% of normal.

Glucose-6-phosphate dehydrogenase deficiency, an X-linked hereditary genetic defect, is the most common human red cell enzyme disorder in the world, affecting over 500 million people (Luzzatto *et al.* 2020). The disorder can present with neonatal jaundice, a chronic non-spherocytic haemolytic anaemia or fulminant acute haemolytic episodes, as described in the patient here. The acute haemolytic

Haematology: From the Image to the Diagnosis, First Edition. Mike Leach and Barbara J. Bain.
© 2022 John Wiley & Sons Ltd. Published 2022 by John Wiley & Sons Ltd.

episodes are typically triggered by infection, drug exposure or fava bean ingestion, which induce red cell oxidative stress. The enzyme catalyses the first reaction of the pentose phosphate pathway, so generating NADPH, which is essential in red cell biosynthetic pathways and in protecting cells from oxidative stress. Fava beans contain a number of glycosides that induce haemolysis (favism) and, whilst G6PD deficiency is a requirement of the condition, the response of G6PD-deficient individuals to ingestion of the bean is inconsistent A large number of mutations in the G6PD gene are recognised and the nature of the mutation is correlated with clinical severity and susceptibility (Luzzatto *et al.* 2020). The condition has likely prevailed due to the relative protection from *Plasmodium falciparum* malaria that it offers and the worldwide distributions of the two conditions show significant concordance. Paradoxically, many drugs used to prevent and treat malaria can also trigger a haemolytic episode in G6PD-deficient individuals. The management in a known affected patient is therefore largely preventative, but a significant number of those without a prior diagnosis present with an acute haemolytic episode. Hemizygous females are largely symptom-free but because of Lyonisation (with an excess of X-inactivated red cells carrying the normal allele) symptomatic haemolytic episodes can still occur.

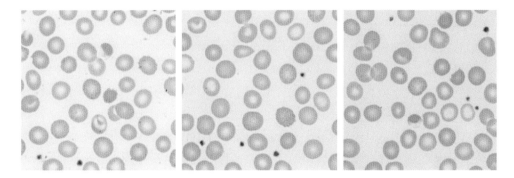

More typically, affected females are homozygotes. Uncommonly, homozygous women have a chronic partially compensated haemolytic anaemia. The images above are from such a patient with a chronic mild anaemia (Hb 100 g/l). Note the hemighosts and bite cells (left and right images ×100) and basophilic stippling (all images). Overall, the morphological features are much less profound when compared with the usual acute presentation.

Reference

Luzzatto L, Ally M and Notaro R (2020) Glucose-6 phosphate dehydrogenase deficiency. *Blood*, **136**, 1225–1240.

MCQ

Heinz bodies:

1 Are removed by the spleen
2 Are specific for defects of the pentose shunt
3 Can be detected during acute haemolytic episodes in G6PD deficiency
4 Can sometimes be identified on an MGG-stained blood film
5 Represent denatured haemoglobin

For answers and discussion, see page 206.

36 Leukaemic presentation of hepatosplenic γδ T-cell lymphoma

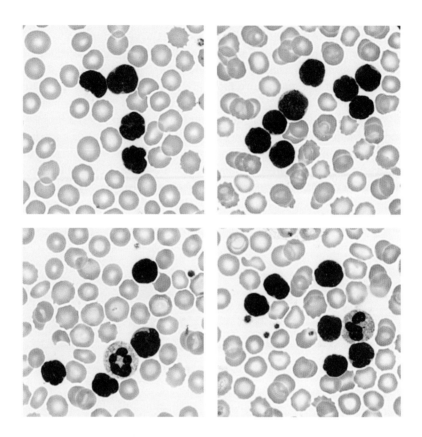

A 5-year-old boy presented with fatigue, anorexia and weight loss. His parents had noted a yellow colour to his skin. On examination he was clearly unwell with marked abdominal distension. His full blood count showed Hb 120 g/l, WBC 180 × 10^9/l and platelets 62 × 10^9/l. His renal function was normal but there was significant hepatic derangement with serum AST 2845 u/l, ALT 1835 u/l, alkaline phosphatase 530 u/l, bilirubin 250 µmol/l and albumin 28 g/l. A whole-body MRI showed significant hepatosplenomegaly but, importantly, there was no lymphadenopathy. The blood film showed a large population of abnormal lymphoid cells, small to medium sized, with prominent narrow nuclear clefts and a largely condensed chromatin pattern (all images ×100 objective). Nucleoli were not apparent. Flow cytometric studies on peripheral blood showed the abnormal cells to have a CD45+, CD3+, CD5+, CD2−, CD7+, CD1a−, CD8+, CD4−, TdT−, CD34− immunophenotype. There was no expression of myeloid antigens. The differential diagnosis lay between a T-lymphoblastic leukaemia (T-ALL) and the leukaemic phase of a T-cell lymphoma, with the former seeming likely.

In T-ALL the order of antigen acquisition is quite predictable, with non-lineage-specific CD7 being seen in early T-cell precursor lymphoblastic/leukaemia lymphoma followed, in cases that can be defined as T-ALL, by T-lineage specific cytoplasmic CD3, then CD5 and CD2, then surface CD3 then CD4 and CD8. Cortical T-ALL is derived from a precursor cell at the thymic stage of maturation.

Haematology: From the Image to the Diagnosis, First Edition. Mike Leach and Barbara J. Bain.
© 2022 John Wiley & Sons Ltd. Published 2022 by John Wiley & Sons Ltd.

These cells have a CD7+, CD5+, CD2+, CD3+, CD1a+ phenotype with no clear commitment to a CD4 or CD8 phenotype (often CD4 partial, CD8 partial or CD4 and CD8 dual positive). In this case T-ALL seemed initially most likely but the morphology, the lack of expected expression of CD2, TdT and CD34, the absence of lymphadenopathy and a hepatosplenic presentation raised the question of a leukaemic presentation of hepatosplenic T-cell lymphoma. The bone marrow trephine biopsy sections showed a heavy infiltration of small to medium sized lymphoid cells, within marrow sinusoids, showing a CD45+, CD7+, CD3+, CD5+, CD2−, partial CD8+ immunophenotype. Importantly, T-cell receptor (TCR) delta was positive whilst CD34, TdT and CD99 were not expressed. The features were therefore of heavy marrow infiltration by a T-cell lymphoma with a γδ phenotype. Cytogenetic analysis on peripheral blood showed 46,XY with isochromosome 7q being shown on FISH. The diagnosis of hepatosplenic T-cell lymphoma was confirmed.

MCQ

Hepatosplenic T-cell lymphoma:

1 Consistently expresses γδ T-cell receptor
2 Has a good prognosis
3 Has a strong association with isochromosome 7q
4 Not infrequently arises in the setting of chronic immune suppression
5 Rarely involves the bone marrow

For answers and discussion, see page 206.

37 Myelodysplastic syndromes

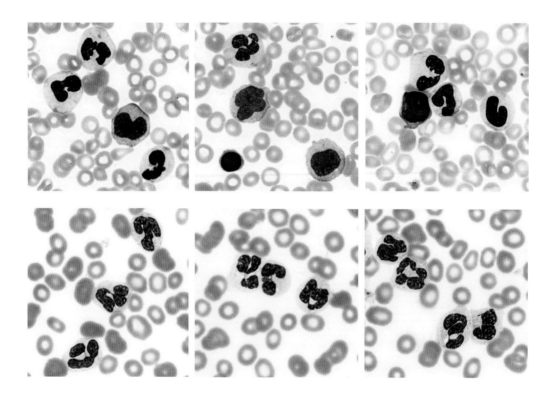

An 80-year-old woman was admitted to hospital with falls. Her full blood count showed Hb 107 g/l, WBC 36.9 × 10^9/l, neutrophils 9.2 × 10^9/l and platelets 50 × 10^9/l. Her blood film was leucoerythroblastic with neutrophils showing profound hypogranularity (top images ×100 objective). Some neutrophils showed Döhle bodies (top left). In addition, there were promonocytes (top left and centre), hypogranular myelocytes (top centre) and myeloblasts (top right). Hypogranular myelocytes can be mistaken for promonocytes; as the latter count as blast equivalents it is important to differentiate the two. Note the abnormal chromatin condensation in the neutrophils. A bone marrow aspirate showed trilineage dysplasia with 12% total blast equivalents (myeloblasts and promonocytes), giving a diagnosis of myelodysplastic syndrome with excess blasts 2 (MDS-EB2). Metaphase cytogenetic analysis showed 46,XX.

A second patient, a 73-year-old man was admitted to hospital with cardiac chest pain. His full blood count showed Hb 101 g/l, WBC 41.6 × 10^9/l, neutrophils 34 × 10^9/l and platelets 57 × 10^9/l. His blood film showed similar features to that of the first patient (leucoerythroblastic with circulating myeloblasts (not shown) with marked abnormalities of neutrophils). In this patient, in addition to hypogranularity of neutrophils, the nuclear segmentation was markedly abnormal (bottom images ×100). Note how nuclear segments are abnormally joined, unlike the typical end to end 'string of sausages' type of arrangement of the normal neutrophil nucleus. His bone marrow aspirate also showed trilineage dysplasia but with 7% myeloblasts. Peripheral blood blast cells were less than 5%, giving a diagnosis of myelodysplastic syndrome with excess blasts 1 (MDS-EB1).

Haematology: From the Image to the Diagnosis, First Edition. Mike Leach and Barbara J. Bain.
© 2022 John Wiley & Sons Ltd. Published 2022 by John Wiley & Sons Ltd.

Cytogenetic analysis showed a complex, poor-risk karyotype: 44,XY,−2,−3,add(4)(q25),del(5)(q22q33)−6,−7,t(12;17)(q13;p13),−16. Note the likely translocation of *TP53* at 17p13 to 12q13.

These two examples of MDS show many similarities and both carry a poor prognosis; both transformed to AML within a few months. The main contrast is in karyotypic studies, with the first case being normal and the second complex with translocation and likely loss of function of *TP53*. Up to 50% of all MDS cases do show a normal karyotype. We are just beginning to understand the important myeloid genetic driver mutations in these normal karyotype cases.

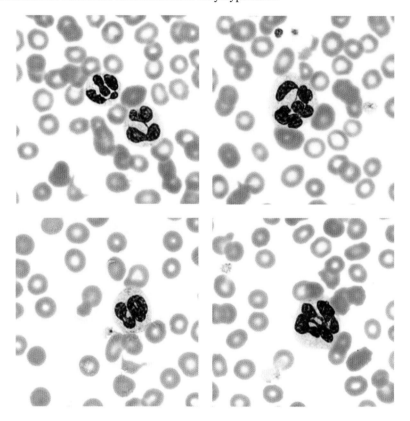

The images above (×100) all show further examples of abnormal neutrophil nuclear segmentation (and hypogranularity) in the second patient with MDS; note the apparent nuclear ring in the neutrophil bottom left. Their size and the number of nuclear lobes in the two neutrophils on the right suggest they may be tetraploid.

MCQ

Hypogranularity of neutrophils can be a feature of:

1 Chédiak–Higashi syndrome
2 Human immunodeficiency virus (HIV) infection
3 Inherited specific granule deficiency
4 Myelokathexis
5 Therapy-related acute myeloid leukaemia

For answers and discussion, see page 206.

38 Pelger–Huët anomaly

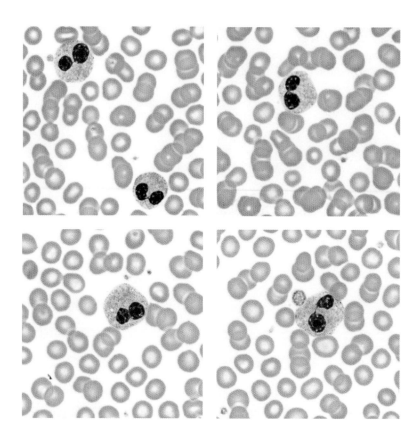

A 30-year-old woman attended a routine obstetric clinic appointment at 30 weeks' gestation. Her full blood count showed Hb 120 g/l, WBC 9×10^9/l, neutrophils 6×10^9/l and platelets 140×10^9/l. A blood film was prepared on account of the borderline thrombocytopenia. This showed neutrophils with distinct bilobed nuclei and a coarse condensed chromatin pattern (all images ×100 objective). All the neutrophils showed the same nuclear characteristics and were normally granulated. No other abnormalities were noted. The platelet count was confirmed.

The Pelger–Huët anomaly is an autosomal dominant inherited condition due to mutations in the lamin B receptor gene (*LBR*) mapping to chromosome 1 (1q42.12). It affects around 1 in 6000 individuals in the United Kingdom and is characterised by distinctive bilobed neutrophil nuclei with a mild coarsening of the nuclear chromatin. Some nuclei are dumbbell or peanut-shaped, rather than having two distinct lobes. Eosinophils and basophils are similarly affected and bone marrow myelocytes and promyelocytes show abnormally coarse chromatin clumping. This anomaly has little if any clinical effect, with the neutrophils generally being considered to have normal migratory, phagocytic and bactericidal activity, although reduced diapedesis has been described in several studies (Cunningham *et al.* 2009).

Karl Pelger, a Dutch specialist in tuberculosis, first described the condition in 1928 and a Dutch paediatrician, G.H. Huët, reported it as an autosomal dominant inherited anomaly 3 years later, his patient being the niece of one of Pelger's two patients (Cunningham *et al.* 2009). Homozygotes have variable somatic abnormalities and their neutrophils have non-lobed (ovoid) nuclei.

The inherited Pelger–Huët anomaly must be distinguished from the morphologically similar acquired or pseudo-Pelger–Huët anomaly, which is clinically much more significant. A distinction must also be made from a left shift of neutrophils, when there is an increase of neutrophils with bilobed nuclei but band forms are also increased and the round lobes and chromatin clumping of the Pelger–Huët anomaly are absent. All relevant information must therefore be considered when assessing the significance of hypolobation of granulocyte nuclei.

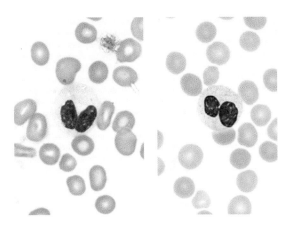

The images above (×100) are from a patient with MDS showing hypogranular neutrophils with pseudo-Pelger nuclear morphology.

Reference

Cunningham JM, Patnaik MM, Hammerschmidt DE and Vercellotti GM (2009) Historical perspective and clinical implications of the Pelger-Huet cell. *Am J Hematol*, **84**, 116–119.

MCQ

The pseudo-Pelger–Huët anomaly can be a feature of:

1 Azathioprine therapy
2 Mycophenolate mofetil therapy
3 Myelodysplastic syndromes
4 Sodium valproate therapy
5 Therapy-related acute myeloid leukaemia

For answers and discussion, see page 206.

39 Russell bodies in lymphoplasmacytic lymphoma

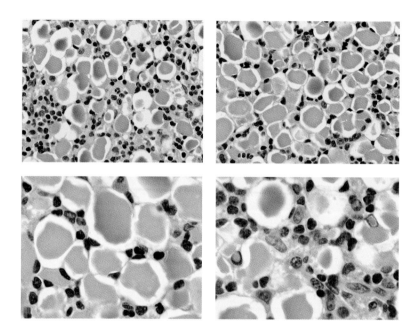

An 80-year-old man presented with fatigue, pallor and bruising. His full blood count showed Hb 100 g/l, WBC 5×10^9/l, neutrophils 2×10^9/l and platelets 22×10^9/l. A coagulation screen was normal. A 12 g/l IgM paraprotein was identified and urinary Bence Jones protein was detected. CT imaging identified a 15 cm spleen but no lymphadenopathy. A bone marrow aspirate showed a population of mature clonal B cells with a CD19+, CD20+, FMC7+, CD79b+, surface kappa-restricted immunophenotype. The working diagnosis was lymphoplasmacytic lymphoma and this was supported by the finding of an L265P mutation in *MYD88*. The bone marrow trephine biopsy sections were remarkable in showing large orange/pink globules throughout the section on H&E staining (top images ×10 objective, bottom images ×50). In addition, an interstitial infiltrate of small lymphoid cells was apparent and many of the globules appear to have arisen from the expanded cytoplasm of these cells. These globules are Russell bodies and correspond to large volumes of paraprotein collecting within the cell. These proteins are not degraded and remain lodged within the cell. Russell bodies are often seen as smaller multiple forms in multiple myeloma or lymphoplasmacytic lymphoma but can also be seen in non-malignant inflammatory conditions.

This case is unusual in that affected cells show a single large form. In addition, two cells show apparently intranuclear globulin inclusions known as Dutcher bodies (bottom right). Dutcher bodies are actually cytoplasmic inclusions that overlie or are invaginated into the nucleus; they are an extension of the same process generating Russell bodies and the two phenomena are often seen together, as in this patient.

Haematology: From the Image to the Diagnosis, First Edition. Mike Leach and Barbara J. Bain.
© 2022 John Wiley & Sons Ltd. Published 2022 by John Wiley & Sons Ltd.

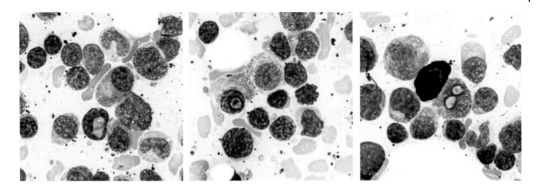

The images above (×100) are of a bone marrow aspirate from another patient with a lymphoplasmacytic lymphoma, showing Dutcher bodies. Note that they are well circumscribed and pale, sometimes multiple (right image) and should not be misinterpreted as nucleoli.

MCQ

Recognised features when neoplastic cells show plasmacytic differentiation include:

1 Auer rods
2 Cytoplasmic crystals
3 Dutcher bodies
4 Flame cells
5 Mott cells

For answers and discussion, see page 206.

40   T-cell prolymphocytic leukaemia

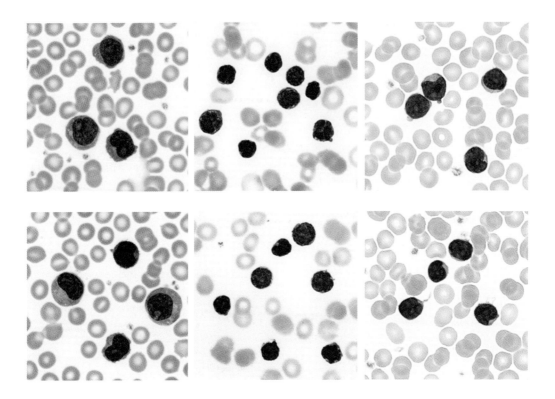

An 82-year-old woman was admitted for investigation of progressive fatigue. She was found to have widespread small-volume lymphadenopathy and splenomegaly. Her blood count showed Hb 72 g/l, WBC 122 × 10⁹/l and platelets 15 × 10⁹/l. The blood film showed medium to large cells with oval, bean-shaped and sometimes clefted nuclei, condensed chromatin, frequent nucleoli and basophilic cytoplasm with occasional tufts and blebs (left images ×100 objective). Flow cytometry showed these cells to have a CD4+, CD7+, CD5+, CD2+ and uniform CD26+ immunophenotype, in keeping with a diagnosis of T-cell prolymphocytic leukaemia (T-PLL). The karyotype was normal but a *TCL1* break-apart probe spanning the *TCL1A/TCL1B* cluster showed a rearrangement in 80% of cells indicating a cryptic t(14;14)(q11.2;q32.1) or inv(14)(q11.2q32.1) which brings the genes into juxtaposition with promoters and enhancers at the TRA locus.

A second patient, a 33-year-old man, presented with progressive erythema and swelling of the skin of his face and torso. His full blood count showed Hb 77 g/l, WBC 344 × 10⁹/l and platelets 117 × 10⁹/l. His blood film showed small to medium sized lymphoid cells with condensed chromatin, multiple nuclear clefts and folds and a thin rim of cytoplasm with occasional blebs (centre images ×100). Nucleoli could be seen in some of the larger cells. The immunophenotype of these cells was identical to that noted above. He had a complex karyotype including an abnormal chromosome 14 with additional material of unknown origin replacing part of the long arm at 14q32.

A third patient, a 70-year-old man, was found to have an abnormal full blood count when attending a surgical clinic with Hb 132 g/l, WBC 84 × 10⁹/l and platelets 169 × 10⁹/l. His blood film

Haematology: From the Image to the Diagnosis, First Edition. Mike Leach and Barbara J. Bain.
© 2022 John Wiley & Sons Ltd. Published 2022 by John Wiley & Sons Ltd.

showed medium sized lymphoid cells with condensed chromatin, single nucleoli and nuclear clefts with cytoplasmic wisps and blebs (right images, facing page ×100) and these cells also had a CD4+ pan-T phenotype including expression of CD7. He had a 47,XY,+8 karyotype.

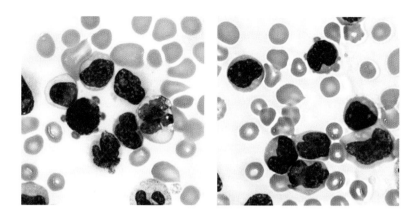

The 33-year-old man (the second patient reported here) was treated intensively but only managed a partial response; his peripheral blood and skin were never cleared of disease. The images above (×100) are of peripheral blood after 12 weeks of therapy; note the change in the prolymphocyte size but many of the typical morphological features are still present.

MCQ

T-cell prolymphocytic leukaemia:

1 Can respond to alemtuzumab, directed at CD52
2 Is aetiologically related to a retroviral infection
3 Is unusual among mature T-cell neoplasms in that both CD4 and CD8 may be expressed
4 Responds well to combination chemotherapy
5 Should be suspected if there is expression of CD7 by a mature T-cell neoplasm

For answers and discussion, see page 206.

41 Myeloid maturation arrest

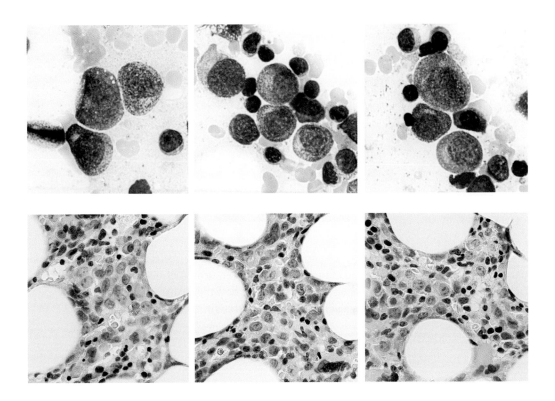

A 52-year-old man had two admissions to the Infectious Disease Unit within a space of 4 weeks, each time after returning from business in the Mediterranean. On both occasions he presented with lethargy, sore throat, myalgia and fever associated with severe neutropenia. No infectious cause was identified despite extensive screens for viral, bacterial and fungal pathogens and no deep-seated infective focus was evident on CT imaging of his neck, chest, abdomen and pelvis. He was treated empirically with broad-spectrum antibiotics during both episodes. The neutropenia resolved spontaneously during the first admission but not during the second when a Haematology opinion was sought. His full blood count at this point showed Hb 131 g/l, WBC 1.14×10^9/l, neutrophils 0×10^9/l and platelets 220×10^9/l. Routine biochemical tests were normal but his CRP was elevated at 88 mg/l. The coagulation screen showed a prolonged APTT that was shown to be due to a lupus anticoagulant. Serological studies showed strong positivity for cytoplasmic antineutrophil cytoplasmic antibodies (cANCA) but perinuclear ANCA (pANCA), MPO and proteinase 3 (PR3) antibodies were not identified. Antinuclear antibodies and rheumatoid factor were not detected and serum complement C3 and C4 levels were normal. The bone marrow aspirate was particulate and cellular and did not show an abnormal infiltrate. It did show a notable myeloid maturation arrest at the promyelocyte/myelocyte stage with no mature neutrophils being identified (top images ×100 objective). Note the arrested myeloid series also in the trephine biopsy sections (the large ovoid cells with reticular nuclei are promyelocytes whilst mature neutrophils are absent) (bottom images, H&E ×50). The erythroid and megakaryocyte lineages showed no

Haematology: From the Image to the Diagnosis, First Edition. Mike Leach and Barbara J. Bain.
© 2022 John Wiley & Sons Ltd. Published 2022 by John Wiley & Sons Ltd.

abnormality but lymphocytes and plasma cells were prominent. He was treated with G-CSF and his neutrophil count recovered over the next 7 days with resolution of fever.

Myeloid maturation arrest, when occurring acutely and in the absence of other bone marrow pathology, is usually the result of some form of toxic insult, most frequently as an idiosyncratic reaction to drugs, but it can also occur with severe sepsis and extensive burns. This patient did not take regular prescribed or 'over the counter' medicines. On questioning about recreational drug use he initially denied any exposure, but on repeat questioning and realising the potential relevance to his hospital admissions, he subsequently admitted to the intermittent use of cocaine, particularly when travelling abroad. Cocaine is a class A recreational neurostimulant drug, which is taken by nasal insufflation, inhalation or injection. In the last few years a common practice among dealers has been to expand the volume of cocaine by cutting it with levamisole, an antihelminthic antibiotic; the latter has a colour and texture similar to cocaine, is much cheaper and also enhances the neurostimulatory effect. Levamisole was withdrawn from the medical market as it causes neutropenia in up to 10% of those exposed, though it is still used in veterinary practice. Cocaine–levamisole also has the potential to cause a leucocytoclastic vasculitis with skin necrosis (Lee *et al.* 2012), sometimes associated with transient positivity for antineutrophil antibodies, anticardiolipin antibodies and lupus anticoagulant. Reported findings on bone marrow morphology in levamisole-induced neutropenia include myeloid hypoplasia, maturation arrest, megakaryocyte hyperplasia and reactive plasmacytosis (Czuchlewski *et al.* 2010).

References

Czuchlewski DR, Brackney M, Ewers C, Manna J, Fekrazad MH, Martinez A *et al.* (2010) Clinicopathologic features of agranulocytosis in the setting of levamisole-tainted cocaine. *Am J Clin Pathol*, **133**, 466–472.
Lee KC, Ladizinski B and Federman DG (2012) Complications associated with the use of levamisole-contaminated cocaine: An emerging public health challenge. *Mayo Clin Proc*, **87**, 581–586.

MCQ

Maturation arrest in the granulocytic series can be a feature of:

1 Acute promyelocytic leukaemia
2 Copper deficiency
3 Drug-induced agranulocytosis
4 Myelokathexis
5 Some types of congenital neutropenia

For answers and discussion, see page 206.

42 MDS/MPN with ring sideroblasts and thrombocytosis

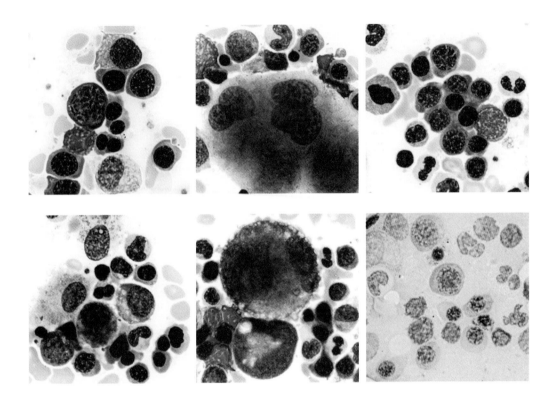

An 83-year-old man was referred for investigation of a persistent normocytic anaemia in the absence of any specific defining features. His full blood count showed Hb 99 g/l, WBC 19.3×10^9/l, neutrophils 14.5×10^9/l and platelets 558×10^9/l. His blood film showed a proportion of hypochromic cells, basophilic stippling, teardrop poikilocytes and pencil cells. There was a mild neutrophilia and the thrombocytosis was confirmed with giant platelets being notable. The serum ferritin was raised at 450 µg/l. Clinical examination was unremarkable and notably his spleen was not palpable. A *JAK2* V617F mutation was identified and a diagnosis of essential thrombocythaemia was considered. The latter is one of the most common MPNs we encounter and is characterised by thrombocytosis without significant abnormality in the red cell or leucocyte lineages; the presence of anaemia should always trigger consideration of another MPN or a coexistent unrelated disorder as a possible explanation. A bone marrow aspirate showed a particulate hypercellular specimen with prominent erythroid precursor activity and moderate dysplasia. Megakaryocytes were prominent and showed separation of nuclear components (top centre) and immature forms (bottom centre, all images ×100 objective). The myeloid series showed full maturation but hypogranularity in the later forms (top centre and right, bottom left and centre). Notably, on Perls staining the erythroid precursors included prominent ring forms (bottom right), accounting for 20% of erythroblasts. The features here are in keeping with an MDS/MPN crossover disorder with characteristics defining a diagnosis of MDS/MPN with ring sideroblasts and thrombocytosis (MDS/MPN-RS-T) in the 2016 WHO classification (Orazi *et al.* 2017).

Haematology: From the Image to the Diagnosis, First Edition. Mike Leach and Barbara J. Bain.
© 2022 John Wiley & Sons Ltd. Published 2022 by John Wiley & Sons Ltd.

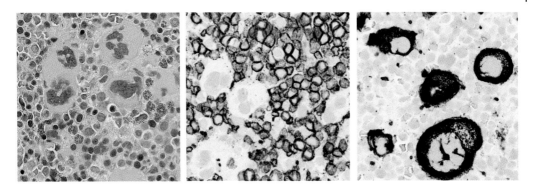

This diagnosis was supported by the morphology of the trephine biopsy sections which showed marked hypercellularity, erythroid expansion and prominent pleomorphic megakaryocytes of various sizes (images above, H&E left, immunoperoxidase for glycophorin centre and for CD42b right ×50). Marrow reticulin was not increased. Standard cytogenetic studies showed a normal karyotype but next generation sequencing (NGS) identified a number of additional relevant mutations: *SF3B1* c.2098A>G, *TET2* c.1471C>T and *TET2* c.1630C>T. The *SF3B1* mutation is strongly associated with the finding of an acquired sideroblastic anaemia and *TET2* mutations are frequently encountered in MDS/MPN. The working diagnosis of MDS/MPN-RS-T was thus confirmed.

Reference

Orazi A, Hasserjian RP, Cazzola M, Theile J and Malcovati L (2017) Myelodysplastic/ myeloproliferative neoplasm with ring sideroblasts and thrombocytosis. *In* Swerdlow SH, Campo E, Harris NL, Jaffe ES, Pileri SA, Stein H and Theile J (Eds) *WHO Classification of Tumours of Haematopoietic and Lymphoid Tissues.* IARC, Lyon, pp. 93–94.

MCQ

Myelodysplastic/myeloproliferative neoplasm with ring sideroblasts and thrombocytosis (MDS/MPN-RS-T) is defined in the WHO classification by:

1   A platelet count of at least 450×10^9/l.
2   At least 5% ring sideroblasts in the bone marrow if an *SF3B1* mutation is present
3   At least 15% ring sideroblasts in the bone marrow
4   Less than 20% bone marrow blast cells
5   No previous exposure to leukaemogenic drugs

For answers and discussion, see page 206.

43 Acute myeloid leukaemia with inv(16)(p13.1q22)

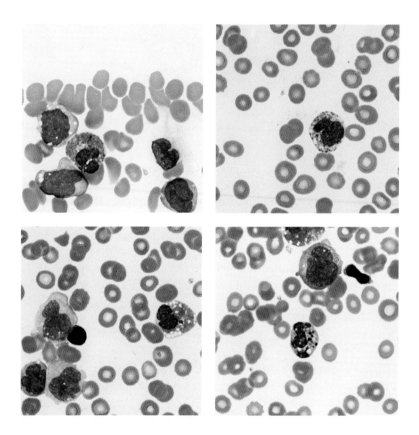

A 34-year old man presented with the recent onset of fatigue. Some bruises were noted on physical examination. His FBC showed WBC 38×10^9/l, Hb 84 g/l and platelet count 13×10^9/l. The differential count showed blast cells plus promonocytes 33%, neutrophils 3%, lymphocytes 10%, monocytes 48% and eosinophils 6%. The images show good examples of promonocytes (top and bottom left, all images ×100 objective). These cells have delicate chromatin and nucleoli are present; they differ from monoblasts in that their nuclei are irregular, grooved, lobated or folded. Distinguishing promonocytes from monoblasts (bottom right) is not clinically important since promonocytes are blast equivalents. However, distinguishing promonocytes from immature monocytes can be very important in order to reliably distinguish acute monoblastic/monocytic leukaemia from chronic myelomonocytic leukaemia. The bottom left image shows, in addition to two promonocytes, an immature monocyte, which is recognised because of its chromatin condensation.

Although eosinophils were only a minor population, many of them showed cytological abnormalities including vacuolation (top and bottom right), hypogranularity (top right, bottom right) and hyperlobation. Some had basophilic granules (bottom), which were sometimes very large (bottom right). The presence of mature eosinophils or eosinophil myelocytes with large basophilic granules is strongly suggestive of AML with inv(16)(p13.1q22).

Haematology: From the Image to the Diagnosis, First Edition. Mike Leach and Barbara J. Bain.
© 2022 John Wiley & Sons Ltd. Published 2022 by John Wiley & Sons Ltd.

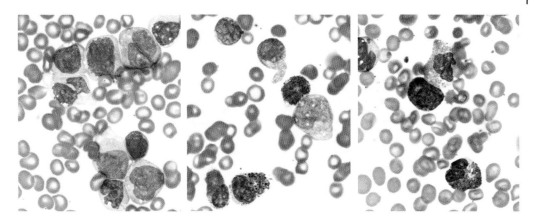

The patient's bone marrow aspirate (images above) showed monoblasts, promonocytes and occasional immature monocytes (left). In addition, there were eosinophil myelocytes with large basophilic granules (centre and right) and mature eosinophils, both morphologically normal and abnormal (centre). These eosinophil myelocytes are very typical but are often only detected in the bone marrow whereas observing abnormal granules in peripheral blood eosinophils can give a rapid indication of the diagnosis. The basophilic granules have nothing to do with the basophil lineage but represent immature granules of the eosinophil lineage. The abnormal granules are particularly prominent in the late eosinophil promyelocyte and myelocyte stages and become less obvious with subsequent eosinophil maturation. Similarly staining granules can be seen in reactive eosinophilia; it is their large size together with their dense basophilic staining characteristics that provides the clue to this clonal condition. Cytogenetic analysis confirmed this diagnosis. Acute myeloid leukaemia with inv(16)(p13.1q22) typically shows myeloid and monocytic proliferation with a morphologically defined abnormal bone marrow eosinophil population. On immunophenotyping, it is important to respond to the morphological assessment and to accurately gate both the myeloblast and monocyte precursor populations. This is very important in diagnosis, but equally so in the assessment of response to treatment.

MCQ

AML with inv(16)(p13.1q22):

1 Can be therapy-related
2 Generally has a good prognosis
3 Has a *RUNX1-RUNX1T1* fusion gene that is demonstrable on FISH analysis
4 Has identical features to AML with t(16;16)(p13.1;q22)
5 Is often complicated by disseminated intravascular coagulation

For answers and discussion, see page 206.

44 Babesiosis

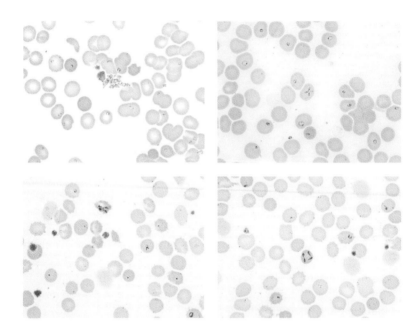

An 83-year-old man who normally resided in the north-eastern United States presented, during a visit to England, with fever, worsening jaundice and acute kidney injury. He had recently been treated for a low-grade lymphoma with rituximab. His FBC showed Hb 80 g/l and platelet count of 42×10^9/l). The total white cell and differential counts were normal. Initially cholecystitis and resultant sepsis were suspected but there was no response to antibiotics. The image above top left (MGG, all images ×100 objective) shows multiple intracellular parasites. These are small, delicate ring forms, resembling those of *Plasmodium falciparum*. However, the patient had not visited any country where malaria was endemic and careful inspection of this image provides a clue that this is not the diagnosis. Near the centre of the image is an aggregate of extracellular parasites, a feature that is not seen in malaria but is often seen in babesiosis. It is important that such parasite aggregates are not mistaken for debris or for platelet clumps. The ring trophozoites with their nuclear dots are apparent on close inspection and the two platelets to the left of the aggregate permit comparison of the different staining characteristics. The top right image (Giemsa) confirms the diagnosis, showing a perfect Maltese cross formation. The final diagnosis was babesiosis due to *Babesia microti*, confirmed by PCR (McGregor *et al.* 2019). Despite intensive treatment, the patient succumbed to the infection.

A second patient, a 72-year-old woman resident in a rural area in England where cattle were known to carry *Babesia divergens*, presented with fever, nausea, abdominal pain and dark urine. Her FBC showed Hb 75 g/l and platelet count 69 × 10^9/l with a normal MCV, WBC and differential count. A blood film was examined because of the anaemia and, particularly, the thrombocytopenia and *Babesia* were recognised. There were pyriform parasites, sometimes in pairs (bottom left), Maltese cross formations (bottom right) and erythrocytes with up to six parasites. *B. divergens* was confirmed by PCR. Rapid diagnosis from the blood film led to appropriate treatment and with vigorous support, despite the patient being seriously ill, recovery occurred (Chan *et al.* 2021).

Features that help to distinguish *Babesia* from *Plasmodium* are the presence of pyriform parasites, which can be in pairs or tetrads (the Maltese cross), multiple parasites in a single red cell (up to eight parasites per erythrocyte), extracellular clumps of parasites, parasites of a variety of shapes, and the absence of Maurer's clefts, Schüffner's dots, haemozoin and decolouration or enlargement of the red cell.

References

Chan WY, Macdonald C, Keenan A, Xu K, Bain BJ and Chiodini PL (2021) Severe babesiosis due to *Babesia divergens* acquired in the United Kingdom. *Am J Hematol*, doi: 10.1002/ajh.26097.

McGregor A, Lambert J, Bain BJ and Chiodini P (2019) Unexpected babesiosis with dramatic morphological features. *Am J Hematol*, **94**, 947–948.

MCQ

Babesiosis:

1   Can be transmitted by blood transfusion
2   Can cause leucopenia, neutropenia and thrombocytopenia
3   Has a similar distribution to malaria
4   Is more likely to be severe in hyposplenic patients
5   Is transmitted by mosquitoes

For answers and discussion, see page 206.

45   Haemoglobin E disorders

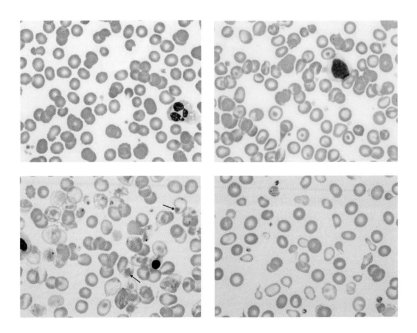

Haemoglobin E is a common variant haemoglobin in Southeast Asia. It is also found, not infrequently, in Bangladesh, north-eastern India, Sri Lanka, Indonesia and southern China. The top left image is from a patient with haemoglobin E heterozygosity (haemoglobin E trait) (all images ×100 objective). There was mild anaemia and microcytosis (Hb 110 g/l, MCV 74 fl and MCH 25.1 pg) with minor blood film abnormalities being apparent. There are several irregularly contracted cells, which lack central pallor but can be distinguished from spherocytes by their irregular outline. Some patients also have occasional target cells. The top right image is from a 10-year-old boy with haemoglobin E homozygosity showing more marked abnormalities. His FBC showed Hb 109 g/l, RBC 6.60×10^{12}/l, MCV 55 fl, MCH 18 pg and MCHC 328 g/l. The film shows anisocytosis, poikilocytosis, microcytosis, target cells and irregularly contracted cells. This condition is often referred to as 'haemoglobin E disease' but this term could be considered inappropriate since most homozygotes are asymptomatic and often do not have anaemia or splenomegaly.

The situation is very different when haemoglobin E is co-inherited with β thalassaemia. The bottom left image is from a compound heterozygote for haemoglobin E and β^0 thalassaemia who is transfusion dependent despite having been splenectomised. The FBC a month post-transfusion showed Hb 93 g/l, RBC 3.99×10^{12}/l, MCV 78.8 fl, MCH 23.3 pg and MCHC 300 g/l. The post-transfusion film is dimorphic and shows features of hyposplenism (acanthocytes and Howell–Jolly bodies). In addition, NRBC are present and α chain inclusions are seen within several hypochromic cells (arrows); Pappenheimer bodies are also evident. The bottom right image is from a compound heterozygote for haemoglobin E and β^+ thalassaemia, who was also transfusion dependent. The FBC showed Hb 85 g/l, RBC 3.7×10^{12}/l, MCV 75.4 fl, MCH 23 pg and MCHC 314 g/l. In this case there is prominent basophilic stippling. Other features noted were NRBC and post-transfusion dimorphism with the patient's own red cells showing hypochromia, microcytosis, poikilocytosis, Pappenheimer bodies and α chain inclusions. Haemoglobin electrophoresis showed 51% haemoglobin F, 42% haemoglobin E plus A_2 and 7% haemoglobin A.

This case series illustrates an important learning point in that the significance of any inherited globin gene mutation can be greatly influenced by co-inheritance of a mutation of the other allele. Co-inheritance of haemoglobin E and β thalassaemia is clinically much more significant than homozygosity for haemoglobin E. This is extremely important in diagnosis, in anticipating disease behaviour and ultimately in enabling informed, carefully considered patient management. This knowledge is also important in antenatal counselling.

MCQ

Haemoglobin E:

1 Can be regarded as a thalassaemic haemoglobinopathy
2 Can cause a mild sickling disorder when co-inherited with haemoglobin S
3 In heterozygotes, constitutes about 50% of haemoglobin
4 Is a high-affinity haemoglobin
5 Is of no significance in heterozygotes

For answers and discussion, see page 206.

46   Juvenile myelomonocytic leukaemia

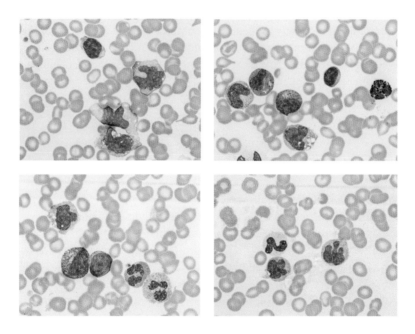

A 4-year-old boy who was known to have neurofibromatosis presented with massive hepatosplenomegaly. His FBC showed Hb 87 g/l, WBC 61.4×10^9/l and platelet count 41×10^9/l. His blood film showed normocytic, sometimes mildly hypochromic, red cells and confirmed the low platelet count. There was prominent monocytosis with mature or immature morphology (top images) and basophilia (top right) (all images ×100 objective). Some neutrophils were normally granulated (bottom left) while others were hypogranular (bottom right). Blast cells, myelocytes and promyelocytes were present. The differential count showed blast cells 4%, promyelocytes 3%, myelocytes 3%, neutrophils 13%, eosinophils 3%, basophils 17%, monocytes 41% and lymphocytes 16%. There were 3 NRBC/100 WBC.

The prominent monocytosis with immature forms, the dysplastic neutrophils and the lack of a distinct myelocyte peak indicated that this was not Philadelphia-positive chronic myeloid leukaemia. The haematological features and the underlying neurofibromatosis strongly suggested a diagnosis of juvenile myelomonocytic leukaemia (JMML), which was confirmed on further investigation. Haemoglobin F was 14%. Such marked basophilia is uncommon in this condition.

JMML (in the WHO classification assigned to the MDS/MPN group of disorders) is characterised by a chronic proliferation in the neutrophil and monocyte lineages (Baumann *et al.* 2017). Typically, the peripheral blood shows a moderate leucocytosis due to an increase in neutrophils and monocytes with some neutrophil precursors. There is a lesser degree, if any, increase in eosinophils and basophils. Blasts and blast equivalents account for less than 20% of nucleated cells in the bone marrow and dysplasia in erythroblasts and megakaryocytes is common. Leukaemic infiltration of the liver and spleen is almost universal, but lymphadenopathy and extranodal disease (including skin involvement) can also occur. The majority of cases are identified in children under 3 years of age, particularly in males. The disease appears to be driven by mutations, either inherited or somatic, in genes involved in RAS pathway signalling. These included *NF1* in cases associated with neurofibromatosis (reported 200–500 times increase in incidence compared to that of the general paediatric population) and *PTPN11* in cases associated with Noonan syndrome, also showing a significantly increased risk but associated with some instances of spontaneous resolution. Other genes that have been incriminated include *KRAS*, *NRAS*, *RRAS*, *SOS1*, *RAF1*, *RIT1* and *CBL*. Targeted gene sequencing can be informative in confirming a diagnosis. Allogeneic stem cell transplantation needs to be considered early in the disease course. This is a fascinating condition with clear somatic predisposition, further informing our understanding of rare disease pathogenesis.

Reference

Baumann I, Bennett JM, Niemeyer CM and Thiele J (2017) Juvenile myelomonocytic leukaemia. *In* Swerdlow SH, Campo E, Harris NL, Jaffe ES, Pileri SA, Stein H and Thiele J (Eds) *WHO Classification of Tumours of Haematopoietic and Lymphoid Tissues.* IARC, Lyon, pp. 89–92.

MCQ

Recognised features of juvenile myelomonocytic leukaemia (JMML) include:

1 Frequent complex chromosomal abnormalities
2 Increased haemoglobin F
3 Reduced erythrocyte carbonic anhydrase
4 Reduced haemoglobin A_2
5 Right shifted oxygen dissociation curve

For answers and discussion, see page 206.

47 Non-haemopoietic tumours

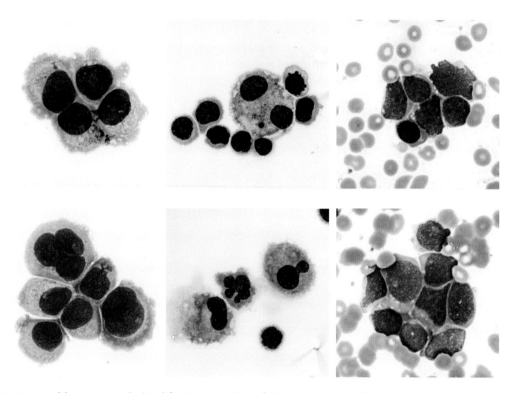

A 55-year-old man was admitted for investigation of the recent onset of anorexia, weight loss and abdominal distension. On examination he appeared unwell and ascites was apparent without obvious organomegaly. The full blood count showed a mild normocytic anaemia, Hb 105 g/l. On CT imaging ascites was confirmed and there was diffuse peritoneal nodularity with multiple low-density lesions in keeping with metastatic tumour. An ascitic fluid sample was taken for cytology and flow cytometry; the latter identified a CD45− population. A cytospin preparation showed a population of large pleomorphic cells with pale, mildly vacuolated cytoplasm (left images) (all images ×100 objective). Immunohistochemistry showed these cells to express epithelial markers (ERA, BerEp4, CK7 and CDX2) with the pattern suggesting a likely upper gastrointestinal tract adenocarcinoma with metastasis to peritoneum and liver.

A second patient, a 66-year-old woman with a history of bladder carcinoma, presented with headaches, recent onset proptosis and confusion. The FBC was normal. MRI imaging of the brain identified a periorbital mass and diffuse meningeal enhancement. A cerebrospinal fluid specimen showed a cell count of 0.041×10^9/l and the cytospin showed prominent small lymphocytes and medium sized cells with convoluted nuclei and frothy blue cytoplasm (centre images). Flow cytometry immunophenotyping showed the latter cells to be CD45−, CD10+, CD33+, CD15+ but no lineage-specific antigens were identified. The small lymphocytes were reactive T cells. A core biopsy of an enlarged groin node showed features of metastatic, poorly differentiated small cell carcinoma; the cells expressed AE1/3, CK7 and GATA3 with the latter, alongside the history, suggesting metastasis from a primary bladder carcinoma.

Haematology: From the Image to the Diagnosis, First Edition. Mike Leach and Barbara J. Bain.
© 2022 John Wiley & Sons Ltd. Published 2022 by John Wiley & Sons Ltd.

A third patient, a 3-year-old girl, was admitted for investigation of lethargy, irritability, headache and right eye pain. On examination the child was clearly unwell and poorly cooperative with clinical examination. Her FBC showed Hb 76 g/l, WBC 11.5×10^9/l, neutrophils 4.1×10^9/l and platelets 122×10^9/l and the blood film was leucoerythroblastic. CT imaging showed abnormal infiltrates around the base of the skull and the orbits and a left pararenal soft tissue mass. A bone marrow aspirate showed clumps of medium to large cells with a primitive chromatin pattern and pale blue cytoplasm (right images, facing page); there were no defining features but the presentation and cell morphology suggested a non-haemopoietic tumour. Flow cytometric analysis showed these cells to have a CD45−, CD56+ phenotype. No lineage-specific markers were expressed. Immunohistochemical studies on the marrow trephine biopsy sections identified a tumour and were in keeping with metastatic neuroblastoma.

In haematological practice it is not uncommon to encounter non-haemopoietic neoplasms. They can be encountered in bone marrow aspirates, trephine biopsy sections, CSF, pleural and peritoneal aspirates and lymph node fine needle aspirates. It is obviously important to recognise them as such. The important morphological features are: (i) lack of recognisable morphological features of normal haemopoietic cells; (ii) cell clumping, particularly in poorly cellular aspirates; and (iii) focal cohesive aggregates of cells in trephine biopsy sections, often with associated fibrosis. These features need additional work-up in terms of flow cytometry of fluid samples, looking for CD45-negative cells but also using extensive immunohistochemistry, firstly to show a non-haemopoietic phenotype but also possibly to delineate the lineage of the primary tumour.

MCQ

Bone marrow infiltration by a non-haemopoietic tumour:

1   Can show cohesive masses of cells in both the aspirate and trephine biopsy sections
2   Can show moulding of cells by adjacent cells
3   Is often associated with fibrosis and osteosclerosis
4   Is strongly suggested if cells show expression of CD10
5   May show increased osteoblasts and osteoclasts in a bone marrow aspirate

For answers and discussion, see page 206.

48 Richter transformation of chronic lymphocytic leukaemia

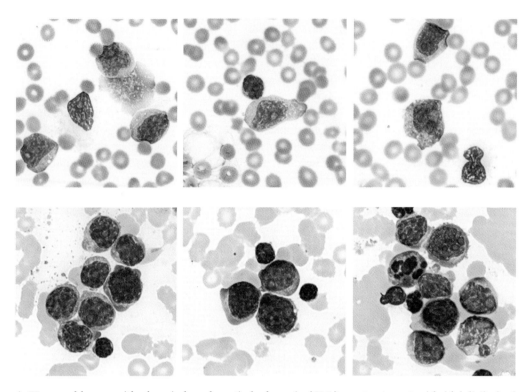

A 77-year-old man with chronic lymphocytic leukaemia (CLL), on treatment with idelalisib, had recurrent treatment interruptions due to infection. He was admitted to hospital with a scalp infection but despite appropriate antibiotic therapy and improvement in the cellulitis, his fever continued. His full blood count showed Hb 86 g/l, WBC 62.6 × 10⁹/l and platelets 17 × 10⁹/l, which was a significant deterioration from the previous assessment. The blood film showed small numbers of residual CLL cells (top centre) but there were now large cells with nucleoli and plentiful, mildly vacuolated basophilic cytoplasm (all top images ×100 objective). Their immunophenotype, gating on the large cells alone, was CD19+, CD20 strong, CD5+, FMC7+, CD23+, CD79b+, HLA-DR+ and surface lambda strong. The remaining CLL cells were CD19+, CD20 weak, CD5+, FMC7−, CD23+, CD79b−, HLA-DR+ and surface lambda weak. This confirmed a phenotypic shift in the larger cells (expression of strong CD20, FMC7 and CD79b) but some CLL phenotypic traits (CD5 positivity) were preserved. The findings are in keeping with a leukaemic phase Richter transformation.

A second patient, a 75-year-old woman with a history of treated CLL was admitted for treatment of disseminated herpes zoster. This responded to therapy, but despite this, she showed an acute clinical decline. Her full blood count showed Hb 114 g/l, WBC 92 × 10⁹/l and platelets 22 × 10⁹/l. Her blood film also showed a population of large pleomorphic cells with condensed chromatin, prominent nucleoli and basophilic cytoplasm whilst residual CLL cells were still present (all lower images ×100 objective). Note the karyorrhectic cell in the bottom right image. The immunophenotype of the large cells was identical to that shown above and showed the same phenotypic shift compared to the background CLL.

Haematology: From the Image to the Diagnosis, First Edition. Mike Leach and Barbara J. Bain.
© 2022 John Wiley & Sons Ltd. Published 2022 by John Wiley & Sons Ltd.

MCQ

Richter syndrome:

1 Can usually be effectively managed with chemoimmunotherapy appropriate for a large cell lymphoma
2 Consistently involves the peripheral blood and bone marrow
3 Describes the development of a large B-cell lymphoma in a patient with chronic lymphocytic leukaemia
4 Has no known aetiological factors
5 Usually represents transformation of a clonal B cell

For answers and discussion, see page 206.

49   Sickle cell–haemoglobin C disease

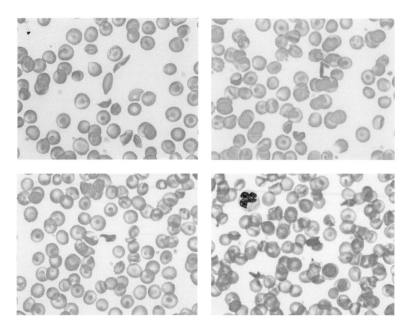

A young man of West African origin presented to the Accident and Emergency department with limb pains. He said that he had sickle cell disease. On examination, he was afebrile and normally hydrated with no abnormal physical findings. His Hb was 124 g/l and MCV 84 fl. The very mild reduction of his Hb suggested that this was not sickle cell anaemia. A sickle solubility test was positive and a blood film was examined.

The blood film showed small numbers of sickle cells (top left, all images ×100 objective), boat-shaped cells, target cells, irregularly contracted cells and occasional Howell–Jolly bodies. In addition, there were cells containing rectangular crystals (top right); these indicated the presence of haemoglobin C. Furthermore, there were cells with a gentle curve and also rectangular projections, indicating polymerisation of haemoglobin S and crystallisation of haemoglobin C within the one cell (lower images). High-performance liquid chromatography confirmed the absence of haemoglobin A and the presence of both haemoglobin S and haemoglobin C. These distinctive cells are known as SC poikilocytes and are present in about half of patients with this compound heterozygous state (Bain 1993).

Sickle cell disease is a somewhat ambiguous term, which is sometimes used as a synonym for sickle cell anaemia and sometimes as a generic term encompassing also compound heterozygous states that similarly lead to a sickling disorder (compound heterozygosity for haemoglobin S and, for example, haemoglobin C, β thalassaemia or haemoglobin D-Punjab). When patients present in an emergency with an unrelated condition requiring anaesthesia and are found to have a positive sickle solubility test and a normal or near normal Hb, it is important to distinguish between sickle cell trait and SC compound heterozygosity. The clinical history is important but blood film examination is also useful since the only abnormality likely to be found in a patient with sickle cell trait is the presence of target cells. This is a further example of where a

Haematology: From the Image to the Diagnosis, First Edition. Mike Leach and Barbara J. Bain.
© 2022 John Wiley & Sons Ltd. Published 2022 by John Wiley & Sons Ltd.

carefully considered morphological assessment can indicate a likely diagnosis, and in an emergency situation can inform an optimal and safe patient pathway. The clinical implications for early patient management of sickle cell trait, haemoglobin SC disease and sickle cell anaemia are significantly different.

Reference

Bain BJ (1993) Blood film features of sickle cell–haemoglobin C disease. *Br J Haematol*, **83**, 516–518.

MCQ

In comparison with sickle cell anaemia, sickle cell–haemoglobin C disease has:

1 A higher haematocrit
2 A higher incidence of retinal disease and bone marrow necrosis
3 A lower oxygen affinity
4 Less evidence of hyposplenism
5 Shorter red cell survival

For answers and discussion, see page 206.

50 T cell/histiocyte-rich B-cell lymphoma

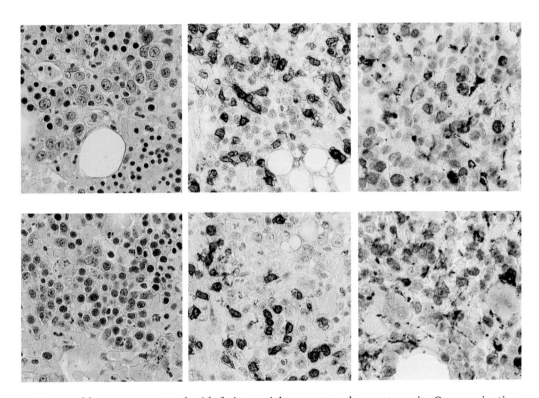

A 55-year-old woman presented with fatigue, night sweats and pancytopenia. On examination, there was no lymphadenopathy or palpable splenomegaly. Her full blood count showed Hb 81 g/l, WBC 2.1 × 10⁹/l, neutrophils 0.6 × 10⁹/l and platelets 106 × 10⁹/l. The blood film showed no informative features and in particular no blasts or abnormal lymphoid cells were seen. Routine biochemistry tests showed a low serum albumin at 25 g/l and an LDH of 1512 iu/l but was otherwise normal. A CT scan showed mild splenomegaly (15 cm long axis) but no lymphadenopathy. A PET-CT scan showed abnormal diffuse bone marrow and splenic fluorodeoxyglucose uptake. A bone marrow aspiration was dry but the trephine biopsy sections were hypercellular at 90% with diffuse and nodular infiltrates. Many cells had the features of histiocytes and small lymphocytes but there were suspicious admixed larger cells of unclear origin (H&E, left images ×50 objective). Staining for CD3 confirmed a pleomorphic reactive T-cell infiltrate (centre images, immunoperoxidase ×50), these being mainly CD8+ cells. A histiocyte population was highlighted using CD68R (right images, immunoperoxidase ×50) and these corresponded to the cells with ovoid nuclei and visible nucleoli in the H&E-stained images. Immunohistochemistry for CD20 highlighted a significant population of large pleomorphic B cells within these nodular areas (images, facing page, immunoperoxidase ×50); these were positive for PAX5, CD75, OCT2 and BCL2 whilst a proportion were positive for CD30. CD10, CD15 and Epstein–Barr virus *in situ* hybridisation were negative. There was no T-cell rosetting of the larger CD20+ B cells.

Haematology: From the Image to the Diagnosis, First Edition. Mike Leach and Barbara J. Bain.
© 2022 John Wiley & Sons Ltd. Published 2022 by John Wiley & Sons Ltd.

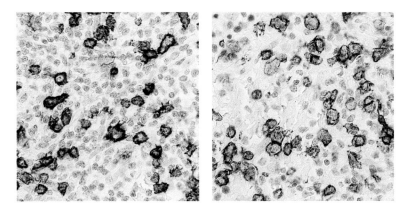

The working diagnosis was now a T cell/histiocyte-rich B-cell lymphoma (THRBCL) and B-cell clonality was confirmed after identifying an IGH rearrangement on marrow tissue. The patient was treated with R-CHOP (rituximab, cyclophosphamide, doxorubicin, vincristine, prednisolone) immunochemotherapy and showed a complete response including recovery of bone marrow function and morphology.

MCQ

T cell/histiocyte-rich B-cell lymphoma (THRBCL):

1 Can occur *de novo* or evolve from nodular lymphocyte predominant Hodgkin lymphoma
2 Is one of the more common types of large B-cell lymphoma
3 Often presents with advanced stage disease
4 Usually expresses CD15 and CD30
5 Usually harbours the Epstein–Barr virus

For answers and discussion, see page 206.

51 Miliary tuberculosis

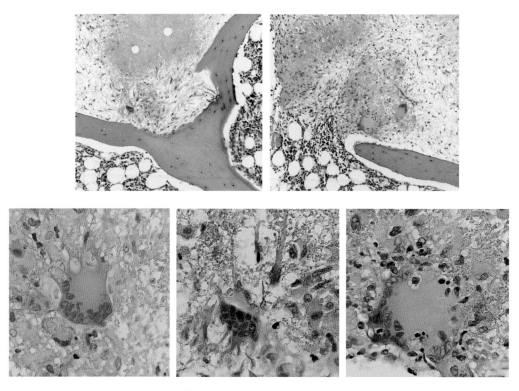

A 20-year-old woman from a socially deprived background was admitted to hospital with weight loss and anorexia. On examination, she appeared grossly undernourished. She had a low-grade intermittent fever but no organ-specific symptoms. The full blood count showed Hb 84 g/l, WBC 12.1×10^9/l, neutrophils 10.9×10^9/l, lymphocytes 0.9×10^9/l and platelets 327×10^9/l. Her blood film did not show any specific diagnostic features. The ESR was 53 mm in 1 h, C-reactive protein 181 mg/l and serum albumin 22 g/l. Her chest X-ray showed a fine pulmonary interstitial nodularity which was confirmed on CT imaging. The clinical and laboratory features all indicated a poorly nourished patient with a chronic disease of an infective, inflammatory or neoplastic nature. The bone marrow aspirate did not show any specific diagnostic features but the trephine biopsy sections showed a single focus of necrotic marrow with an adjacent granulomatous reaction (top images ×10 objective, bottom images ×50). Note the bone marrow necrosis in the upper parts of the top images. In view of the necrotising granulomatous reaction, miliary tuberculosis was suspected and a Ziehl–Neelsen stain on a marrow trephine biopsy section confirmed the diagnosis (images, facing page ×100). Compare the images here with those in Theme 6. Note the subtle scarce bacteria staining red with this stain. Remarkably, despite the widespread dissemination of this advanced variant of tuberculosis, the bacteria themselves are quite difficult to positively identify.

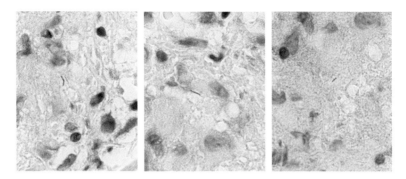

Tuberculosis is a mycobacterial infection that has caused serious morbidity and mortality for thousands of years. It can be a surprisingly difficult condition to diagnose, even in patients with disseminated infection, as in this case. The organism is slow to grow even in specialised culture media and the bacterium is notoriously difficult to demonstrate with direct staining of infected tissues. A provisional diagnosis is often made through interpretation of clinical circumstances and pathological findings with rapid molecular tests now being available for confirmation (WHO 2017).

Reference

World Health Organization (2017) Algorithm for laboratory diagnosis and treatment-monitoring of pulmonary tuberculosis and drug-resistant tuberculosis using state-of-the-art rapid molecular diagnostic technologies. https://www.euro.who.int/__data/assets/pdf_file/0006/333960/ELI-Algorithm.pdf

MCQ

Tuberculosis:

1 Can be complicated by haemophagocytic lymphohistiocytosis
2 Can be excluded if there are tissue granulomas but the Ziehl–Neelsen stain is negative
3 Can cause anaemia of chronic disease
4 Can cause bone marrow necrosis
5 Is often associated with more numerous bacteria in bone marrow lesions than are found in atypical mycobacterial infection

For answers and discussion, see page 206.

52 Pure red cell aplasia

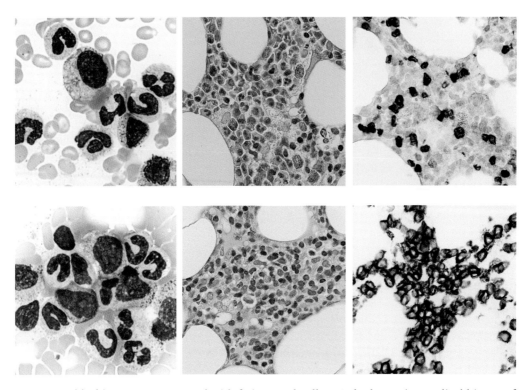

A 68-year-old Chinese man presented with fatigue and pallor. He had no prior medical history of note, took no regular medication and was otherwise well. His full blood count showed Hb 50 g/l, WBC 5.5 × 10^9/l, neutrophils 3.2 × 10^9/l and platelets 320 × 10^9/l. The reticulocyte count was 2 × 10^9/l. Serum ferritin, folate and vitamin B12 levels were within the normal range. There was no elevation of inflammatory markers and routine biochemical tests were normal. The blood film did not show any specific features. The bone marrow aspirate showed an almost complete absence of red cell precursors (left images ×100 objective) while the trephine biopsy sections showed only mature red cells within the marrow vasculature (top centre, H&E ×50 and top right, glycophorin C, immunoperoxidase ×50). Notably, reactive CD4- and CD8-positive T cells were prominent throughout the sections and formed focal aggregates in places (bottom centre, H&E ×50 and bottom right, CD3, immunoperoxidase ×50). The findings confirm a diagnosis of acquired pure red cell aplasia whilst the T-cell infiltrate might be implicated in the pathophysiology. A chest X-ray was normal. A CT scan was performed looking for evidence of an underlying lymphoma or solid tumour. This showed a well-circumscribed mass with partial calcification in the anterior mediastinum (image, facing page), compatible with a thymoma; this was confirmed after the tumour was fully resected at thoracotomy (type A/B1 histology).

Haematology: From the Image to the Diagnosis, First Edition. Mike Leach and Barbara J. Bain.
© 2022 John Wiley & Sons Ltd. Published 2022 by John Wiley & Sons Ltd.

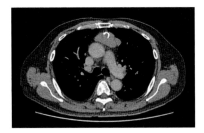

The patient remained transfusion dependent for 3 months post-surgery, at which point a small dose of ciclosporin was introduced. Within 2 weeks he developed a brisk reticulocytosis; further transfusion was not necessary and his Hb has now normalised.

MCQ

Chronic red cell aplasia can be a feature of:

1 ABO-incompatible allogeneic stem cell transplantation
2 Autologous stem cell transplantation
3 Development of an anti-erythropoietin antibody
4 Parvovirus infection in an immunodeficient patient
5 Systemic lupus erythematosus

For answers and discussion, see page 206.

53 Lymphoblastic transformation of follicular lymphoma

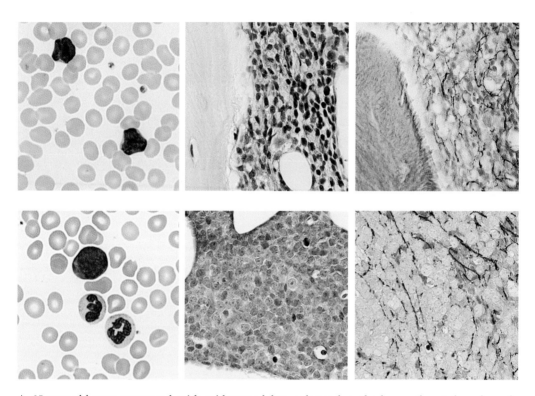

A 65-year-old man presented with widespread low-volume lymphadenopathy. A lymph node biopsy showed grade 2 follicular lymphoma and t(14;18)(q32;q21) was identified using an IGH/*BCL2* dual fusion probe. Small numbers of follicular lymphoma cells were identified in the blood film (top left image ×100 objective) and this was confirmed by immunophenotyping with a CD19+, CD20+, FMC7+, CD10+, HLA-DR+, CD22+, CD79b+, surface kappa-restricted population being identified. Note that the cells are cytologically very typical of follicular lymphoma cells, being small and angular with scanty cytoplasm, very dense chromatin and a nuclear cleft apparent in the top cell. Bone marrow trephine biopsy sections showed paratrabecular infiltrates of small mature B cells (top centre, H&E ×50) with the same immunophenotype and associated grade 1/3 fibrosis (top right, reticulin stain ×50). He initially underwent a period of observation as he had no systemic upset and had a normal full blood count. Within 6 months he developed progressive lymphadenopathy, occasional night sweats and abdominal discomfort so he was commenced on R-CVP (rituximab, cyclophosphamide, vincristine, prednisolone) chemoimmunotherapy. He completed six cycles with a good clinical and radiological response.

Six months later he developed progressive leucocytosis and thrombocytopenia with bone pain. The full blood count now showed Hb 101 g/l, WBC 21×10^9/l, neutrophils 1.1×10^9/l and platelets 32×10^9/l. The blood film appearances had changed significantly as blast cells were now evident (bottom left ×100). Immunophenotyping now showed the neoplastic cells to have a CD19+, CD20−, FMC7−, CD10+, HLA-DR+, CD22+, CD79b−, surface kappa negative, CD79a+, TdT+ immunophenotype in keeping with transformation to a precursor B-cell neoplasm. A repeat

Haematology: From the Image to the Diagnosis, First Edition. Mike Leach and Barbara J. Bain.
© 2022 John Wiley & Sons Ltd. Published 2022 by John Wiley & Sons Ltd.

trephine biopsy showed a diffuse infiltrate of cells with blastoid morphology (bottom centre, H&E ×50) with associated grade 1 diffuse fibrosis (bottom right, facing page, reticulin stain ×50). An IGH/*BCL2* fusion was again detected in 78.5% of nuclei. No rearrangement of *MYC* or *TP53* was identified. The findings now are in keeping with lymphoblastic lymphoma/leukaemia transformation of follicular lymphoma.

MCQ

Follicular lymphoma can transform into:

1 B lymphoblastic leukaemia/lymphoma
2 Burkitt lymphoma
3 Diffuse large B-cell lymphoma
4 Lymphoma with features intermediate between Burkitt lymphoma and diffuse large cell lymphoma
5 Mantle cell lymphoma

For answers and discussion, see page 206.

54 Primary hyperparathyroidism

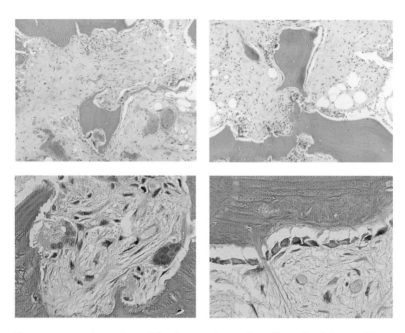

A 67-year-old woman was investigated for hypercalcaemia, adjusted calcium 2.98 mmol/l, phosphate 0.83 mmol/l and parathyroid hormone (PTH) 23.6 pmol/l (NR 1.6–7.5). The bone texture was abnormal on MRI and there was concern with regard to a haematological disorder. The blood film and bone marrow aspirate were not informative. The bone marrow trephine biopsy was abnormal, showing marked remodelling of the trabeculae with bone resorption (top images, H&E ×10 objective) and obvious Howship's lacunae (bottom left, H&E ×50) with active osteoclasts cutting bony hollows. Furthermore, and in adjacent parts of the biopsy sections, linear teams of osteoblasts were actively generating new bone (bottom right, H&E ×50). Note the deposition of collagenous tissue within the bone marrow spaces. The laboratory features suggested a diagnosis of primary hyperparathyroidism, which usually results from a benign parathyroid adenoma. This was confirmed in this case. The marrow trephine biopsy features are in keeping with this diagnosis as the high PTH activates osteoclasts liberating bone-derived calcium. The osteoclast-related trabecular changes then lead to secondary increased osteoblast activity striving to respond through active bone repair. These endocrine changes with their effect on bone can cause radiographic bone changes on plain radiography, CT or MRI examination. Alterations of bone texture, cysts, lytic lesions and sclerosis are all reported radiological manifestations of hyperparathyroidism.

Osteoclasts are multinucleated cells derived from bone marrow haemopoietic stem cells. They are important cells to identify in bone marrow trephine biopsy sections and should not be mistaken for the giant cells of granulomas. They play an essential role in calcium homeostasis, bone remodelling and bone marrow function. Inherited disorders of osteoclasts have serious clinical consequences (see Theme 22).

Haematology: From the Image to the Diagnosis, First Edition. Mike Leach and Barbara J. Bain.
© 2022 John Wiley & Sons Ltd. Published 2022 by John Wiley & Sons Ltd.

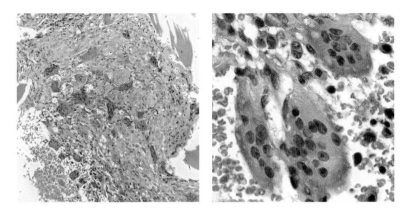

The images above (left, H&E ×10, right, H&E ×50) are of an osteoclastoma. This was found incidentally when undertaking a staging bone marrow biopsy in a patient with lymphoma. Also known as giant cell tumour, osteoclastomas are benign but locally aggressive tumours, which typically involve long bones. They cause localised bone destruction, appear as lytic lesions on plain X-ray or CT imaging and predispose to pathological fractures. When encountered incidentally, they are important to identify.

MCQ

The histological changes of hyperparathyroidism can be seen in the bone marrow as a result of:

1 Chronic renal insufficiency
2 Osteopetrosis
3 Osteosclerosis
4 Paget disease
5 Parathyroid adenoma

For answers and discussion, see page 206.

55 Gamma heavy chain disease

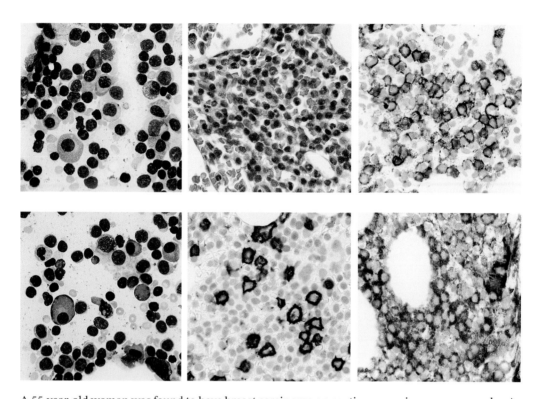

A 55-year-old woman was found to have breast carcinoma on routine screening mammography. As part of her work-up and staging she was noted to have small 1 cm pulmonary nodules on CT imaging and biopsy showed AL amyloidosis without evidence of an associated lymphoid or plasma cell disorder. She had a history of recurrent respiratory infections and bronchiectasis. She was referred to Haematology and on further CT imaging she had low-volume lymphadenopathy and mild splenomegaly. Serum immunoglobulin assays showed IgG 32.4 g/l (NR 6–16), IgA 0.16 g/l (NR 0.8–4) and IgM 0.43 g/l (NR 0.4–2.4). An IgG paraprotein, 4 g/l, was identified and serum free light chain analysis showed free kappa light chain 79.9 mg/l (NR 3.3–19.4 mg/l) and free lambda light chain 20.3 mg/l (NR 5.7–26.3) with a $\kappa{:}\lambda$ ratio of 3.9 (NR 0.26–1.65). In view of the apparent discrepancy between the increase in total IgG and the concentration of the IgG paraprotein, further immunological assessment was requested and this was informative. There was a low concentration of both an intact IgG kappa paraprotein and of polyclonal IgG and also a significant concentration of free gamma heavy chains quantitated at 21 g/l. The latter were not initially appreciated as there was a diffuse abnormal zone (rather than a discrete band) on electrophoresis but was confirmed and quantified using rocket immunoselection. These are highly unusual findings, which are suggestive of gamma heavy chain disease.

The patient had a normal full blood count. Nevertheless, bone marrow aspiration and trephine biopsy were performed. The aspirate showed a significant lymphoid infiltrate (left images) (all images ×50 objective) with plasmacytoid lymphocytes and plasma cells, some showing peripheral eosinophilic cytoplasmic staining, known as flame cells (bottom left). The trephine biopsy sections

Haematology: From the Image to the Diagnosis, First Edition. Mike Leach and Barbara J. Bain.
© 2022 John Wiley & Sons Ltd. Published 2022 by John Wiley & Sons Ltd.

showed a diffuse and nodular lymphocytic infiltrate (top centre, facing page, H&E), with some cells showing Dutcher bodies, some cells expressing CD20 (top right, facing page, immunoperoxidase) and some cells showing plasmacytic differentiation and expressing CD138 (bottom centre, facing page, immunoperoxidase). The neoplastic cells also expressed cytoplasmic gamma heavy chain (bottom right, facing page, immunoperoxidase). *In situ* hybridisation for kappa and lambda light chains showed a mild kappa excess but the cells expressing light chain were at a much lower percentage than the total B-cell population. The majority of cells were therefore expressing free gamma heavy chains but without light chains. No *MYD88* L265P mutation was identified. There was no evidence of bone marrow amyloid deposition.

These features are all in keeping with gamma heavy chain disease which is now recognised as a specific entity in the 2016 WHO classification of tumours of haemopoietic and lymphoid tissues (Cook *et al*. 2017).

Reference

Cook JR, Harris NL, Isaacson PG and Jaffe ES (2017) Heavy chain diseases. *In* Swerdlow SH, Campo E, Harris NL, Jaffe ES, Pileri SA, Stein H and Thiele J (Eds) *WHO Classification of Tumours of Haematopoietic and Lymphoid Tissues*. IARC, Lyon, pp. 237–240.

MCQ

Gamma heavy chain disease:

1 Almost always involves the bone marrow
2 Can involve Waldeyer's ring
3 Histologically does not differ from multiple myeloma
4 Shows an association with autoimmune disease
5 Usually involves liver, spleen and lymph nodes

For answers and discussion, see page 206.

56   Acute promyelocytic leukaemia with t(15;17)(q24.1;q21.2)

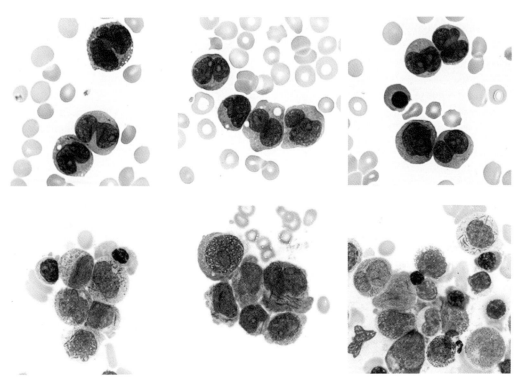

A 52-year-old man presented to his GP with fatigue, gum bleeding and widespread ecchymoses. The automated full blood count showed Hb 86 g/l, WBC 5.4×10^9/l, neutrophils 0.6×10^9/l, monocytes 2.3×10^9/l and platelets 80×10^9/l. Note the significant bleeding history at presentation despite only mild thrombocytopenia, suggesting a coexistent coagulopathy. The coagulation screen showed PT 16 s, APTT 30 s, thrombin time 19 s, fibrinogen 0.7 g/l and D dimer 1649 ng/ml. The blood film (top images ×100 objective) showed abnormal promyelocytes characterised by bilobed nuclei, nucleoli (unusually prominent in this case), prominent cytoplasmic granules and Auer rods. Note that monocytes are not present and the automated monocyte count is erroneous, resulting from promyelocytes that had similar forward and side light scatter properties. The bone marrow aspirate (bottom images ×100) showed a large population of granulated promyelocytes with many showing multiple Auer rods, known as faggot cells) (best example bottom centre). Note that the heavy granulation appears to be condensing to form Auer rods in some cells. Note also that the nuclear clefting is less apparent but the Auer rod formation more obvious in the bone marrow promyelocytes, as is often the case. Flow cytometry showed a typical acute promyelocytic leukaemia (APL) phenotype: CD34−, HLA-DR−, CD13+, CD33+, CD15−, CD64+, CD14−, MPO+. Note that typically CD13 expression is heterogeneous and CD33 expression strong and homogeneous in APL. No T- or B-lineage markers were evident. Note that hypogranular APL is sometimes misinterpreted as acute monocytic leukaemia; the promonocytes characteristic of the latter condition express HLA-DR and CD11b, in distinct contrast to APL. Urgent FISH studies identified a *PML-RARA* fusion gene due to a later confirmed t(15;17)(q24.1;q21.2) translocation. The patient

Haematology: From the Image to the Diagnosis, First Edition. Mike Leach and Barbara J. Bain.
© 2022 John Wiley & Sons Ltd. Published 2022 by John Wiley & Sons Ltd.

was treated with intensive blood product support and the non-chemotherapy combination of arsenic trioxide and all-*trans*-retinoic acid and remains well and in remission 7 years later.

Acute promyelocytic leukaemia is a haematological emergency since, in addition to the usual features of acute leukaemia, there is often a significant coagulopathy (combined DIC and excessive fibrinolysis) where patients have a high risk of serious bleeding. These patients have a good prognosis but there is still a significant early mortality, often before attending hospital, from bleeding complications. A rapid diagnosis is essential and a morphological diagnosis should be possible in the vast majority of cases. Typically, the hypergranular variant presents with a low white cell count so careful scrutiny of the blood film and early examination of the bone marrow is absolutely essential. Immunophenotyping can give rapid support for the diagnosis, but with morphology as unequivocal as this case initiation of treatment need not await confirmatory tests.

MCQ

Acute promyelocytic leukaemia:

1 Always has abnormal promyelocytes in the peripheral blood film when a careful search is done
2 Can be complicated by thrombosis
3 Can be reliably diagnosed when a case of acute myeloid leukaemia does not express CD34 or HLA-DR
4 Is more common in the elderly
5 Morphologically, can simulate acute megakaryoblastic leukaemia

For answers and discussion, see page 206.

57 AA amyloidosis

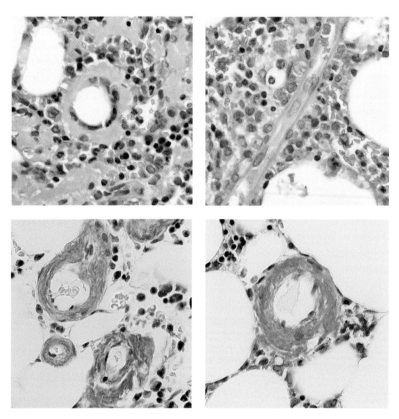

A 70-year-old woman with a long history of rheumatoid arthritis presented with fatigue, dyspnoea and leg oedema. On examination she was pale and had an irregular pulse, features of bilateral pleural effusions and pitting oedema to the knees. Her full blood count showed Hb 80 g/l, MCV 75 fl, WBC 10×10^9/l, neutrophils 7×10^9/l and platelets 450×10^9/l. The ESR was 80 mm in 1 h, serum ferritin 120 µg/l, serum creatinine 200 µmol/l, serum albumin 15 g/l and urinary protein 5 g in 24 h. Immunoglobulins were polyclonally elevated. A clinical diagnosis of nephrotic syndrome was made. A bone marrow aspirate and trephine biopsy were undertaken. The aspirate was unremarkable morphologically and stainable iron was present. The trephine biopsy sections were largely normocellular but the blood vessels showed intimal thickening with an amorphous pink material (transverse vessel, top left image and longitudinal vessel, top right image, H&E, all images × 50 objective). Further staining with Sirius red (bottom images) showed prominent uptake in the bone marrow blood vessels in keeping with a diagnosis of amyloidosis. This material also showed apple-green birefringence when examined under polarised light. In context this was likely to represent AA amyloidosis and this was confirmed on immunohistochemistry. This finding also made it extremely likely that the nephrotic syndrome was due to renal AA amyloidosis and a renal biopsy was not deemed necessary.

Haematology: From the Image to the Diagnosis, First Edition. Mike Leach and Barbara J. Bain.
© 2022 John Wiley & Sons Ltd. Published 2022 by John Wiley & Sons Ltd.

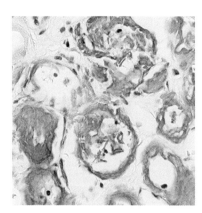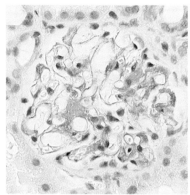

The images above, from another patient, show renal tubular (left) and glomerular (right) involvement by AA amyloid (Sirius red stain ×50). Once established, these amyloid fibrils are resistant to removal or remodelling and they normally continue to accumulate whilst the underlying disease remains active. Notably, the identification of conditions responsible for AA amyloidosis continues to grow and obesity has now been identified as a significant risk factor for a proportion of patients with the hitherto described 'idiopathic' AA amyloidosis (Blank *et al.* 2018).

Reference

Blank N, Hegenbart U, Dietrich S, Brune M, Beimler J, Rocken C *et al.* (2018) Obesity is a significant susceptibility factor for idiopathic AA amyloidosis. *Amyloid*, **25**, 37–45.

MCQ

Recognised causes of AA amyloidosis include:

1 Crohn's disease
2 Familial amyloidosis due to mutation in the transthyretin gene (*TTR*)
3 Familial Mediterranean fever
4 Osteomyelitis
5 Plasma cell myeloma

For answers and discussion, see page 206.

58   Acquired sideroblastic anaemia

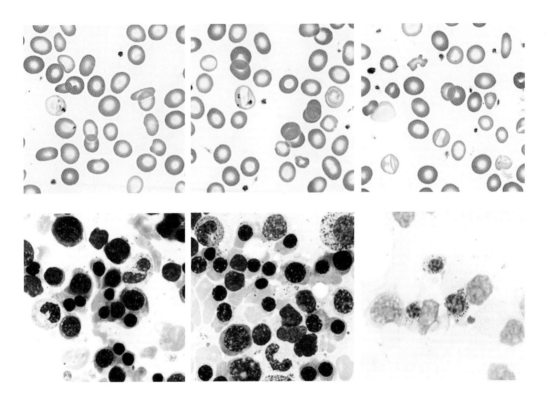

A 76-year-old man presented with fatigue due to significant anaemia. His full blood count showed Hb 62 g/l, MCV 77 fl, MCH 25 pg, WBC 4.9×10^9/l, neutrophils 3.2×10^9/l and platelets 303×10^9/l. The reticulocyte count was 13×10^9/l. Serum ferritin was 127 µg/l. The blood film was abnormal, showing a dimorphic red cell population with a subpopulation of hypochromic microcytes (top images) (all images ×100 objective) and prominent dense Pappenheimer bodies (top left and centre). There were occasional elliptocytes. A disorder of failed iron utilisation was suspected. The bone marrow aspirate showed erythroid hyperplasia with a prevalence of later erythroid forms. Some late erythroblasts showed defective haemoglobinisation but otherwise dysplasia was minimal. There was no excess of blast cells either morphologically or on flow cytometric immunophenotyping. A marrow iron stain showed prominent ring sideroblasts accounting for 25% of erythroid precursors (bottom right, Perls stain). These findings are in keeping with a diagnosis of a myelodysplastic syndrome with ring sideroblasts and single lineage dysplasia (MDS-RS-SLD). Cytogenetic studies showed a normal karyotype but myeloid gene sequencing demonstrated a mutation of *SF3B1*. We are increasingly noting, in diagnostic haematopathology, that standard metaphase cytogenetic and FISH studies set a baseline and that subsequent targeted investigations, such as myeloid next generation sequencing, further refine the diagnosis, treatment options and prognosis.

The directed investigations here are relevant to the presentation and are informative. The morphological diagnosis is MDS-RS-SLD and this is in keeping with all the presentation data. Furthermore, the *SF3B1* mutation identified on myeloid sequencing independently strongly

Haematology: From the Image to the Diagnosis, First Edition. Mike Leach and Barbara J. Bain.
© 2022 John Wiley & Sons Ltd. Published 2022 by John Wiley & Sons Ltd.

supports this and permits the diagnosis to be made with a lower percentage of ring sideroblasts than the conventional 15%. The patient was commenced on pyridoxine therapy and his haemoglobin concentration and reticulocyte count have normalised. This response has been sustained for over a year with Hb 124 g/l, MCV 103 fl and MCH 35 pg. The dimorphic blood film appearance has resolved.

MCQ

Sideroblastic erythropoiesis is a feature of:

1 *ALAS2* mutation
2 Copper deficiency
3 GATA1 deficiency
4 Pearson syndrome
5 Zinc deficiency

For answers and discussion, see page 206.

59 Diffuse large B-cell lymphoma

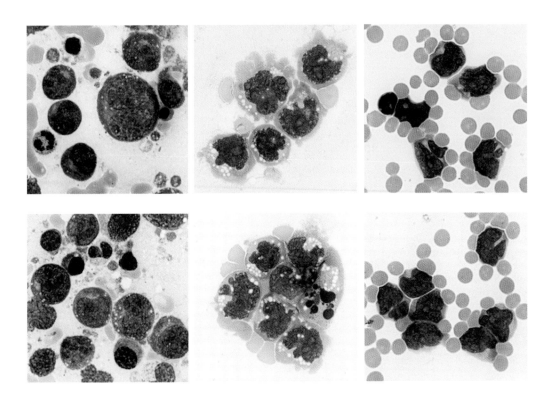

A 70-year-old man presented with fatigue and progressive dyspnoea. On examination he had reduced air entry in the right lung and basal dullness, suggesting a pleural effusion. No lymphadenopathy was apparent but his liver was clearly palpable. CT scanning showed an intrapulmonary mass with lymphangitis, right pleural effusion and enlarged mediastinal and para-aortic lymph nodes. His full blood count showed Hb 129 g/l, WBC 18.3 × 10⁹/l, neutrophils 18.3 × 10⁹/l, lymphocytes 1.7 × 10⁹/l and platelets 58 × 10⁹/l. The blood film showed a reactive neutrophilia and thrombocytopenia but no specific features. PET-CT imaging confirmed FDG uptake in all the above disease sites but in addition showed widespread uptake in bone marrow, including the iliac crests. A bone marrow aspirate and a trephine biopsy were taken and aspirate films are illustrated (left images) (all images ×100 objective). Note the population of large cells with round ovoid or irregular nuclei with condensed chromatin, obvious nucleoli and vacuolated basophilic cytoplasm. Some very large cells were binucleated (top left image) and had a diameter three to four times that of a neutrophil. Flow cytometry showed these cells to have a CD19+, CD20+, CD79b+, FMC7+, CD10−, surface lambda-restricted immunophenotype. The bone marrow trephine biopsy sections showed extensive replacement by large immunoblastic cells with a CD20+, CD10−, BCL2+, BCL6+, MUM1− immunophenotype, in keeping with a non-germinal centre-derived diffuse large B-cell lymphoma (DLBCL). No *MYC* or IGH/*MYC* rearrangements were identified.

A second patient, a 62-year-old woman, presented with persistent cough and dyspnoea. On examination she had features suggestive of a large right pleural effusion. On CT imaging the

Haematology: From the Image to the Diagnosis, First Edition. Mike Leach and Barbara J. Bain.
© 2022 John Wiley & Sons Ltd. Published 2022 by John Wiley & Sons Ltd.

effusion was confirmed but no mediastinal or pleural-based abnormality was apparent. She had extensive abnormal soft tissue in the retroperitoneum encasing the aorta and inferior vena cava. Her full blood count was normal. A therapeutic pleural fluid aspiration was performed and this showed high levels of LDH at 1707 iu/l (NR blood <250) and Ca125 (cancer antigen 125) at 377 ku/l (NR <35). A cytospin of the pleural fluid showed prominent large cells with convoluted nuclei, nucleoli and pale blue vacuolated cytoplasm (centre images, facing page) with some cells showing karyorrhexis. The cells had a CD19+, CD20+, CD79b+, FMC7+, CD10+ phenotype but surface light chains were not expressed. The cells in pleural fluid were made into a clot preparation and paraffin embedded. They showed a CD20+, CD10+, BCL6+, BCL2+, MUM1+ phenotype; CD34 and TdT were not expressed. Both *MYC* and IGH/*BCL2* rearrangements were detected by FISH, giving a final diagnosis of high-grade B-cell lymphoma with *MYC* and *BCL2* rearrangement, also sometimes referred to as 'double hit' lymphoma.

A third patient, a previously well 66-year-old man, presented with progressive right arm pain and weakness with sensory loss in the right trigeminal nerve distribution. On examination he had right-sided mixed motor and sensory impairment at C5–C8, suggestive of brachial plexus pathology. MRI showed no mass lesion but did show abnormal enhancement and oedema along the distal plexus trunks, whilst brain imaging was normal. A CSF specimen was blood stained but showed a population of large pleomorphic cells with prominent nuclear folds and nucleoli (right images); these also had a mature CD10+ B-cell phenotype without precursor antigen expression by flow cytometry and immunohistochemistry. Importantly, these cells were not present in blood, indicating true CSF and likely peripheral nerve involvement by DLBCL.

MCQ

Diffuse large B-cell lymphoma:

1 Can be a feature of the acquired immune deficiency syndrome (AIDS)
2 Can result from Epstein–Barr virus or human herpes virus 8 infection
3 Can result from immune suppression following transplantation
4 Consistently shows a germinal centre immunophenotype
5 Is the most frequently observed non-Hodgkin lymphoma

For answers and discussion, see page 206.

60 Hickman line infection

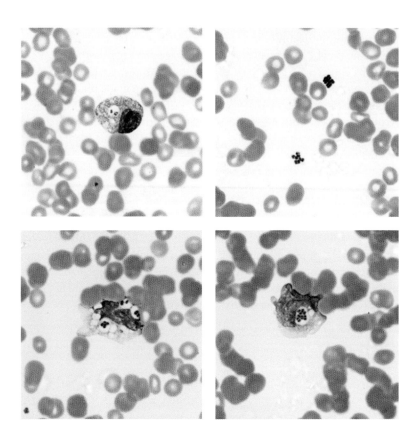

A 40-year-old man undergoing an autologous stem cell transplant for relapsed diffuse large B-cell lymphoma became acutely unwell on day 10 of the procedure with fever, hypotension and hypoxaemia within minutes of his Hickman line being accessed. The full blood count at the time showed Hb 80×10^9/l, WBC 0.2×10^9/l, neutrophils 0×10^9/l and platelets 15×10^9/l. Blood cultures were immediately taken from both the line and a peripheral vein and broad-spectrum antibiotic therapy was started. Careful review of the blood film from the original FBC specimen showed phagocytosed cocci in scarce, left shifted neutrophils (top left images) (all images ×100 objective) and monocytes (bottom images) and also free bacteria (top right). Blood cultures grew *Staphylococcus epidermidis* sensitive to piperacillin and teicoplanin. The patient made a steady recovery over the next 24 hours and remained afebrile until neutrophil recovery at day 14.

Hickman lines are temporary subcutaneously tunnelled silicone venous catheters which are commonly used in patients with haematological disorders requiring prolonged periods of treatment and needing reliable vascular access. The tunnelling substantially increases the distance between the skin surface and the central vein, lessening the risk of infection and so improving the durability of the catheter. Multiple complications can occur but all are uncommon or rare (Kornbau *et al.* 2015). The benefits outweigh the risks but infection, particularly in the context of neutropenia, remains a constant threat.

Haematology: From the Image to the Diagnosis, First Edition. Mike Leach and Barbara J. Bain.
© 2022 John Wiley & Sons Ltd. Published 2022 by John Wiley & Sons Ltd.

Reference

Kornbau C, Lee KC, Hughes GD and Firstenberg MS (2015) Central line complications. *Int J Crit Illn Inj Sci*, **5**, 170–178.

MCQ

Recognised complications of indwelling central venous lines include:

1 Bacterial infection
2 Cardiac arrhythmia
3 Fungal infection
4 Pneumothorax
5 Venous thrombosis

For answers and discussion, see page 206.

61 Monocytes and their precursors

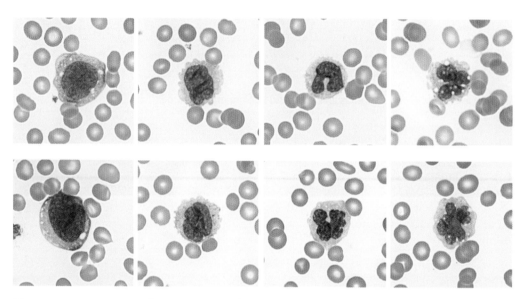

The accurate assessment of monocyte morphology is absolutely key in relation to the diagnosis of a number of haematological diseases. There are four main stages of maturation that need to be reliably identified. Monoblasts are large cells with a round or occasionally ovoid nucleus, nucleoli and finely granular blue cytoplasm on an MGG stain (left images) (all images ×100 objective). Promonocytes are medium to large cells with an irregularly shaped, convoluted, folded, grooved or cleft nucleus, occasional nucleoli and finely granular pale blue cytoplasm (centre left images). Both monoblasts and promonocytes have delicate chromatin without condensation. Immature monocytes have more condensed nuclear chromatin, a more complex nuclear shape (often horse-shoe like), absent nucleoli and sky-blue cytoplasm often without vacuoles (centre right images). Mature monocytes have a more complex nuclear outline with multiple lobes and pale blue cytoplasm, often with obvious vacuoles (right images). Both mature and immature monocytes have some chromatin condensation. Promonocytes are considered to be blast equivalents and when monoblasts plus promonocytes are 20% or more in the peripheral blood or bone marrow a mono-blastic leukaemia (majority are monoblasts) or monocytic leukaemia (majority are promonocytes) is diagnosed. This is not necessarily straightforward when the differential diagnosis is between a *de novo* presentation of acute leukaemia (monoblasts and promonocytes) and chronic myelomono-cytic leukaemia (immature and mature monocytes). Misdiagnosis of chronic myelomonocytic leu-kaemia as acute monocytic leukaemia sometimes occurs. Recognising promonocytes and immature monocytes is of critical importance in making this distinction and requires a careful assessment of chromatin characteristics. In patients with chronic myelomonocytic leukaemia all stages of matu-ration can be present in the blood or bone marrow simultaneously.

Since promonocytes and immature monocytes have different diagnostic implications, difficulty in their morphological identification and hence quantitation in blood and bone marrow aspirate films is problematic. Furthermore, they are very difficult to identify in bone marrow trephine biopsy sections as their immunophenotype is not unique and the subtle features of their morphol-ogy are not easy to identify.

Haematology: From the Image to the Diagnosis, First Edition. Mike Leach and Barbara J. Bain.
© 2022 John Wiley & Sons Ltd. Published 2022 by John Wiley & Sons Ltd.

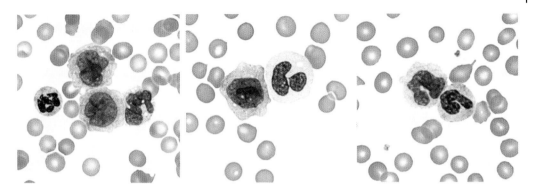

The images above illustrate some of the potential difficulties. The left image shows two central promonocytes, an immature monocyte and a dysplastic neutrophil. The centre image shows a promonocyte and a dysplastic neutrophil with hypogranularity and abnormal segmentation. The right image shows an immature monocyte (left in the image) alongside a dysplastic hypogranular band cell; note the subtle difference in cytoplasmic colour which if not appreciated could lead to misclassification of cell lineage.

MCQ

Promonocytes:

1   Can be distinguished from monoblasts by their lack of expression of CD34
2   Can be present in acute myeloid leukaemia with t(9;11) and *KMT2A* rearrangement
3   Can be readily differentiated from monocytes on immunophenotyping
4   Often express CD11b, CD11c, CD14 and CD64
5   Sometimes show chromatin condensation.

For answers and discussion, see page 206.

62 Paroxysmal cold haemoglobinuria

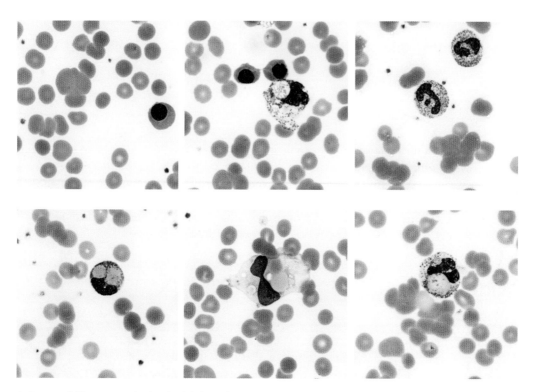

A 3-year-old boy was admitted with jaundice and pallor following a febrile illness over the preceding 5 days. His full blood count showed Hb 41 g/l, MCV 104 fl, WBC 22.8 × 10⁹/l, neutrophils 18 × 10⁹/l and platelets 398 × 10⁹/l. The reticulocyte count was 350 × 10⁹/l, serum bilirubin was 80 μmol/l, AST 90 u/l, ALT 45 u/l and LDH 520 u/l whilst haptoglobin was absent. A direct antiglobulin (Coombs) test showed positivity for C3d only. His blood film showed spherocytes, polychromasia, nucleated red cells (including a pair showing cytoplasmic bridging) and red cell agglutinates (all images ×100 objective). Furthermore, red cell phagocytosis was prominent, involving both neutrophils and monocytes (lower images). Also, there were neutrophils containing partly digested red cells (top centre image). The blood film appearances strongly supported a diagnosis of paroxysmal cold haemoglobinuria (PCH) and this was confirmed with a positive Donath–Landsteiner test.

Paroxysmal cold haemoglobinuria is an uncommon acquired immune haemolytic anaemia typically affecting children and young adults. It is often precipitated by a viral infection. The implicated autoantibody is a biphasic IgG complement-binding antibody that binds to red cells at cooler body temperatures in the peripheries but activates complement on warming centrally. This is the basis of the Donath–Landsteiner test where donor red cells are only lysed when incubated with patient serum at 18°C then at 37°C, in the presence of complement; if the dual phases are not undertaken or complement is not available then red cell lysis is not seen. This antibody is unusual for an IgG antibody in that it is able to cause red cell agglutination. The antibody- and complement-coated red cells are particularly attractive to neutrophils and monocytes and erythrophagocytosis is the classic

Haematology: From the Image to the Diagnosis, First Edition. Mike Leach and Barbara J. Bain.
© 2022 John Wiley & Sons Ltd. Published 2022 by John Wiley & Sons Ltd.

consequence. If this diagnosis is being considered, it is important to search the blood film looking for this phenomenon. Treatment is largely supportive, sometimes requiring blood transfusion, but the condition is often self-limiting after a period of 7–14 days.

MCQ

Paroxysmal cold haemoglobinuria:

1 Can be caused by syphilis
2 Is associated with intravascular haemolysis
3 Is caused by an antibody directed at the P antigen
4 Is caused by an IgG antibody so that IgG is usually detected when a direct antiglobulin tests is done
5 Occurs most often in children

For answers and discussion, see page 206.

63   Transient abnormal myelopoiesis

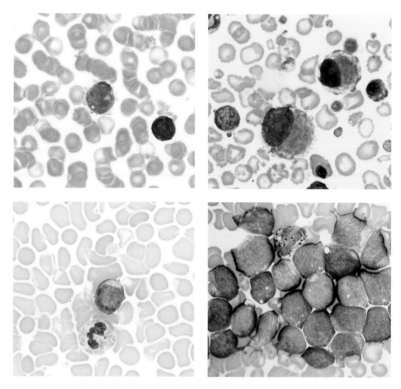

A significant proportion of neonates with Down syndrome suffer from transient abnormal myelopoiesis (TAM), also known as transient leukaemia of Down syndrome.

The top left image is from a neonate with known Down syndrome (all images ×100 objective).
His FBC showed Hb 167 g/l, WBC 30.8 × 10^9/l and platelet count 39 × 10^9/l. A blood film showed
35% blast cells, some with cytoplasmic protrusions, suggesting they were of megakaryocyte lineage
(image) and this was confirmed by immunophenotyping. In addition, there were some morphologically normal platelets and other irregular, agranular fragments of megakaryocyte cytoplasm.
Spontaneous remission occurred but during infancy the baby developed myelodysplastic features
and subsequently acute megakaryoblastic leukaemia.

The top right image is from a premature neonate (31 weeks' gestation) with dysmorphic features, hepatosplenomegaly and unexpected hydrops fetalis. The direct antiglobulin test was negative. There was impaired liver function, hypoalbuminaemia and abnormal coagulation. The total
nucleated cell count was 132 × 10^9/l, Hb 95 g/l and platelet count 447 × 10^9/l. The blood film
showed marked anisocytosis, poikilocytosis, nucleated red blood cells and blast cells, some with
cytoplasmic blebs. In addition there were numerous micromegakaryocytes, some fully mature
with dense chromatin and granular cytoplasm (top right in the image) and others with less chromatin condensation (bottom left in the image). The blood film features led to the suspicion of
Down syndrome and this was confirmed by demonstration of trisomy 21. Spontaneous remission
occurred. With cytological features such as these there is no need for immunophenotyping for
confirmation.

Haematology: From the Image to the Diagnosis, First Edition. Mike Leach and Barbara J. Bain.
© 2022 John Wiley & Sons Ltd. Published 2022 by John Wiley & Sons Ltd.

The bottom left image is from a baby with known Down syndrome. The FBC showed Hb 232 g/l, MCV 110 fl, WBC 11.5×10^9/l and platelet count 198×10^9/l. The blood film showed 17% blast cells and hypogranular platelets. The blast cells did not have any distinctive features but were confirmed as megakaryoblasts on immunophenotyping. They expressed CD42a, CD61 and CD117. A third of them were CD34-positive and some expressed CD7, CD33, CD71 and HLA-DR. Spontaneous remission occurred.

The bottom right image is from a baby born with hydrops fetalis and an Hb of 70 g/l. The white cell count was very high and there was severe thrombocytopenia. The blood film showed 88% blast cells. An unusual feature was that there was some differentiation to basophils (image). The blast cells showed expression of CD7, CD13, CD33, CD34, CD38, CD105 and CD117 and weak expression of CD42a, CD61 and myeloperoxidase. The baby died at 72 hours of age.

These four babies show the spectrum of features of TAM, ranging from an asymptomatic condition, which may have preservation of the Hb and the platelet count, to a life-threatening condition in which there may be hydrops fetalis, liver failure and disseminated intravascular coagulation. Blast cells are usually megakaryoblasts but there can also be prominent primitive erythroid cells and basophil precursors.

MCQ

Transient abnormal myelopoiesis of Down syndrome:

1 Can occur in mosaic Down syndrome
2 Generally requires chemotherapy to lower the white cell count
3 Is associated with a *GATA1* mutation
4 On cytogenetic analysis, shows only trisomy 21
5 Represents a leukaemoid reaction

For answers and discussion, see page 206.

64 Systemic lupus erythematosus

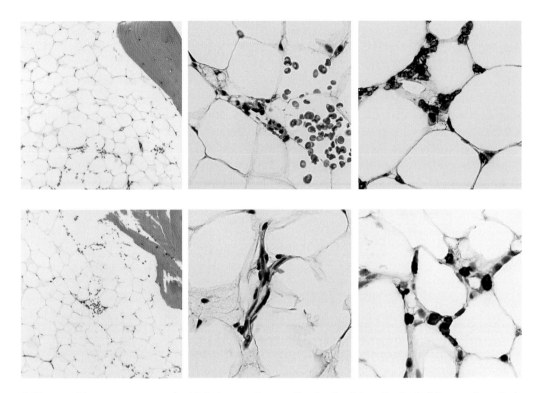

A 55-year-old woman presented with fatigue and generalised arthralgias. She had a history of psoriasis but the symmetrical distribution of pain and the involvement of larger joints were not typical of psoriatic arthropathy. The full blood count showed Hb 84 g/l, WBC 1.1×10^9/l, neutrophils 0.8×10^9/l and platelets 20×10^9/l. The ESR was 52 mm in 1 h but CRP was only mildly elevated at 25 mg/l on a background of a polyclonal increase in immunoglobulins. The direct Coombs test was positive for IgG only. Renal function was preserved with serum creatinine 47 µmol/l but the urine protein/creatinine ratio was elevated at 86 mg/mmol creatinine (NR <20). Liver enzyme levels were normal but the serum albumin was reduced at 30 g/l. The antinuclear antibody titre was 1/2560, rheumatoid factor was negative and anti-DNA antibody levels were markedly elevated at >379 iu/ml (NR <10). The blood film showed no abnormal cells. A bone marrow aspirate was profoundly hypocellular and trephine biopsy sections showed extreme hypocellularity (<5%) with a severe depletion of all marrow elements and no abnormal infiltrate (images, H&E, left ×10 objective and centre ×50). There were only small numbers of residual erythroid precursors (top right image, immunoperoxidase for glycophorin ×50) and normal T lymphocytes (bottom right image, immunoperoxidase for CD3 ×50). The features were of aplastic anaemia in the context of a new diagnosis of systemic lupus erythematosus.

Systemic lupus erythematosus is a serious autoimmune disorder where the target of autologous cytotoxic T cells appears to be cellular DNA. It has protean manifestations affecting many organs (skin, kidneys, joints, brain and blood vessels) and haematological complications are not unusual. An interesting laboratory phenomenon seen in SLE is that polyclonal immunoglobulins are often elevated with an associated high ESR but CRP levels are often only mildly elevated. This contrasts with many other active connective tissue disorders.

Haematology: From the Image to the Diagnosis, First Edition. Mike Leach and Barbara J. Bain.
© 2022 John Wiley & Sons Ltd. Published 2022 by John Wiley & Sons Ltd.

MCQ

Haematological manifestations of systemic lupus erythematosus (SLE) include:

1 Autoimmune neutropenia
2 Autoimmune thrombocytopenia ('ITP')
3 Cold haemagglutinin disease
4 Evans syndrome
5 Pure red cell aplasia

For answers and discussion, see page 206.

65 Granular blast cells in acute lymphoblastic leukaemia

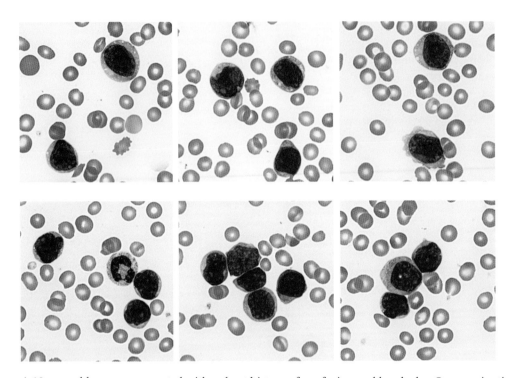

A 19-year-old woman presented with a short history of confusion and headache. On examination, her Glasgow Coma Scale score was 9 (normal 15) and she had a partial left third cranial nerve palsy. Her conscious level continued to decline and within hours she needed intubation and ventilation. The full blood count showed Hb 72 g/l, WBC 216 × 10⁹/l and platelets 68 × 10⁹/l. The coagulation profile showed PT 18 s, APTT 28 s, fibrinogen 1.1 g/l and D dimer 7440 ng/ml (NR <500). The blood film showed a large population of blast cells, which were medium size to large with prominent nucleoli. A proportion of these showed fine cytoplasmic granules (granular blasts shown in each image) (all images ×100 objective) but there was no significant neutrophil dysplasia. An acute myeloid leukaemia was suspected with an associated coagulopathy due to disseminated intravascular coagulation (DIC), though the morphology was not in keeping with acute promyelocytic leukaemia. An urgent CT of the brain showed multiple foci of intracerebral haemorrhage with intraventricular bleeding and features of raised intracranial pressure (shown below).

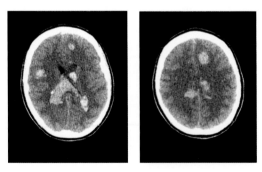

Haematology: From the Image to the Diagnosis, First Edition. Mike Leach and Barbara J. Bain.
© 2022 John Wiley & Sons Ltd. Published 2022 by John Wiley & Sons Ltd.

Flow cytometric studies on peripheral blood showed all the blasts to express weak CD45, CD19, TdT, HLA-DR, CD79a and CD15. No other myeloid antigens were expressed; cytoplasmic MPO, CD34, CD117 and CD10 were all negative. The phenotype is that of a pro-B ALL; the aberrant expression of CD15 often correlates with a *KMT2A* translocation and this was confirmed, karyo-typic analysis showing 47,XX,+X,t(4;11)(q21;q23.3) in 9 out of 10 cells examined.

For the morphologist, there are a number of features which, in assessing an acute leukaemia, can support a diagnosis of AML. The presence of cytoplasmic granules, Auer rods, monocyte precursors and dysplasia in erythroid, myeloid and megakaryocyte lineages are all regular features of AML. Auer rods, of course, are only seen in myeloid lineage and mixed phenotype neoplasms and cytoplasmic granules, when carefully sought, are usually indicative of AML or MDS with excess blasts. There are reports, however, of cytoplasmic granulation in a subset of ALL cases. This is more often seen in childhood cases (only 2–7%) and is rare in adults (Pitman and Huang 2007). These blasts stain negatively for myeloperoxidase and with Sudan black B. They do not express MPO by flow cytometry. Ultrastructural studies indicate that these inclusions are the result of abnormal organelle formation and are quite different from the typical MPO-positive granules seen in cells of myeloid lineage. Flow cytometric studies are key in defining cell lineage and excluding mixed phenotype acute leukaemia (MPAL) in these patients.

Furthermore, this patient had features of clinical and laboratory DIC at presentation with catastrophic intracerebral bleeding. Again, DIC is typically a feature of AML, with acute promyelocytic leukaemia being the usual culprit. However, DIC does occur in ALL and may be triggered or exacerbated by induction chemotherapy (Sarris *et al.* 1996). This patient was managed with full blood product support in an attempt to stabilise the situation but sadly she deteriorated and died before induction chemotherapy could be instituted.

References

Pitman SD and Huang Q (2007) Granular acute lymphoblastic leukemia: A case report and literature review. *Am J Hematol*, **82**, 834–837.
Sarris A, Cortes J, Kantarjian H, Pierce S, Smith T, Keating M *et al.* (1996) Disseminated intravascular coagulation in adult acute lymphoblastic leukaemia: frequent complications with fibrinogen levels less than 100 mg/dl. *Leuk Lymphoma*, **21**, 85–92.

MCQ

Rearrangement of *KMT2A*:

1 Can be associated with lineage switch at relapse, from acute lymphoblastic leukaemia (ALL) to acute monoblastic leukaemia (AMoL) or mixed phenotype acute leukaemia (MPAL)
2 Can be therapy-related
3 Generally has a good prognosis
4 In ALL, is usually associated with a common ALL immunophenotype
5 Is occasionally found in congenital ALL

For answers and discussion, see page 206.

66 Chronic myelomonocytic leukaemia

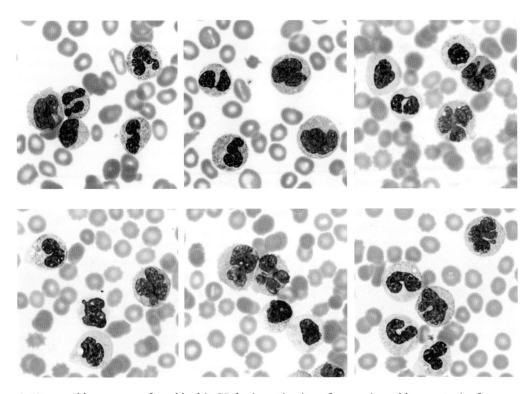

A 69-year-old man was referred by his GP for investigation of anaemia and leucocytosis after pre-senting with fatigue, sweats and weight loss. On examination he was pale and thin with some abdominal distension and an easily palpable spleen. His full blood count showed Hb 67 g/l, MCV 114 fl, WBC 64.5 × 10⁹/l, neutrophils 40 × 10⁹/l, monocytes 22 × 10⁹/l and platelets 176 × 10⁹/l. His blood film confirmed neutrophilia and monocytosis. The neutrophils were variably granulated (hypogranular forms, top right, bottom left and centre images) (all images ×100 objective) and showed frequent abnormal nuclear segmentation (all images). The monocytes were either mature (top right and bottom) or immature (top left, bottom centre and right) but a small population of promonocytes was evident (top centre). The morphological diagnosis is chronic myelomonocytic leukaemia (CMML). A bone marrow aspirate showed 8% promonocytes yielding a more specific diagnosis of CMML with excess blasts 1 (CMML EB1). The karyotype was 47,XY,+21 and next generation sequencing identified pathological mutations: *SRSF2* c.284C>A, *ASXL1* C.2324del and *TET2* c.4210C>T.

Chronic myelomonocytic leukaemia is a disease belonging to the subgroup of myelodysplastic/myeloproliferative neoplasms within the WHO classification. As the name implies it has both pro-liferative (neutrophilia, monocytosis and sometimes thrombocytosis, particularly if *JAK2* is mutated) and dysplastic features (erythroid and neutrophil dysplasia). Cytogenetic studies in this case confirmed a clonal disorder but a significant proportion of cases have a normal karyotype. The diagnosis is usually clear but patients with deep-seated chronic bacterial infections, such as empyema, hepatic abscess or diverticular abscess, can develop similar blood counts though

Haematology: From the Image to the Diagnosis, First Edition. Mike Leach and Barbara J. Bain.
© 2022 John Wiley & Sons Ltd. Published 2022 by John Wiley & Sons Ltd.

typically without the dysplastic features shown here. Next generation sequencing can aid in the diagnosis of CMML in patients with low-level persistent monocytosis, as can flow cytometry (see below) where the proportions of classical CD14+CD16− (Q4), intermediate CD14+CD16+/− (Q2) and non-classical monocytes CD14−CD16+ (Q1) are significantly disturbed. Note the change in distribution of each population below in CMML (left image) where non-classical monocytes are depleted and the classical population is increased, compared with a normal control (right image).

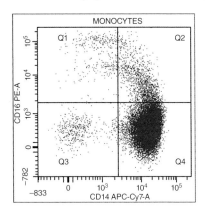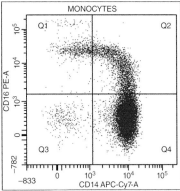

Next generation sequencing can also give prognostic information: *TET2* mutations are common and some are prognostically favourable (Coltro et *al.* 2020), whilst an increasing number of mutations are prognostically adverse. *ASXL1* mutations may indicate a more progressive disease course and this was observed in the patient described here with early evolution to acute monocytic leukaemia that proved refractory to therapy.

Reference

Coltro G, Mangaonkar AA, Lasho TL, Finke CM, Pophali P, Carr R *et al.* (2020) Clinical, molecular, and prognostic correlates of number, type, and functional localization of *TET2* mutations in chronic myelomonocytic leukemia (CMML) – a study of 1084 patients. *Leukemia*, **34**, 1407–1421.

MCQ

Chronic myelomonocytic leukaemia:

1 By definition, in the WHO classification, cannot be therapy-related
2 Can have an associated proliferation of plasmacytoid dendritic cells
3 Has an abnormal karyotype in 20–40% of patients
4 Is associated with an increase in haemoglobin F
5 Shows *BCR-ABL1* in a minority of patients

For answers and discussion, see page 206.

67   Burkitt lymphoma/leukaemia

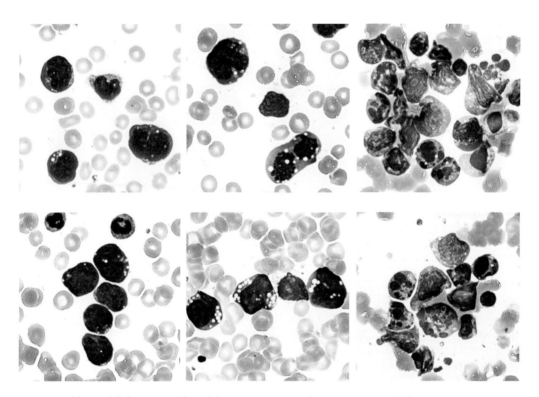

A 4-year-old Scottish boy was referred for investigation of acute-onset right facial swelling, sweats and lethargy. On examination he was pale and unwell with swelling over the right maxilla and mandible; there was no lymphadenopathy or organomegaly. His automated full blood count showed Hb 101 g/l, WBC 43 × 10^9/l, neutrophils 14 × 10^9/l, lymphocytes 15.4 × 10^9/l, monocytes 12.9 × 10^9/l and platelets 146 × 10^9/l. His blood film (left images ×100 objective) showed large pleomorphic lymphoid cells with nucleoli and intensely basophilic cytoplasm with vacuoles. These features are suggestive of Burkitt leukaemia/lymphoma which would be in keeping with the clinical presentation. Flow cytometric studies showed the large cells to have a CD19+, CD20+, FMC7+, CD79b+, CD10+ and surface kappa+ immunophenotype, which is compatible with this diagnosis. This was confirmed by FISH studies, which showed an IGH/*MYC* rearrangement, subsequently confirmed to be due to t(8;14)(q24;q32). Serum LDH was massively elevated at 25 171 iu/l (NR for age 170–380). Whole body MRI showed an abnormal signal and soft tissue oedema within the right maxilla and mandible; there was no lymphadenopathy but the spleen was enlarged and both kidneys were diffusely enlarged with an abnormal parenchymal signal. Renal function, however, was preserved.

A second patient, an 11-year-old boy, also Scottish, presented with a prolonged epistaxis. His full blood count showed Hb 111 g/l, WBC 40.5 × 10^9/l and platelets 31 × 10^9/l. His blood film showed abnormal vacuolated lymphoid cells but a bone marrow aspirate specimen was sent for examination (centre images ×100). This showed a population of medium to large malignant lymphoid cells, with characteristics very similar to those seen in patient 1. Note the malignant cell in mitosis in the top centre image. Again, Burkitt leukaemia/lymphoma seemed a likely diagnosis and t(8;14) (q24;q32) was again identified on cytogenetic analysis. In addition, some cells showed that the short arm of the derivative chromosome 14 was involved in an unbalanced translocation with the long arm of chromosome 1, resulting in trisomy for the long arm of chromosome 1. Structural rearrangements of the long arm of chromosome 1, resulting in a partial trisomy of 1q, are found in 30% of Burkitt lymphoma cases.

A third patient, a 27-year-old woman without a prior medical history, presented with pallor fatigue and night sweats. No additional features were apparent on examination but her full blood count showed Hb 91 g/l, WBC 10.4×10^9/l, neutrophils 2.8×10^9/l, lymphocytes 6.3×10^9/l and platelets 118×10^9/l. Her blood film also showed abnormal large lymphoid cells with vacuolated cytoplasm. Her bone marrow aspirate was highly abnormal, being populated by large numbers of largely karyorrhectic and degenerate lymphoid cells with little residual normal haemopoiesis (right images, facing page ×100). Flow cytometric immunophenotyping was able to confirm a mature B-cell neoplasm, despite the limitations, with a CD10+ pan-B phenotype in keeping with Burkitt lymphoma. This was confirmed by a karyotype showing t(8;14)(q24;q32). Further testing showed her to be human immunodeficiency virus (HIV) positive with a CD4 count of 10 cells/ mm^3 (NR 540–1660).

Burkitt lymphoma or leukaemia presents the ultimate haematological emergency. This high-grade mature B-cell neoplasm has an acute onset; the blood and bone marrow, lymph nodes and spleen are often involved. The disease has an affinity for tissues of the gastrointestinal tract but can involve almost any extranodal site including the CNS. The disease is frequently sporadic but also presents as an immunodeficiency-related lymphoma, as described in the third patient in this series. The disease is highly sensitive to chemotherapy and cure rates are high, even in those with advanced stage disease at presentation, but careful early management is key. The gravity of the tumour lysis syndrome due to massive cell kill presents its own specific clinical challenges but the use of copious hydration, uricolytic agents, careful management of electrolyte imbalance and renal support including haemofiltration or even haemodialysis are essential components if a successful outcome is to be achieved.

MCQ

Burkitt lymphoma/leukaemia:

1 Can involve the breasts and ovaries
2 Has a proliferation fraction approaching 100%
3 Is consistently associated with t(8;14)(q24;q32)
4 Is of marginal zone origin
5 Occurs in endemic, sporadic and immunodeficiency-related forms

For answers and discussion, see page 206.

68 Gaucher disease

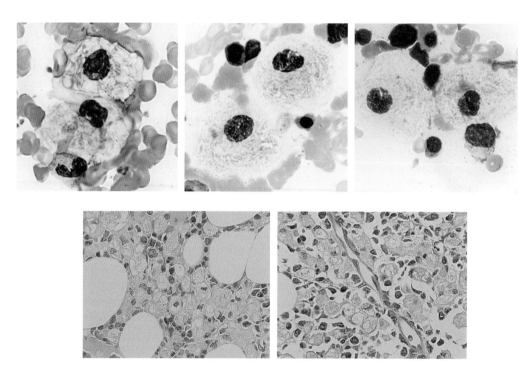

A 57-year-old woman was referred between haematologists in two separate health boards after she relocated her family home. She had a working diagnosis of immune thrombocytopenia but the thrombocytopenia was moderate and had not required therapy.

The full blood count now showed Hb 121 g/l, WBC 4.6×10^9/l, neutrophils 3.2×10^9/l and platelets 30×10^9/l. A serum ferritin was elevated at over 2000 µg/l. Renal and liver function tests were normal. On clinical assessment, the patient was noted to have significant splenomegaly and this was confirmed on radiological imaging. The spleen was 24 cm in long axis and showed a number of filling defects. A lymphoma was suspected so a bone marrow aspiration and trephine biopsy were performed. The aspirate was cellular, but prominent macrophages with an expanded cytoplasm with a texture resembling crushed tissue paper or cotton wool were present throughout (top images ×100 objective). The trephine biopsy showed large numbers of the same cells which were present throughout the marrow interstitium (bottom images ×50). The morphological features were highly suggestive of Gaucher disease.

Gaucher disease is an autosomal recessive inherited disorder due to mutations in the *GBA* (beta-glucosidase) gene, which is characterised by lysosomal β glucocerebrosidase deficiency; this enzyme is responsible for the breakdown of glucocerebroside, which is a constituent of cell membranes. This accumulates and is phagocytosed by macrophages but cannot be broken down. Affected macrophages show expansion of the cytoplasm and features of activation with corresponding elevations of immunoglobulins and serum ferritin. They accumulate in liver, spleen, bones and bone marrow, generating cytopenias due to hypersplenism and marrow compromise. Splenic involvement is typically diffuse but focal nodular infiltrates occur in some patients and this

Haematology: From the Image to the Diagnosis, First Edition. Mike Leach and Barbara J. Bain.
© 2022 John Wiley & Sons Ltd. Published 2022 by John Wiley & Sons Ltd.

may be apparent on imaging. Skeletal involvement is common, with the long bones and vertebrae being particularly affected; osteopenia, osteonecrosis, lytic lesions/endosteal scalloping or pathological fractures may be apparent on plain X-ray. The most common milder type I non-neuronopathic form often shows some residual enzyme activity and is not infrequently diagnosed in adults. The type II and III forms are diagnosed in children and young adults and have serious neurological sequelae.

MCQ

Gaucher disease:

1 Can cause osteolytic bone lesions
2 Is associated with an increased incidence of multiple myeloma and lymphoplasmacytic lymphoma
3 Is associated with increased serum ferritin, indicative of iron overload
4 Has a high prevalence in Ashkenazi Jews
5 Requires a biopsy for diagnosis

For answers and discussion, see page 206.

69   Myelodysplastic syndrome with haemophagocytosis

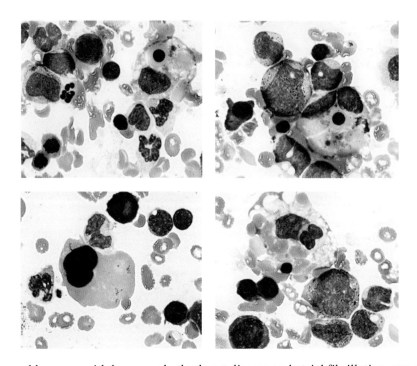

An 83-year-old woman with known valvular heart disease and atrial fibrillation was admitted after suffering a fall at home that had led to extensive bruising. The full blood count showed Hb 65 g/l, MCV 96 fl, WBC 6.6 × 10^9/l, neutrophils 4.7 × 10^9/l and platelets 11 × 10^9/l. Her blood film showed a small number of circulating myeloblasts. The bone marrow aspirate was abnormal, showing trilineage dysplasia and an excess of myeloblasts at 8% of all nucleated cells. In addition, there was prominent haemophagocytosis with macrophages displaying ingested red cells, red cell precursors and nuclear debris (top left and right, bottom right images). Note the bizarre massive late normoblast with Pappenheimer bodies (bottom left) (all images ×100 objective). Metaphase cytogenetic preparations showed a highly complex karyotype 47,XX,−3,−5,del(17)(p11.2),−20,−20,−22 and numerous other abnormalities. The patient was managed with supportive therapy.

   The diagnosis here is clearly of a myelodysplastic syndrome requiring transfusion support with a complex karyotype and a poor prognosis. The haemophagocytosis is a curiosity and should not detract from the primary diagnosis. In the myelodysplastic syndromes there is ineffective haemopoiesis; the increased rate of death of precursor cells leads to increased phagocytic activity. In this patient, not only is there cell debris within the macrophages but also intact cells. One might postulate that it results from an alteration in the surface membrane of defective haemopoietic cells, attracting monocyte/macrophage activity and so likely contributing to the ineffective haemopoiesis and resultant cytopenias. This should not be misinterpreted as a haemophagocytic syndrome, which is characterised by systemic decline, fever, cytopenias, hyperferritinaemia, hypertriglyceridaemia and organomegaly. Of these features only cytopenias were present in this

Haematology: From the Image to the Diagnosis, First Edition. Mike Leach and Barbara J. Bain.
© 2022 John Wiley & Sons Ltd. Published 2022 by John Wiley & Sons Ltd.

patient and these can be explained by the serious marrow disorder. A haemophagocytic syndrome is a life-threatening condition with specific triggers, normally either infective or neoplastic when encountered in the adult population. When seen in children and infants a genetic predisposition is often present (see Theme 90).

MCQ

In the myelodysplastic syndromes an adverse prognosis is associated with:

1 A complex karyotype
2 Del(5q)
3 Del(20q)
4 Monosomy 7
5 −Y

For answers and discussion, see page 206.

70 Primary oxalosis

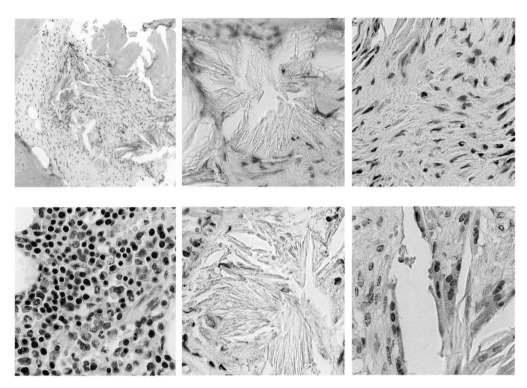

A 55-year-old woman with end-stage renal failure on haemodialysis was referred on account of anaemia and thrombocytopenia. She was receiving full-dose erythropoietin replacement. Her full blood count showed Hb 68 g/l, WBC 3.3×10^9/l, neutrophils 2×10^9/l and platelets 95×10^9/l. The blood film showed teardrop poikilocytes but no other specific features. Bone marrow was not aspirable but the bone marrow trephine biopsy sections were informative. There was extensive collagen fibrosis throughout the marrow space and large fractured crystals were evident; crystals were deposited in the typical fan-shaped formation (top left image ×10 objective, centre images ×50). Some small pockets of normal haemopoiesis remained (bottom left image ×50) but note the dense collagenous fibrosis in other areas (right images ×50) adjacent to the crystal deposition.

The patient had a diagnosis of type 1 primary hyperoxaluria. This rare autosomal recessive disorder of oxalate metabolism leads to high serum and urinary oxalate levels, predisposing to kidney stones, nephrocalcinosis and progressive renal failure. Systemic deposition of calcium oxalate can also occur in the heart, bone, blood vessels, joints and eyes. Deposition of oxalate in the bone marrow leads to an inflammatory reaction with resultant progressive fibrosis and anaemia that is resistant to erythropoietin. Trephine biopsy sections can also show a granulomatous response to the oxalate crystals, together with increased bone remodelling with thickened trabeculae. Note the crystals are far too large to be scavenged by macrophages as in some other metabolic disorders. Here the oxalate crystals precipitate in the bone marrow interstitium and in multiple other tissues. The only potential curative therapy is a combined liver and renal transplant.

Haematology: From the Image to the Diagnosis, First Edition. Mike Leach and Barbara J. Bain.
© 2022 John Wiley & Sons Ltd. Published 2022 by John Wiley & Sons Ltd.

MCQ

Haematological features of oxalosis can include:

1 A leucoerythroblastic blood film
2 Oxalate crystals, osteoblasts, osteoclasts and multinucleated giant cells in bone marrow aspirates
3 Pancytopenia
4 Susceptibility to myeloid neoplasms
5 Thrombocytopenia

For answers and discussion, see page 206.

71 Acute myeloid leukaemia with inv(3)(q21.3q26.2)

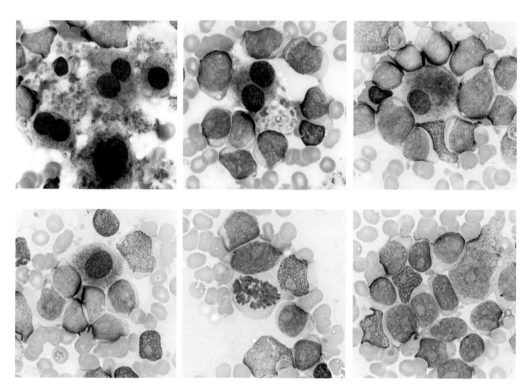

A 25-year-old man presented with fatigue and bruising. His full blood count showed Hb 70 g/l, MCV 105 fl, WBC 0.5×10^9/l, neutrophils 0.1×10^9/l and platelets 200×10^9/l. His blood film (not illustrated) showed small numbers of myeloblasts. The bone marrow aspirate was hypercellular with 60% myeloblasts (CD34+, CD117+, CD41−, CD61−) showing prominent nucleoli and minimal differentiation (top left) (all images ×100 objective). Notably, there was also a large population of abnormal megakaryocytes, including micromegakaryocytes, some binucleated or with non-lobated or bilobed nuclei, many of which were actively shedding platelets (top and bottom left). Note the myeloblast population showing no differentiation and prominent nucleoli. A micromegakaryocyte should have a non-lobated nucleus and be of a similar size to a promyelocyte (bottom left image is typical). Metaphase cytogenetic analysis showed inv(3)(q21.3q26.2). The patient sadly failed multiple lines of induction chemotherapy and each phase of chemotherapy-related cytopenia was followed by a rapid early rebound (10 days) in the platelet count. Normally platelet recovery suggests clearance of an acute leukaemia following induction chemotherapy but in this context it is a sinister sign as the 'recovering' platelets are a manifestation of persistence of abnormal clonal megakaryocytes. Unusually in acute myeloid leukaemia, cases with inv(3) or t(3;3), often show preservation of the platelet count at presentation (as in this patient) or even an increased platelet count.

Inversion (3)(q21.3q26.2) and t(3;3)(q21.3;q26.2) occur in only 1–2% of cases of myelodysplastic syndrome and AML. Both rearrangements result in an abnormal juxtaposition of *MECOM* (previously known as *EVI1*) at 3q26.2 to *GATA2* (a transcription factor encoding gene) at 3q21.3. Even when *de novo*, these leukaemias carry a very poor prognosis.

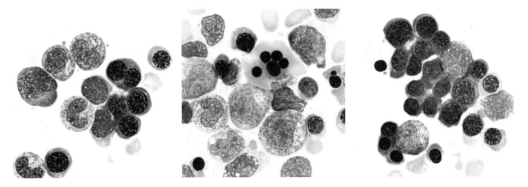

Curiously, some cases also show monosomy 7 and for reasons as yet unexplained these patients often develop diabetes insipidus. These patients can also present with MDS, including MDS with excess blasts (MDS-EB), as well as acute leukaemia. The images above are from such a patient with MDS-EB1. Note the predominant erythroid dysplasia with clusters of mainly basophilic normo-blasts which appear to be arrested at this stage of maturation (right image). He presented with very problematic diabetes insipidus. This additional complication adds significantly to the burden of management of patients through induction chemotherapy. This cytogenetic abnormality, which carries a poor prognosis, is disease-defining, so an intensive approach to treatment in fit patients, even those with MDS, is justified.

MCQ

The inv(3)(q21.3q26.2) and t(3;3)(q21.3;q26.2) cytogenetic abnormalities:

1 Are associated with an appreciably better prognosis in MDS than in AML
2 Can occur in myeloid blast crisis of *BCR-ABL1*-positive chronic myeloid leukaemia
3 Can occur in therapy-related AML
4 Lead to formation of a fusion gene that is responsible for leukaemogenesis
5 Permit a diagnosis of MDS in a cytopenic patient without significant dysplasia

For answers and discussion, see page 206.

72   Autoimmune haemolytic anaemia

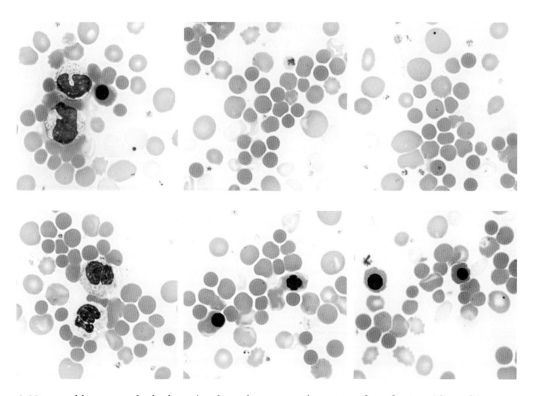

A 38-year-old woman who had previously undergone a splenectomy for refractory idiopathic warm autoimmune haemolytic anaemia (AIHA) with an ongoing transfusion requirement, re-presented with profound fatigue and jaundice. Her full blood count showed Hb 62 g/l, WBC 10.9 × 10⁹/l and platelets 461 × 10⁹/l with reticulocyte count 503 × 10⁹/l (NR 50–100). The direct Coombs test was positive for IgG only. Serum ferritin was 1508 μg/l with a transferrin saturation of 76% (NR 25–50). Serum bilirubin was 116 μmol/l, AST 282 u/l, ALT 69 u/l, albumin 30 g/l and LDH 5571 iu/l. Haptoglobin was absent. The blood film was leucoerythroblastic with prominent nucleated red cells, polychromasia and spherocytes together with Pappenheimer bodies and Howell–Jolly bodies (all images ×100 objective). Note the dysplastic nucleus in the late normoblast (bottom centre), which has resulted from marrow stress due to the fulminant haemolysis. Note also that the polychromatic macrocytes, representing reticulocytes (all images), have not yet become spherocytic.

A diagnosis of AIHA should always prompt investigation for an underlying cause. A minority of cases are idiopathic but the majority of patients will have an associated disorder, either autoimmune or neoplastic. The clinician should undertake a search for B-cell lymphoproliferative disorders such as chronic lymphocytic leukaemia, small lymphocytic lymphoma and splenic marginal zone lymphoma. Even monoclonal B lymphocytosis, which may not be apparent from the full blood count, can underlie AIHA. Importantly, the autoantibody is polyclonal in nature and not directly derived from the B-cell clone; the autoantibody is thought to result from immune dysregulation that accompanies these diseases. T-cell lymphoproliferative disorders can also be responsible, with angioimmunoblastic T-cell lymphoma and large granular lymphocytic leukaemia being

Haematology: From the Image to the Diagnosis, First Edition. Mike Leach and Barbara J. Bain.
© 2022 John Wiley & Sons Ltd. Published 2022 by John Wiley & Sons Ltd.

most often implicated. Autoimmune diseases such as systemic lupus erythematosus (which may precede the diagnosis), solid tumours, viral infections and various medications are also associated (Jager *et al.* 2020). Chemotherapeutic agents such as fludarabine may be implicated due to depletion of T regulatory cells.

Reference

Jager U, Barcellini W, Broome CM, Gertz MA, Hill A, Hill QA *et al.* (2020) Diagnosis and treatment of autoimmune haemolytic anemia in adults: Recommendations from the First International Consensus Meeting. *Blood Rev*, **41**, 100648. doi: 10.1016/j.blre.2019.100648.

MCQ

Warm autoimmune haemolytic anaemia:

1 Can result from inherited immunodeficiency
2 Causes only extravascular haemolysis
3 Has a recognised association with levodopa therapy
4 Is more common in women than men
5 Is sometimes a complication of allogeneic haemopoietic stem cell transplantation

For answers and discussion, see page 206.

73 Chronic eosinophilic leukaemia with *FIP1L1-PDGFRA* fusion

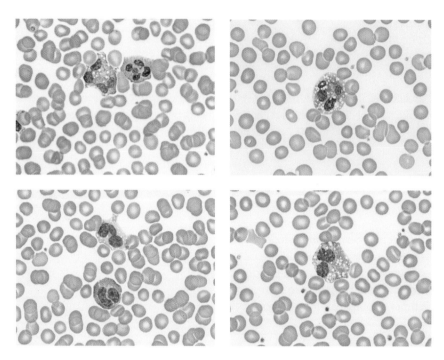

A 56-year-old man presented with an intractable cough of 2 years' duration. He had suffered significant weight loss in the previous 2 years, night sweats and episodic diarrhoea. Physical examination was normal. His WBC, Hb and platelet count were normal but the eosinophil count was 1.85×10^9/l. Respiratory function tests were normal. Immunoglobulin E was normal and investigation for parasitic infection and autoimmunity was negative. CT of the chest showed thickening of intrapulmonary airways but no lymphadenopathy. CT of the abdomen showed hepatosplenomegaly. A haematological neoplasm was suspected.

Examination of the blood film (all images ×100 objective) showed some cytologically normal eosinophils but many were vacuolated and hypogranular and some had hypersegmented nuclei. There were no blast cells, eosinophil precursors or lymphoma cells. A bone marrow aspirate showed increased eosinophils and precursors together with increased mast cells but without any increase of blast cells. Cytogenetic analysis was normal but nested PCR and FISH analysis showed the presence of *FIP1L1-PDGFRA*. A diagnosis of myeloid neoplasm with *PDGFRA* rearrangement was made.

When investigating chronic eosinophilia it is important to consider connective tissue disorders, helminth infection, neoplasia and allergy. Of the neoplastic disorders these may be solid tumours, with reactive eosinophilia (see Theme 23) or primary haematological diseases. Of the latter, the eosinophilia may be a component of an acute leukaemia (see Themes 26 and 43), of chronic myeloid leukaemia (see Theme 34), a part of a mast cell disorder or a part of a clonal proliferation due to specific groups of disease defined by characteristic genetic aberrations. Chronic eosinophilic leukaemias due to *PDGFRA* rearrangement, as described here, falls into this WHO-defined group. Also in this category are clonal eosinophilias associated with *PDGFRB* and *FGFR1* rearrangement plus the more recently defined entity of myeloid neoplasms associated with *PCM1-JAK2*. It is therefore clear that due to the multitude of causes, chronic eosinophilia needs careful sequential thoughtful investigation. In haematology practice our experience suggests that clinicians sometimes investigate eosinophilia in a slightly random opportunistic manner, with the rare clonal disorders sometimes being sought first. There is little doubt that the magnitude of eosinophilia is correlated with the likelihood of finding a specific cause (mild chronic non-progressive eosinophilia is relatively common) but all aspects of the clinical and laboratory investigation are important in this context.

Another patient, a 60-year-old female was referred for investigation of an isolated eosinophilia of $10 \times 10^9/l$. The rest of the full blood count was normal and the blood film showed unremarkable morphology. A detailed history and careful general examination did not show any light on the matter but whilst going through the electronic patient record it was noted that the patient had been referred to Gynaecology for investigation following an abnormal cervical smear cytology report. Further investigation confirmed a diagnosis of cervical carcinoma, one of the solid tumours which can have a propensity for driving a reactive eosinophilia.

MCQ

The most appropriate treatment for the first patient described is:

1 Corticosteroids
2 Imatinib
3 Midostaurin
4 Ruxolitinib
5 Vemurafenib

For answers and discussion, see page 206.

74 Leukaemic phase of follicular lymphoma

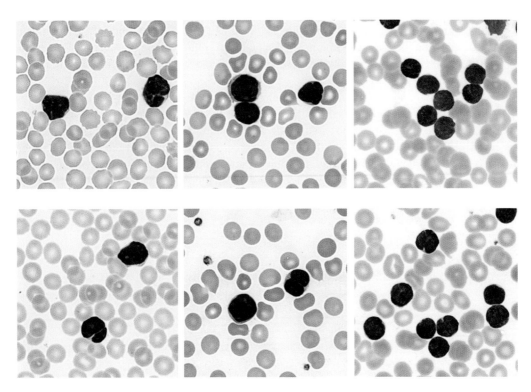

A 53-year-old man was referred for investigation of cervical lymphadenopathy. He had no past history of note and pathological nodes were palpable bilaterally in his neck. His full blood count showed Hb 143 g/l, WBC 24 × 10^9/l, neutrophils 3.6 × 10^9/l, lymphocytes 19.4 × 10^9/l and platelets 110 × 10^9/l. His blood film showed small to medium sized lymphoid cells with a very high nuclear/ cytoplasmic ratio, condensed chromatin and nuclear clefts (some traversing the whole width of the nucleus) (left images) (all images ×100 objective). Flow cytometry showed these cells to have a surface kappa-restricted, CD19+, CD20+, CD10+, CD79b+, HLA-DR+, FMC7+ immunopheno-type indicating a germinal centre-derived neoplasm. The morphology and immunophenotype suggested peripheral blood involvement by follicular lymphoma. This was confirmed on lymph node biopsy, which showed grade 1 histology.

A second patient, a 61-year-old woman, also presented with cervical lymphadenopathy. Her full blood count showed Hb 114 g/l, WBC 57 × 10^9/l, neutrophils 3.6 × 10^9/l, lymphocytes 52 × 10^9/l and platelets 161 × 10^9/l. Her blood film showed very similar features to those described above (centre images). Again, note the prominent deep nuclear clefts. Flow cytometry again showed a CD10+ mature B-cell neoplasm and a lymph node biopsy showed a grade 2 follicular lymphoma.

A third patient, a 65-year-old man, was referred from another haematologist for ongoing management of a presumptive new diagnosis of chronic lymphocytic leukaemia. The flow cytometry Matutes CLL score, however, was 1/5 and CD10 was not expressed. He had widespread lymphadenopathy and his automated full blood count showed Hb 118 g/l, WBC 267 × 10^9/l, neutrophils 8.1 × 10^9/l, lymphocytes 256 × 10^9/l, monocytes 2.9 × 10^9/l and platelets 191 × 10^9/l. His blood film

Haematology: From the Image to the Diagnosis, First Edition. Mike Leach and Barbara J. Bain.
© 2022 John Wiley & Sons Ltd. Published 2022 by John Wiley & Sons Ltd.

showed small compact lymphoid cells with condensed chromatin, multiple nuclear clefts and a fine rim of cytoplasm (right images, facing page). Although the high leucocyte count would be more in keeping with CLL, the lymphoid morphology was not. Repeat flow cytometry was performed with particular attention being paid to CD10 expression: the immunophenotype now shown was CD19+, CD20+, CD10+, CD79b+, HLA-DR+, FMC7+, CD23− and CD5− with weak surface lambda. The prior CD10 assessment was clearly now a false negative (as the same monoclonal antibody–fluorochrome combination had been used) and a diagnosis of follicular lymphoma was now supported. The bone marrow trephine biopsy sections showed diffuse involvement with paratrabecular accentuation by a low grade B-lymphoid neoplasm expressing CD20, CD10, BCL6, CD75 and BCL2. Analysis of 100 nuclei from peripheral blood using an IGH (14q32)/*BCL2* (18q21) probe showed a fusion signal in 95% of cells. Despite the very high white cell count, the diagnosis is leukaemic phase of follicular lymphoma.

Follicular lymphoma accounts for 20–30% of non-Hodgkin lymphoma diagnoses. It is generally an indolent disease affecting lymph nodes and spleen but it often shows an advanced stage at presentation. Other than involvement of the bone marrow and spleen, extranodal disease is unusual. A leukaemic phase is often seen in heavily pre-treated patients at the time of disease progression. A *de novo* leukaemic presentation, as described in the three cases reported here, is unusual and there are limited published data to address the issue. This is confounded by the fact that blood involvement is not captured as part of the FLIPI score and that a lymphocytosis (even with confirmed blood involvement) is not always apparent. There is evidence, however, that a leukaemic phase at presentation is associated with a higher tumour burden and an earlier time to first treatment (Al-nawakil *et al.* 2011, Beltran *et al.* 2013). There is as yet no additional immunophenotypic, cytogenetic or molecular abnormality identified that correlates with such disease behaviour.

References

Al-nawakil C, Kosmider O, Stern MH, Manie E, Bardet V, Leblond V *et al.* (2011) Leukemic phase of follicular lymphomas: an atypical presentation. *Leuk Lymphoma*, **52**, 1504–1508.

Beltran BE, Castillo JJ, Quiñones P, Morales D, Alva JC, Miranda RN *et al.* (2013) Follicular lymphoma with leukaemic phase at diagnosis: An aggressive disease. Report of seven cases and review of the literature. *Leuk Res*, **37**, 1116–1119.

MCQ

Follicular lymphoma:

1 Can be detected reliably by bone marrow aspiration and immunophenotyping when the bone marrow is infiltrated
2 Consistently shows a translocation involving *BCL2*
3 Is cytologically difficult to distinguish from chronic lymphocytic leukaemia
4 Is of germinal centre origin, as shown by expression of CD19 and CD20
5 Typically shows paratrabecular infiltration in the bone marrow

For answers and discussion, see page 206.

75 Megaloblastic anaemia

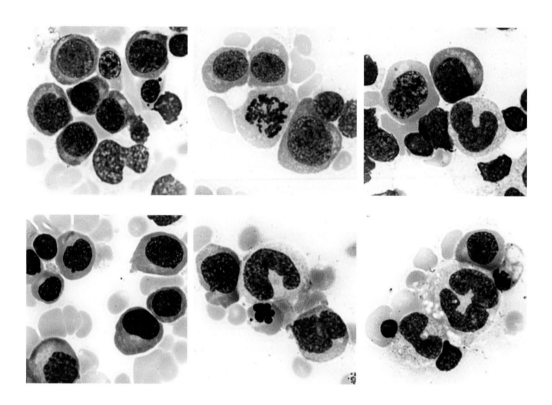

A 70-year-old woman presented with fatigue, anorexia, altered taste and weight loss. On examination she was noted to be pale and icteric. A full blood count showed Hb 42 g/l, MCV 120 fl, WBC 1.3×10^9/l, neutrophils 0.4×10^9/l and platelets 99×10^9/l. The reticulocyte count was 10×10^9/l. The blood film (not illustrated) showed marked anisopoikilocytosis, oval macrocytes, basophilic stippling and left shift. Serum ferritin was 549 µg/l, serum folate 2.1 µg/l (NR 3.1–20) and serum vitamin B12 104 ng/l (NR 200–883). The liver enzyme profile was normal but serum bilirubin was 55 µmol/l; LDH was 1994 iu/l. The haematinic levels were noted but in view of the systemic upset a bone marrow aspirate was taken. This showed classic features of a megaloblastic bone marrow. Note the erythroid hyperplasia and dysplasia with left shift, a mitotic figure (top centre), markedly delayed erythroid nuclear maturation (all images) and prominent giant metamyelocytes (top left, top right, bottom centre, bottom right) including a binucleated giant metamyelocyte (bottom right) (all images ×100 objective).

The diagnosis was megaloblastic anaemia likely due to vitamin B12 deficiency resulting from pernicious anaemia. Vitamin B12 and folic acid are essential for replication of DNA in bone marrow cells and all lineages are affected, resulting in a macrocytic pancytopenic presentation in advanced cases (as reported here). The failure of cell replication results in intramedullary cell death leading to release of free haemoglobin, causing jaundice and marked elevation in serum LDH.

Late presenting patients can show marked systemic symptoms with anorexia, weight loss and diarrhoea; this is thought to be due to abnormalities of gastrointestinal absorption as the gut epithelial cells are also affected by vitamin B12 deficiency. These features can distract from the true diagnosis for those not familiar with other systemic manifestations. Importantly, neurological manifestations with features of a peripheral neuropathy, ataxia and impaired proprioception due to dorsal column involvement can be disabling and may be the first clinical manifestation, even in the absence of anaemia, though an evolving macrocytosis is usually present.

This patient was treated with parenteral vitamin B12 and oral folate replacement and the reticulocyte count rose promptly to 155×10^9/l on day 5 of therapy. She made a full recovery and the full blood count returned to normal.

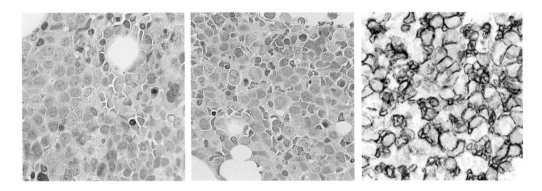

The images above (×50) are of bone marrow trephine biopsy sections from a patient with megaloblastic anaemia (H&E, left and centre; immunoperoxidase for glycophorin C, right). Note the apparent blastoid morphology of the sheets of early erythroid precursors; this could be mistaken for a high-grade neoplasm on H&E staining but the lineage of these large cells is apparent from immunohistochemistry. Even so, a pure erythroid leukaemia might be considered. Careful examination of the aspirate morphology is critical. This is another example of where reporting of the aspirate and trephine biopsy together is essential in making the correct diagnosis.

MCQ

Severe megaloblastic anaemia due to vitamin B12 or folate deficiency is characterised by:

1 Dysplastic haemopoiesis
2 Increased conjugated bilirubin
3 Increased macrophage iron
4 Increased reticulocyte count
5 Ineffective haemopoiesis

For answers and discussion, see page 206.

76   Reactive bone marrow and an abnormal PET scan

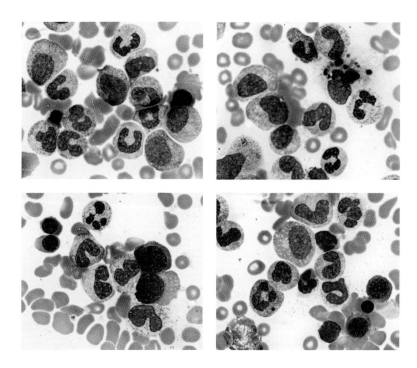

A 55-year-old man with a diagnosis of stage 3A diffuse large B-cell lymphoma was responding well to R-CHOP chemoimmunotherapy according to an interim CT scan after three cycles of treatment. He was, however, developing a progressive normocytic anaemia, requiring blood transfusion during cycles 3 and 4. In addition he had recurrent admissions for investigation of pyrexia, typically between day 12 and day 21 of each cycle, which had hitherto been unexplained. A further admission was necessary due to fever and anaemia following course 5. All bacterial cultures and viral studies were negative. He reported no specific symptoms apart from fatigue which had previously been attributed to his chemotherapy. The full blood count on this admission showed Hb 88 g/l, WBC 12.2 × 10^9/l, neutrophils 9.4 × 10^9/l and platelets 137 × 10^9/l. The ESR was significantly elevated at 98 mm in 1 h. A bone marrow aspirate showed no evidence of lymphoma. There was myeloid hyperplasia without morphological abnormality and also haemophagocytosis (top left image) but erythroid activity was reduced (all images ×100 objective). The clinical and laboratory features could not be explained by the known lymphoma, which was apparently responding well to treatment. An unrelated inflammatory disorder, partly abated by the corticosteroid treatment, was suspected. A PET/CT scan was requested and relevant images are shown on the facing page.

Haematology: From the Image to the Diagnosis, First Edition. Mike Leach and Barbara J. Bain.
© 2022 John Wiley & Sons Ltd. Published 2022 by John Wiley & Sons Ltd.

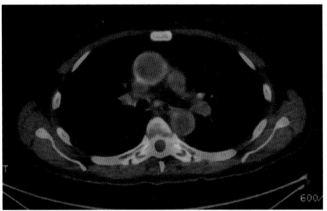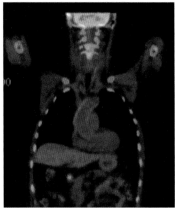

The PET/CT shows increased ^{18}F-fluorodeoxyglucose (FDG) uptake in the root and arch of the aorta, highly suggestive of a diagnosis of giant cell arteritis. There was no isotope uptake in the sites previously involved by lymphoma. The patient was treated with continuous corticosteroid therapy throughout the remainder of chemotherapy and for 6 months following completion. The full blood count and ESR normalised within 2 months. He remains free from both conditions 7 years later.

In this patient the image that led to the diagnosis was the PET scan with the bone marrow showing only non-specific changes of inflammation. In patients undergoing treatment for lymphoma, anaemia and fever are usually the result of the lymphoma or complicating infection. In this patient fatigue, fever, anaemia and an increased ESR were due to an unrelated inflammatory vasculitis.

MCQ

The erythrocyte sedimentation rate (ESR) is:

1 Consistently increased in multiple myeloma
2 Higher in women than in men and higher still in pregnancy
3 Important in the diagnosis of temporal arteritis
4 Increased by a high plasma fibrinogen
5 Increased in polycythaemia

For answers and discussion, see page 206.

77 Acute megakaryoblastic leukaemia

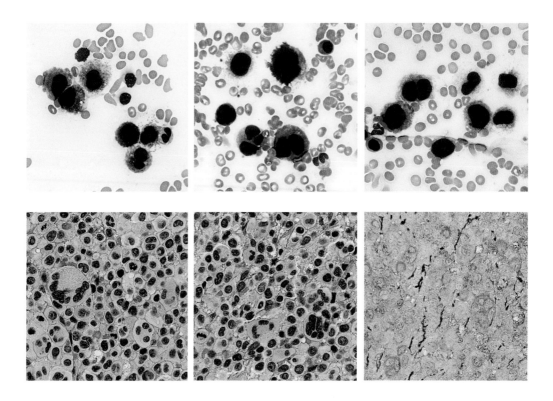

A previously well 69-year-old man presented with fatigue. His full blood count showed Hb 73 g/l, WBC 4.9×10^9/l, neutrophils 3.7×10^9/l and platelets 75×10^9/l. A blood film showed no specific features. His bone marrow aspirate was particulate and hypercellular. Notably, there was a large population of megakaryoblasts showing non-lobated or bilobed nuclei with irregular granular cytoplasm with indistinct margins (top images) (all above images ×50 objective). Flow cytometry studies showed these cells to express CD117, CD13, CD33, CD41 and CD61. CD34 and HLA-DR were not expressed. The bone marrow trephine biopsy sections showed a diffuse large cell infiltrate with almost complete loss of normal haemopoiesis but with some cells resembling megakaryocytes (bottom left and centre images, H&E). Unusually, there was no reticulin excess (which frequently accompanies megakaryocyte proliferations), which certainly allowed an informative, cellular marrow aspirate (bottom right image, reticulin stain). The case described here is unusual in that the blasts are showing morphological characteristics we often associate with megakaryocytes, making them instantly recognisable.

Acute megakaryoblastic leukaemia is an uncommon acute leukaemia accounting for less than 5% of cases. When seen in adults it often evolves from a pre-existent myeloproliferative neoplasm (MPN) and therefore carries a poor prognosis. In children it does occur *de novo* but in neonates it also needs to be differentiated from transient abnormal myelopoiesis associated with Down syndrome (see Theme 63). Megakaryoblasts can be morphologically difficult to differentiate from myeloblasts but some cases do show nuclear lobation, cytoplasmic tufts and blebs and very

Haematology: From the Image to the Diagnosis, First Edition. Mike Leach and Barbara J. Bain.
© 2022 John Wiley & Sons Ltd. Published 2022 by John Wiley & Sons Ltd.

minimal cytoplasm; these features can all be a subtle clue to megakaryocyte lineage (images from another case below ×100). Sometimes megakaryoblasts are of a similar size to small lymphocytes (images below) and dysplastic large platelets are often present.

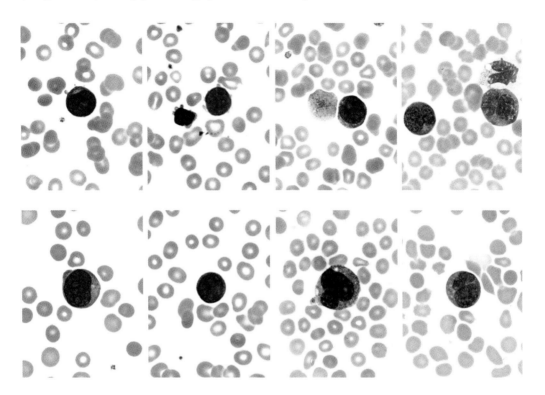

Acute megakaryoblastic leukaemia represents one of the AML subtypes that can show absence of both CD34 and HLA-DR expression and cytoplasmic myeloperoxidase is also negative. Expression of one or more of CD41 (glycoprotein IIb/IIIa), CD42b (glycoprotein Ib) and CD61 (glycoprotein IIIa) confirms the diagnosis. Other myeloid markers, such as CD13 and CD33, are also often positive whilst aberrant expression of CD7 is relatively common. We were interested in the cytogenetic profile of this case but unfortunately the analysis failed.

MCQ

Characteristic cytogenetic abnormalities in acute megakaryoblastic leukaemia include:

1 t(1;22)(p13;q13.1)
2 t(3;3)(q21.3;q26.2)
3 t(8;21)(q22;q22.1)
4 t(9;11)(p21.3;a22)
5 t(9;22)(q34.1;q11.2)

For answers and discussion, see page 206.

78 Erythrophagocytosis and haemophagocytosis

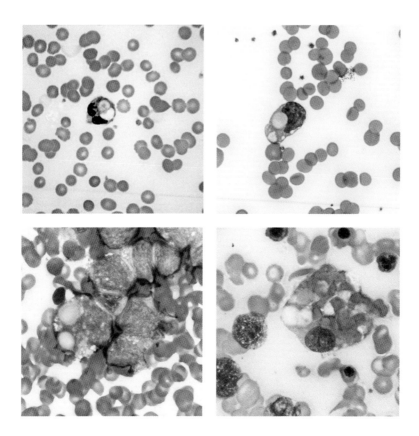

Erythrophagocytosis can be an isolated phenomenon or part of the syndrome of haemophagocytosis. The phagocytosing cells can be neutrophils, monocytes or macrophages. Observation of this phenomenon in the peripheral blood or bone marrow can be an important clue to the underlying diagnosis.

The top left image is from the blood film of an 8-year-old boy who presented with acute mixed warm and cold antibody-mediated autoimmune haemolytic anaemia (Wilding *et al.* 2021). The presence of spherocytes and polychromatic macrocytes is indicative of the haemolytic anaemia. There were also red cell agglutinates, reflecting the presence of an IgM cold autoantibody in addition to an IgG warm autoantibody. A much less frequent feature, illustrated here, was the presence of monocytes that had phagocytosed erythrocytes (top image) (all images ×100 objective). This is likely to reflect the acuteness of the process, the Hb having fallen from 116 to 53 g/l in 48 hours.

The top right image is of the blood film of a 3½-year-old girl with a 2-day history of fever and an upper respiratory tract infection. She was found to have leucocytosis and an Hb of 81 g/l with an MCV of 80 fl and MCHC increased to 370 g/l (Bharadwaj *et al.* 2011). The image shows spherocytosis (correlating with the raised MCHC) and a neutrophil that has ingested an erythrocyte and, in addition, has a second large vacuole, which probably represents a phagocytic vacuole. The blood film also showed small red cell agglutinates. The unusual combination of erythrophagocytosis by neutrophils, spherocytosis and red cell agglutination is strongly suggestive of paroxysmal cold haemoglobinuria (PCH). This provisional diagnosis was confirmed by the observation that the direct antiglobulin test was strongly positive for complement and the Donath–Landsteiner test was positive. Paradoxically, although the anti-P autoantibody that causes haemolysis in PCH is an IgG antibody, it is usual to detect only complement on the red cells.

The bottom left image (facing page) is of the bone marrow film of a 43-year-old man with acute myeloid leukaemia with t(8;16)(p11;p13). He presented with marked bruising and haematuria and was found to have a WBC of 32.4×10^9/l and a platelet count of 97×10^9/l but with a normal Hb (Hastings *et al.* 2021). Coagulation studies showed disseminated intravascular coagulation (DIC). His bone marrow aspirate led to a diagnosis of acute monoblastic leukaemia. Some of the blast cells showed erythrophagocytosis (image ×100) with a smaller number showing phagocytosis of neutrophils or platelets. The unusual combination of DIC and haemophagocytosis led to the suspicion of AML with t(8;16), which was confirmed on cytogenetic analysis.

The bottom right image (facing page) is from an adult male patient with both sickle cell anaemia and miliary tuberculosis complicated by haemophagocytic lymphohistiocytosis. His FBC showed WBC 9.2×10^9/l, Hb 82 g/l, platelet count 61×10^9/l, neutrophils 0.6×10^9/l and lymphocytes 0.8×10^9/l. The bone marrow showed phagocytosis of erythrocytes and sometimes erythroblasts. Note that the image also shows two sickle cells.

References

Bharadwaj V, Chakravorty S and Bain BJ (2011) The cause of sudden anemia revealed by the blood film. *Am J Hematol*, **87**, 520.

Hastings A, Apperley JF, Nadal-Melsio E, Brown L and Bain BJ (2021) Acute myeloid leukemia with a severe coagulopathy and t(8;16)(p11;p13). *Am J Hematol*, **96**, 163–164.

Wilding C, Pelling D, Lund K and Bain BJ (2021) Erythrophagocytosis by monocytes – an unusual observation in autoimmune hemolytic anemia. *Am J Hematol*, doi: 10.1002/ajh.25966 (online ahead of print).

MCQ

Diagnostic criteria for haemophagocytic lymphohistiocytosis include:

1 Haemophagocytosis in any organ
2 Increased erythrocyte sedimentation rate
3 Increased plasma fibrinogen
4 Increased serum ferritin
5 Increased serum triglycerides

For answers and discussion, see page 206.

79 Hyposplenism

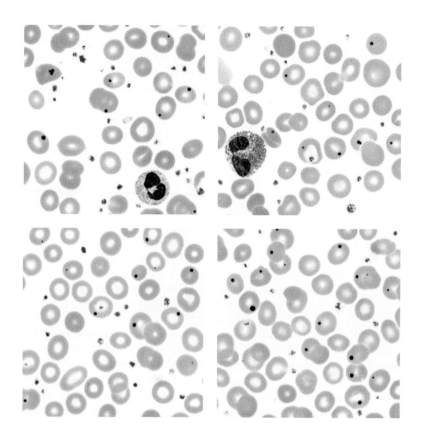

A 34-year-old man with a long history of ulcerative colitis and sclerosing cholangitis attended a routine gastroenterology clinic. His full blood count showed Hb 99 g/l, WBC 8.21 × 10⁹/L, neutrophils 2.1 × 10⁹/l, monocytes 1.2 × 10⁹/l, eosinophils 1 × 10⁹/l and platelets 1028 × 10⁹/l. The blood film showed large numbers of Howell–Jolly bodies suggesting a hyposplenic state. Target cells, acanthocytes and other forms of poikilocyte were surprisingly scarce. The patient gave no history of splenic surgery. An ultrasound scan showed a small, 4 cm spleen.

A hyposplenic state is most commonly seen following splenectomy. It can also occur as a result of splenic infiltration by lymphoma, deposition of amyloid, following episodes of fulminant sepsis, due to vascular occlusion in sickling syndromes or after treatment with chemotherapy and radiotherapy. Splenic atrophy is seen in a number of medical conditions, although the aetiology is currently unclear, including coeliac disease, Crohn's disease and ulcerative colitis, the latter being the proposed mechanism in this case. Congenital absence of the spleen also occurs. Recognition of the morphological features of hyposplenism is therefore important in patient management; it can alert clinicians to the impact of established disease but may prompt consideration of other medical conditions and, importantly, highlights the significant infection risk associated with this condition (William and Corazza 2007, William *et al.* 2007). In addition to the red cell changes, hyposplenism is typically associated with a mild leucocytosis, lymphocytosis, monocytosis, eosinophilia and

Haematology: From the Image to the Diagnosis, First Edition. Mike Leach and Barbara J. Bain.
© 2022 John Wiley & Sons Ltd. Published 2022 by John Wiley & Sons Ltd.

thrombocytosis. Howell–Jolly bodies were unusually frequent in this patient. This observation should raise the suspicion of underlying megaloblastosis but in this case the MCV was normal, as were assays of vitamin B12 and folic acid. The marked thrombocytosis shown in this case persisted for many years. These recognised features of hyposplenism are important in elucidating a cause for blood count abnormalities. In some cases the morphological features of hyposplenism can prompt consideration of other medical conditions that hitherto had not been considered and diagnosed.

References

William BM and Corazza GR (2007) Hyposplenism: A comprehensive review. Part 1: Basic concepts and causes. *Hematology*, **12**, 1–13.
William BM, Thawani N, Sae-Tia S and Corazza GR (2007) Hyposplenism: A comprehensive review. Part 2: Clinical manifestations, diagnosis and management. *Hematology*, **12**, 89–98.

MCQ

Hyposplenism is associated with an increased risk of:

1 Autoimmune haemolytic anaemia
2 Babesiosis
3 *Capnocytophaga canimorsus* infection
4 Pneumococcal infection
5 Thrombotic thrombocytopenic purpura

For answers and discussion, see page 206.

80 Acquired haemoglobin H disease

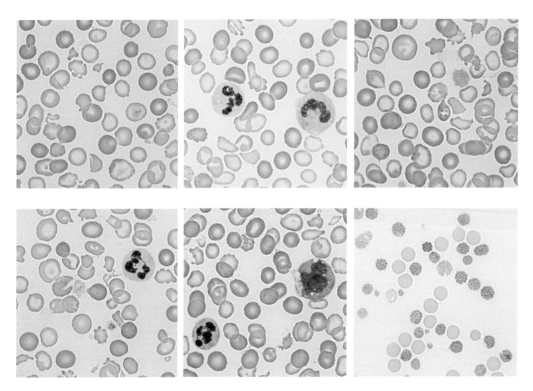

A 68-year-old man presented with a lower respiratory tract infection. He had no medical history of note and was taking no regular medication. His full blood count showed Hb 87 g/l, MCV 69 fl, WBC 9.8×10^9/l, neutrophils 7.7×10^9/l, monocytes 0.9×10^9/l and platelets 375×10^9/l. The reticulocyte count was 20×10^9/l and serum ferritin was 197 μg/l. Routine biochemical tests were normal. His blood film showed a large number of abnormalities. The red cells were dimorphic with a population of well-haemoglobinised cells, contrasting with a larger population of hypochromic cells (left and centre images) (all images ×100 objective). The latter population also showed polychromasia, target cells, anisopoikilocytosis and Pappenheimer bodies. A proportion of neutrophils were markedly hypogranular (top centre and bottom left images). There was marked variation in platelet size, with some platelets also showing hypogranularity (top right image). The morphological features here are of a myelodysplastic syndrome and the dimorphism and microcytosis are suggestive of acquired haemoglobin H disease. This was confirmed using brilliant cresyl blue staining with typical haemoglobin H inclusions being demonstrated (bottom right image). A high-performance liquid chromatography (HPLC) trace showed an early peak consistent with haemoglobin H accounting for 32.9% of total haemoglobin. Despite the dimorphism and Pappenheimer bodies, refractory anaemia with ring sideroblasts would have been a much less likely diagnosis since in that condition the MCV is normal or increased.

Haemoglobin H disease is usually an inherited red cell disorder resulting from deletion of three alpha genes, leading to serious reduction in alpha globin chain synthesis and alpha/beta chain imbalance. It generates a chronic microcytic anaemia, sometimes with transfusion dependence,

Haematology: From the Image to the Diagnosis, First Edition. Mike Leach and Barbara J. Bain.
© 2022 John Wiley & Sons Ltd. Published 2022 by John Wiley & Sons Ltd.

splenomegaly and iron overload. The acquired form can occur in patients with myelodysplastic and myelodysplastic/myeloproliferative syndromes and in acute myeloid leukaemia, particularly erythroleukaemia. Ring sideroblasts are often a feature. It results from acquired somatic mutations in the *ATRX* gene located at Xq21.1, which results in down regulation of alpha globin synthesis. Its location on the X chromosome explains why acquired haemoglobin H disease is predominantly seen in male patients.

MCQ

Features that favour acquired rather than inherited haemoglobin H disease include:

1 Dimorphic blood film
2 Dysplasia in non-erythroid lineages
3 Normal number of alpha genes
4 Occurrence in a female
5 Unusually high percentage of haemoglobin H

For answers and discussion, see page 206.

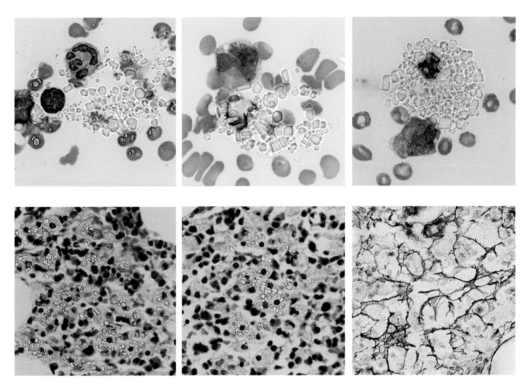

81 Cystinosis

A 14-year-old boy with progressive renal failure and a Fanconi renal profile due to cystinosis was referred to Haematology on account of a mild pancytopenia. His full blood count showed Hb 80 g/l, WBC 3 × 10^9/l, neutrophils 1.5 × 10^9/l and platelets 90 × 10^9/l. The blood film showed no specific features. The bone marrow aspirate showed prominent macrophages laden with colourless crystals; these were mainly hexagonal but some rectangular forms were visible (top images ×100 objective). Note that the macrophage cytoplasm is disrupted by the spreading process but the nucleus is visible. The trephine biopsy specimen also showed increased macrophage numbers with the same prominent intracytoplasmic crystals (bottom images ×50). Furthermore, the crystal phagocytosis and macrophage activity had generated focal bone marrow fibrosis (bottom right image, reticulin stain, focal grade 2/3).

Cystinosis is an autosomal recessive disorder affecting the metabolism of the amino acid cystine. Mutations in the *CTNS* gene, which encodes the protein cystinosin, lead to accumulation of cystine within lysosomes. This in turn affects cell metabolism, leading to autophagy and apoptosis. In the nephropathic forms of the disease an early consequence is damage to renal tubules, leading to renal tubular acidosis with excess urinary loss of glucose, potassium and phosphate (Fanconi syndrome) with progressive renal failure. The condition is usually identified by examining the cornea for crystal precipitates or measuring leucocyte cystine levels, but bone marrow examination can also be diagnostic.

Haematology: From the Image to the Diagnosis, First Edition. Mike Leach and Barbara J. Bain.
© 2022 John Wiley & Sons Ltd. Published 2022 by John Wiley & Sons Ltd.

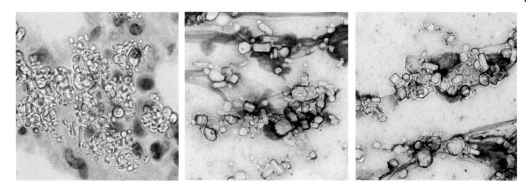

The additional images above (×100) demonstrate the diversity and the ironic pathogenic beauty of cystine crystal morphology. This is a rare disease, the morphology of which is unique. The diagnostic importance is high and once seen the condition should never be forgotten.

MCQ

Factors that can contribute to anaemia in cystinosis include:

1 Bone marrow fibrosis
2 Haemolysis
3 Hypersplenism
4 Hyperthyroidism
5 Renal impairment

For answers and discussion, see page 206.

82 Familial platelet disorder with a predisposition to AML

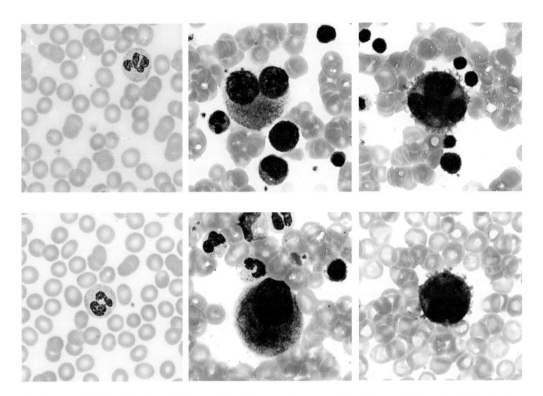

An 8-year-old girl with a long history of bruising and mucosal bleeding, noted particularly during infections, was referred on account of thrombocytopenia. There was no family history of a bleeding disorder. The full blood count showed Hb 115 g/l, WBC 3.8×10^9/l, neutrophils 2.0×10^9/l and platelets 70×10^9/l. The blood film confirmed a true thrombocytopenia; the platelets were generally small (left images ×100 objective) but there was no other abnormality. Platelet aggregometry testing was inconclusive. The bone marrow aspirate showed normal erythroid and myeloid maturation with no excess of blast cells. The megakaryocytes, however, were small and immature with non-lobated or bilobed nuclei (centre images ×100). Many showed poor cytoplasmic granularity with prominent basophilic tufts or blebs as seen in early megakaryocytes (right images ×100). DNA analysis detected a 1.5 Mb deletion within the long arm of chromosome 21 (q21.11 to q22.12) including the *RUNX1* gene.

Familial platelet disorder with germline *RUNX1* mutation or loss is an autosomal dominant condition which generates a quantitative and qualitative platelet disorder with up to 40% lifetime risk of MDS or AML. Platelet aggregation with collagen and adrenaline can be reduced. *RUNX1*, in addition to acting as a tumour suppressor gene, regulates megakaryocyte myosin IIA and IIB expression; mutations in the gene result in reduced nuclear ploidy and abnormal proplatelet formation. Peripheral blood platelets are generally normal in size and without defining characteristics. The thrombocytopenia tends to be mild but patients can have significant haemorrhagic features. Although rare, it is important to consider this condition in the appropriate clinical context when hypolobated, low ploidy megakaryocytes are encountered

Haematology: From the Image to the Diagnosis, First Edition. Mike Leach and Barbara J. Bain.
© 2022 John Wiley & Sons Ltd. Published 2022 by John Wiley & Sons Ltd.

(Kanagal-Shamanna *et al.* 2017). Furthermore, in patients with established AML, and when allogeneic transplantation options are being considered, it is important to exclude this condition in potential sibling donors.

Reference

Kanagal-Shamanna R, Loghavi S, DiNardo CD, Medeiros LJ, Garcia-Manero G, Jabbour E *et al.* (2017) Bone marrow pathologic abnormalities in familial platelet disorder with propensity for myeloid malignancy and germline RUNX1 mutation. *Haematologica*, **102**, 1661–1670.

MCQ

The *RUNX1* gene is involved in:

1 Acute lymphoblastic leukaemia with t(12;21)(p13.2;q22.2)
2 Acute lymphoblastic, myeloid or mixed phenotype leukaemia with t(4;11)(q21;q23.3)
3 Acute myeloid leukaemia with inv(16)(p13.1q22)
4 Acute myeloid leukaemia with t(8;21)(q22;q22.1)
5 The grey platelet syndrome

For answers and discussion, see page 206.

83 Nodular lymphocyte predominant Hodgkin lymphoma

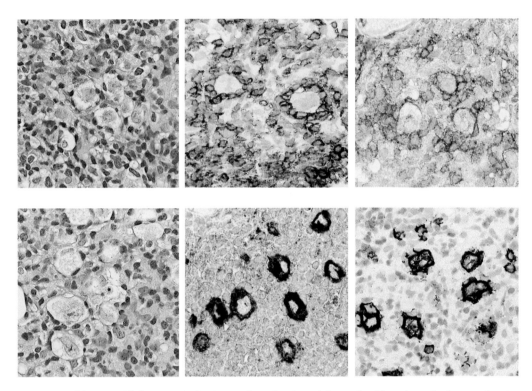

A 68-year-old man with known cirrhosis was found to have bilateral axillary lymphadenopathy. CT imaging showed additional low-volume lymphadenopathy bilaterally in cervical, supraclavicular, para-aortic and inguinal regions. The full blood count showed Hb 126 g/l, WBC 6.3 × 10⁹/l, neutro-phils 1.5 × 10⁹/l and platelets 66 × 10⁹/l. A lymph node biopsy was requested but in the interim a bone marrow biopsy was performed. The bone marrow aspirate showed no specific abnormality but flow cytometric studies identified an activated CD4+ HLA-DR+ T-cell population with rever-sal of the marrow CD4:CD8 ratio at 4:1 (normal 1:2). The marrow trephine biopsy sections showed focal areas with prominent large cells with convoluted nuclei with nucleoli; these were surrounded by small lymphocytes and a few histiocytes (left images, H&E) (all images ×50 objective). Eosinophils were not prominent. Immunohistochemistry showed that the small lymphocytes were mainly expressing CD4 (top centre), PD-1 (CD279) (top right) and CD57 and formed rosettes around the large cells which were shown to express the B-cell markers CD75 (bottom centre) and CD20 (bottom right). Note a population of small mature B cells also (bottom right). The features here are of bone marrow involvement by nodular lymphocyte predominant Hodgkin lymphoma, which was also demonstrated on lymph node biopsy.

Nodular lymphocyte predominant Hodgkin lymphoma is a rare, often indolent lymphoma typi-cally presenting with early-stage disease without B symptoms and with a male to female ratio of 3:1. Bone marrow involvement is unusual. The neoplastic cells, known as LP cells, were previously called lymphocytic and histiocytic (L+H cells) and prior to that 'popcorn cells' for obvious reasons, and are clonal B cells. The tumour cells attract a reactive T-cell population with the phenotype noted above. The T cells often form rosettes around the neoplastic cells, which can help highlight their presence.

Haematology: From the Image to the Diagnosis, First Edition. Mike Leach and Barbara J. Bain.
© 2022 John Wiley & Sons Ltd. Published 2022 by John Wiley & Sons Ltd.

MCQ

Nodular lymphocyte predominant Hodgkin lymphoma:

1 Can relapse as diffuse large B-cell lymphoma
2 Differs from classical Hodgkin lymphoma in that the neoplastic cells have a more clearly B-lineage immunophenotype
3 Is often related to the Epstein–Barr virus
4 Shows an increased incidence in family members
5 Usually shows expression of CD15 and CD30

For answers and discussion, see page 206.

84 Acute monocytic leukaemia with *NPM1* mutation

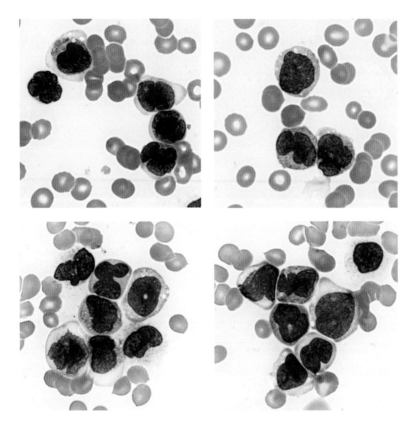

A 67-year-old man who had completed treatment one year previously for *NPM1*-mutated, normal karyotype, acute myeloid leukaemia re-presented with fatigue, dizziness and abdominal pain. His full blood count showed Hb 78 g/l, WBC 80 × 10^9/l and platelets 82 × 10^9/l. His blood film showed large numbers of promonocytes (all images ×100 objective). Note the variation in nuclear form and cytoplasmic granulation between different promonocytes and also the cell with a ring nucleus (bottom left). Immunophenotyping showed these cells to have a CD34−, CD117−, CD13+, CD33+, CD11b+, CD15+, CD14+ and CD64+ phenotype. This indicated relapse of acute monocytic leukaemia (WHO classification acute myeloid leukaemia with mutated *NPM1*) (Arber *et al.* 2017). Note the promonocyte morphology with a round or ovoid, frequently cleft nucleus with non-condensed chromatin, occasional nucleoli and sky-blue cytoplasm with fine pink granules.

See also Theme 61 Monocytes and their precusors, Theme 66 Chronic myelomonocytic leukaemia and Theme 33 Acute monoblastic leukaemia with t(9;11)(p21.3;q23.3).

NPM1-mutated AML with a normal karyotype and without *FLT3* mutation has a favourable prognosis. This entity tends to develop *de novo* and often shows monocytic differentiation. The coexistence of *NPM1* and *FLT3* internal tandem duplication (ITD) is less favourable but these patients still appear to have a better outcome than those with *FLT3*-ITD and wild-type *NPM1*. The early relapse in this patient was treated with a combination of venetoclax and low-dose cytarabine and a second remission was achieved. *NPM1*-mutated AML appears particularly sensitive to venetoclax both in terms of reinduction of remission at relapse and also in achieving measurable residual disease (MRD) negativity after repeated cycles of chemotherapy have failed to do so (Tiong *et al.* 2020).

References

Arber DA, Brunning RD, Le Beau MM, Falini B, Vardiman JW, Porwit A *et al.* (2017) Acute myeloid leukaemia with recurrent genetic abnormalities. *In* Swerdlow SH, Campo E, Harris NL, Jaffe ES, Pileri SA, Stein H and Thiele J. *WHO Classification of Tumours of Haematopoietic and Lymphoid Tissues.* IARC, Lyon, pp. 130–145.
Tiong IS, Dillon R, Ivey A, Teh TC, Nguyen P. Cummings N *et al.* (2020) Venetoclax induces rapid elimination of NPM1 mutant measurable disease in combination with low-intensity chemotherapy in acute myeloid leukaemia. *Br J Haematol*, **192**, 1026–1030.

MCQ

NPM1-mutated AML:

1 According to the WHO classification, can be therapy-related
2 Cannot be diagnosed if multilineage dysplasia is present
3 Is often associated with unbalanced chromosomal rearrangement
4 Shows aberrant cytoplasmic expression of NPM1
5 Shows a specific association with cup-shaped nuclei

For answers and discussion, see page 206.

85 Adult T-cell leukaemia/lymphoma

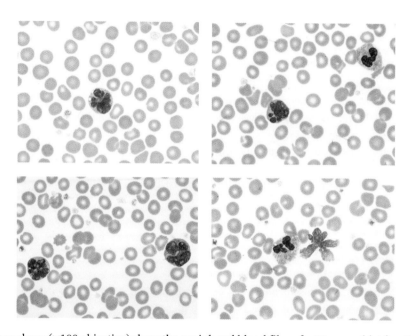

The images above (×100 objective) show the peripheral blood film of a 39-year-old Afro-Caribbean man who had just commenced treatment for adult T-cell leukaemia/lymphoma (ATLL). His FBC showed Hb 124 g/l, MCV 77 fl, WBC 16.5×10^9/l and platelet count 92×10^9/l. Lactate dehydrogenase was increased to 1100 iu/l but serum calcium was normal. The blood film shows typical 'flower cells' – lymphocytes with lobulated nuclei that resemble the radiating petals of a flower (top images and bottom left). There were other highly abnormal neoplastic cells with lobulated nuclei and visible nucleoli (bottom left). The cytoplasm was moderately basophilic and in some cells there was cytoplasmic vacuolation (top left). It is of interest that the radiating 'petals' were also detectable in smear cells (bottom right). The cytological features of ATLL are distinctive and in an appropriate clinical setting are virtually diagnostic of this condition.

This is an aggressive lymphoma characterised morphologically by pleomorphic neoplastic multilobated cells including flower cells. About 90% of patients present with leukaemia, the other 10% with lymphoma. There is usually lymphadenopathy and hepatosplenomegaly and often skin infiltration. Other typical features include frequent hypercalcaemia, due to osteoclast activation, and opportunistic infections including *Pneumocystis jirovecii* pneumonia, candidiasis, *Strongyloides stercoralis* hyperinfection, cryptococcosis and molluscum contagiosum. The neoplastic cells are CD2+, CD3+, CD4+ and CD5+. CD7 is expressed in only a minority of cases. There is almost always expression of CD25 and HLA-DR. The human lymphotropic virus 1 (HTLV-1), which is clonally integrated in neoplastic cells, is an essential aetiological factor in ATLL but the lifetime risk for this disease, which usually occurs in adults, is estimated to be 2.5%. The disease has a long latency but HTLV-1 infection alone is clearly not sufficient to cause the disease.

Haematology: From the Image to the Diagnosis, First Edition. Mike Leach and Barbara J. Bain.
© 2022 John Wiley & Sons Ltd. Published 2022 by John Wiley & Sons Ltd.

MCQ

Human lymphotropic virus 1 (HTLV-1):

1 In carriers, is associated with a low percentage of atypical lymphocytes with lobulated nuclei
2 Is endemic in Japan and the Caribbean
3 Is not transmitted by breastfeeding so antenatal screening is not important
4 Is the cause of tropical spastic paraparesis
5 Leads to immunodeficiency

For answers and discussion, see page 206.

86 Hereditary elliptocytosis and pyropoikilocytosis

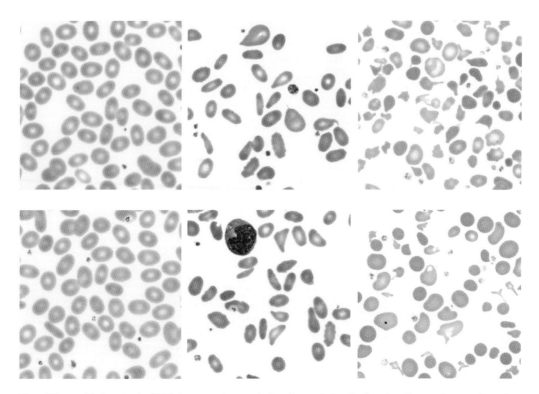

Hereditary elliptocytosis (HE) is an autosomal dominant inherited red cell membrane disorder, which has a variable phenotype. Most frequently it generates a mild, well-compensated haemolytic disorder with normal haemoglobin concentration, which may only be discovered during intercurrent illness due to a haemolytic exacerbation, or when a blood film is made for another reason (left images) (all images ×100 objective). Note that all cells are mildly elliptical with minimal anisopoikilocytosis. The full blood count in this case was normal.

A subset of cases, however, show more pleomorphic morphology, more significantly shortened red cell lifespan and chronic haemolytic anaemia. Such patients are more prone to gallstones and splenomegaly. The centre images are from a 20-year-old man who presented with gallstone cholecystitis. His full blood count showed Hb 107 g/l, WBC 11.4×10^9/l and platelets 257×10^9/l; the reticulocyte count was 170×10^9/l. He had 17 cm splenomegaly. Note the elliptical, pencil- and teardrop-shaped red cells and the polychromasia.

A third patient presented in childhood with a severe chronic haemolytic anaemia with an Hb ranging between 60 and 70 g/l. She underwent splenectomy and now has a stable, partially compensated chronic haemolytic anaemia; full blood count showed Hb 90 g/l, MCV 62 fl, WBC 9.5×10^9/l and platelets 981×10^9/l. In the images (right), note the extreme anisopoikilocytosis with spherocytes, elliptocytes and bizarre poikilocytes with needle-like projections. Note the prominence of micropoikilocytes, which are responsible for the markedly reduced MCV. The features here are of hereditary pyropoikilocytosis, which usually results from compound heterozygosity for HE. The name is derived from *pyros* (Greek for 'fire') as the cells are prone to fragmentation when

Haematology: From the Image to the Diagnosis, First Edition. Mike Leach and Barbara J. Bain.
© 2022 John Wiley & Sons Ltd. Published 2022 by John Wiley & Sons Ltd.

exposed to heat and the morphology resembles that seen when normal red cells are exposed to extreme heat. The images below are from a patient who suffered extensive burns. Note the similarities, with prominent microspherocytes of variable size and frequent tiny membrane fragments. There are also 'microdiscocytes' – red cell fragments with a circular outline but preserved central pallor.

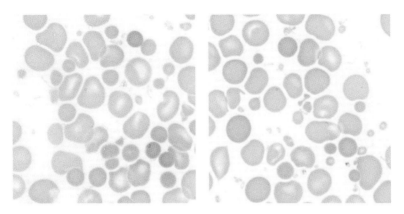

MCQ

Hereditary pyropoikilocytosis:

1. Can result from co-inheritance in *cis* to a mutation that usually causes hereditary elliptocytosis and an alpha spectrin low-expression allele, alpha spectrin[Lely]
2. In the neonatal period, can be confused with hereditary elliptocytosis
3. Is more severe in the neonatal period than later in life
4. Is uniformly associated with hereditary elliptocytosis in both parents
5. Shows reduced eosin-5-maleimide (EMA) binding

For answers and discussion, see page 206.

87 Sézary syndrome

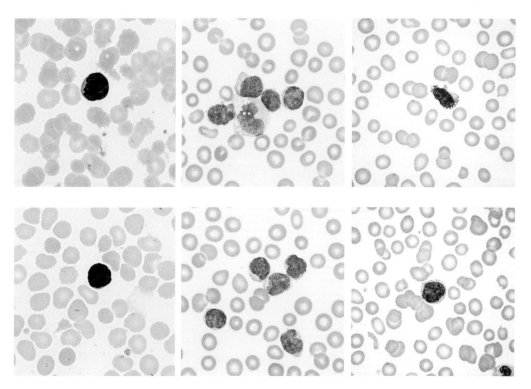

Sézary syndrome is a cutaneous T-cell lymphoma characterised by erythroderma, palmar and plantar hyperkeratosis, hair loss and often lymphadenopathy. Histologically there is infiltration in the dermis and epidermis, the latter designated Pautrier's microabscesses. Circulating lymphoma cells can be infrequent or numerous. Although Pautrier's microabscesses are characteristic, they are not always present and are not pathognomonic since they can also be seen not only in the closely related condition of mycosis fungoides but also in adult T-cell leukaemia/lymphoma. Sézary syndrome is an aggressive disease with a median survival of less than 3 years; the erythroderma and constant pruritus can be quite disabling.

The left images (all images ×100 objective) are from a patient with generalised erythroderma with a full blood count showing a mild leucocytosis (15.7×10^9/l) due to lymphocytosis. The Sézary cells often have a high nuclear/cytoplasmic ratio and show multiple subtle complex nuclear clefts which could be easily overlooked.

The centre images are from a patient who was unusual in having a very high white cell count (100×10^9/l) together with anaemia (Hb 57 g/l) and thrombocytopenia (platelet count 50×10^9/l). The top centre image shows a monocyte and four Sézary cells. Overlapping and entwining nuclear lobes and small nucleoli are apparent in both the centre images. Nuclei such as these are described as cerebriform.

The right images are from another patient, who had much less numerous Sézary cells. In addition to nuclear grooves, they show cytoplasmic vacuoles arranged in a ring around the nucleus. These have been likened to rosary beads. They are positive on periodic acid–Schiff staining.

Haematology: From the Image to the Diagnosis, First Edition. Mike Leach and Barbara J. Bain.
© 2022 John Wiley & Sons Ltd. Published 2022 by John Wiley & Sons Ltd.

MCQ

On immunophenotyping, Sézary cells show:

1 Consistent expression of CD7
2 Expression of CD3
3 Expression of CD4
4 No expression of CD26
5 Usually expression of CD8

For answers and discussion, see page 206.

88 Spherocytic red cell disorders

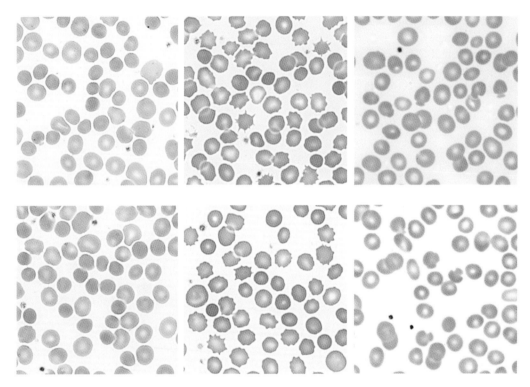

The spherocytic red cell, by its very nature and easily recognisable characteristics, with a shift from the normal biconcave disc to a cell approximating a sphere, is one of the early pathological red cell forms appreciated by haematology trainees and biomedical scientists learning morphology. By shifting toward a sphere, the cell diameter is reduced, the central pallor is lost and the intensity of haemoglobin staining is increased. The mean cell haemoglobin concentration (MCHC) is usually increased when spherocytes are prominent. Spherocytes also carry high diagnostic specificity as they are encountered in relatively few haematological conditions. The images above (all images ×100 objective) are from three patients with different forms of hereditary spherocytosis (HS). The left images are typical of ankyrin-deficient HS, showing regular, fairly uniform spherocytes and polychromasia. The centre images are of beta spectrin-deficient HS, showing spherocytes, acanthocytes and spheroacanthocytes. Note that the acanthocytic features can sometimes distract the morphologist from a diagnosis of HS but in the appropriate clinical context these findings are actually supportive of the diagnosis (see also Theme 9, acanthocytic red cell disorders). The right images show band 3-deficient HS, with very few spherocytes but prominent 'mushroom' or 'pincered' cells; this condition tends to have a milder clinical phenotype and can be identified incidentally later in life (the patient in this example was 85 years old). Mushroom cells are present in all forms of HS but they are more prominent in band 3 disease. Spherocytes can also be prominent in non-HS inherited red cell membrane disorders (see Theme 86).

Haematology: From the Image to the Diagnosis, First Edition. Mike Leach and Barbara J. Bain.
© 2022 John Wiley & Sons Ltd. Published 2022 by John Wiley & Sons Ltd.

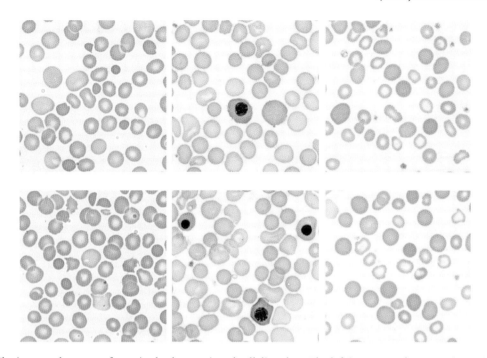

The images above are of acquired spherocytic red cell disorders. The left images are from a patient with haemolytic uraemic syndrome (HUS) following *E. coli* 0157 infection. Note the microspherocytes but also the polychromatic macrocytes and fragments. These features indicate a microangiopathic haemolytic anaemia and the spherocytes are a feature of tearing and remodelling of fragmented red cells; the spherocytes are a secondary phenomenon. The centre images are from a neonate with haemolytic disease of the newborn due to IgG anti-A allo-antibodies. Note the nucleated red cells, a common reaction to stress in the neonate, plus spherocytes and polychromasia. The right images are from a patient who had presented 2 weeks previously with iron deficiency anaemia due to acute on chronic bleeding from a duodenal ulcer. He was transfused 3 units of red cells. Two weeks later he was readmitted with anaemia and jaundice. Note the prominent transfused red cells now appearing as spherocytes, which contrast nicely with the native microcytic hypochromic cells. A direct Coombs test was positive for IgG and his serum showed new anti-c+E and anti-Jk^a antibodies; the latter antibody was eluted from his cells, confirming a delayed haemolytic transfusion reaction. Spherocytes are believed to appear in immune-mediated conditions due to removal of portions of antibody-coated red cell membrane by the spleen, so reducing the surface area without loss of cell contents (see also Theme 72).

MCQ

Microspherocytes can be a feature of the blood film in:

1 Burns
2 Hereditary pyropoikilocytosis
3 Mechanical haemolytic anaemia
4 Pyrimidine 5′ nucleotidase deficiency
5 Thrombotic thrombocytopenic purpura

For answers and discussion, see page 206.

89 Acute myeloid leukaemia and metastatic carcinoma

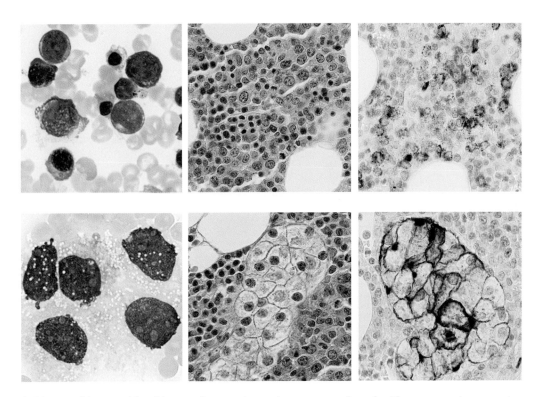

A 70-year-old man with a history of prostatic carcinoma was referred with a progressive pancyto-penia. His full blood count showed Hb 95 g/l, WBC 2.9×10^9/l, neutrophils 1.3×10^9/l and platelets 26×10^9/l. The blood film did not show any specific informative features. A bone marrow aspirate showed a significant myeloblast population (top left ×100 objective) at 30% of events with a CD34+, CD117+, CD13+, CD33+, HLA-DR+, MPO+ and TdT+ immunophenotype. In addition, a sepa-rate population of large, partially disrupted cells with prominent lilac nucleoli and foamy cyto-plasm was present (bottom left ×100). The trephine biopsy sections showed an interstitial increase in blast cells (H&E, top centre, histology images ×50 objective) staining positively with CD34 (top right, immunoperoxidase). The trephine biopsy complemented the aspirate findings, sections showing focal aggregates of large cohesive cells (bottom centre, H&E), which stained positively for cytokeratin (bottom right, immunoperoxidase). The features were in keeping with two separate bone marrow pathologies which are independent of each other: acute myeloid leukaemia and metastatic prostatic carcinoma. The patient was managed with best supportive care.

It is important when analysing bone marrow aspirate and trephine biopsy sections to keep an open mind on potential findings, as sometimes more than one pathology is present. These may be related conditions, such as MDS evolving to AML or diffuse large B-cell lymphoma evolving from follicular lymphoma (both of which have prognostic and therapeutic implications) or unrelated as in the patient described here. The potential management of each tumour is significantly influ-enced by the second pathology. This also demonstrates the importance of assessing the aspirate films and trephine biopsy sections together at the microscope. The traumatised clumps of

Haematology: From the Image to the Diagnosis, First Edition. Mike Leach and Barbara J. Bain.
© 2022 John Wiley & Sons Ltd. Published 2022 by John Wiley & Sons Ltd.

carcinoma cells in the aspirate might have been overlooked in the circumstances, but careful scrutiny of the biopsy sections looking for focal aggregates of non-haemopoietic cells confirmed the suspicion and the different phenotypes of the two populations could easily be confirmed using immunohistochemistry. Finally, this case also illustrates the importance of taking a careful clinical history. Sometimes the history of treatment many years previously for breast cancer or melanoma, for example, might not seem important but these tumours not infrequently show late relapse. Furthermore, the treatment delivered previously, particularly chemotherapy or radiotherapy, could be relevant to the aetiology of a newly diagnosed MDS or AML.

MCQ

Bone marrow infiltration by prostatic cancer can be associated with:

1 Cytokeratin expression
2 Fibrosis
3 Haemophagocytic syndrome
4 Intravascular infiltration
5 Osteosclerosis

For answers and discussion, see page 206.

90 Chédiak–Higashi syndrome

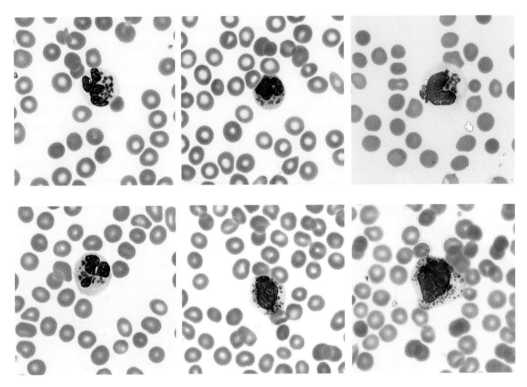

A 7-year-old girl with albinism was referred for assessment by a bone marrow transplant unit. She had a history of recurrent bacterial infections, mouth ulcers and easy bruising. Notably, she had suffered an episode of life-threatening haemophagocytic syndrome one year previously. Her full blood count showed Hb 100 g/l, WBC 2×10^9/l, neutrophils 0.7×10^9/l and platelets 90×10^9/l. The blood film showed markedly abnormal giant coalesced granules in leucocytes: neutrophils (left images) (all images ×100 objective), lymphocytes (centre images) and monocytes (right images). These features are typical of Chédiak–Higashi syndrome, which is a rare autosomal recessive lysosomal disorder characterised by recurrent infection from impaired neutrophil chemotaxis and phagocytosis, oculocutaneous albinism from aberrant melanosome formation, bleeding due to impaired platelet dense body formation and neurodegeneration with the mechanism currently not understood (Nowicki 2019). A morphological diagnosis in the appropriate clinical context should be possible as the leucocyte granule abnormalities are unique. Although this condition is very rare, an appreciation of the condition is important, as it can have catastrophic consequences for patients, and early diagnosis and recognition of potential complications can influence plans for subsequent management. Furthermore, it can supplement our understanding of the importance of lysosomal function in a variety of tissues. We can often learn about the key mechanisms of normal cellular processes by studying the consequences of functional loss in inherited diseases interrupting these pathways. Importantly, the disease often enters an accelerated phase in childhood or early adolescence with a life-threatening episode of haemophagocytic syndrome, which is often fatal if not rapidly identified and treated.

The genetic hallmark is mutation in the *LYST* (*CHS1*) gene at 1q42.3. The gene encodes a lysosomal trafficking regulator that influences cellular granule formation in multiple different tissues. The syndrome often results in death before adulthood, usually as a consequence of infection, bleeding or the aforementioned haemophagocytic syndrome. Allogeneic stem cell transplantation can be successful in correcting multiple facets of the disease but, despite this, progressive neurological dysfunction still occurs in some cases. Patients with deletions in the *LYST* gene tend to have a severe phenotype with multiple complications in childhood whilst missense mutations can lead to a milder phenotype and presentation as young adults, with absence of a complicating haemophagocytic syndrome and neuropathy.

The condition was first described in 1943 by a Cuban paediatrician, Antonio Béguez César, but the eponymous credit goes to Moisés Chédiak Ahuayda, a Cuban haematologist, and Otokata Higashi, a Japanese paediatrician who described patients in 1952 and 1954, respectively.

Reference

Nowicki RJ (2019) Chediak–Higashi syndrome. https://emedicine.medscape.com/article/1114607-overview#a2

MCQ

Abnormally large neutrophil granules can be a feature of:

1 Acute myeloid leukaemia
2 Chronic neutrophilic leukaemia
3 May–Hegglin anomaly
4 Mucopolysaccharidoses (Alder–Reilly anomaly)
5 Myelodysplastic syndrome

For answers and discussion, see page 206.

91 Cortical T-lymphoblastic leukaemia/lymphoma

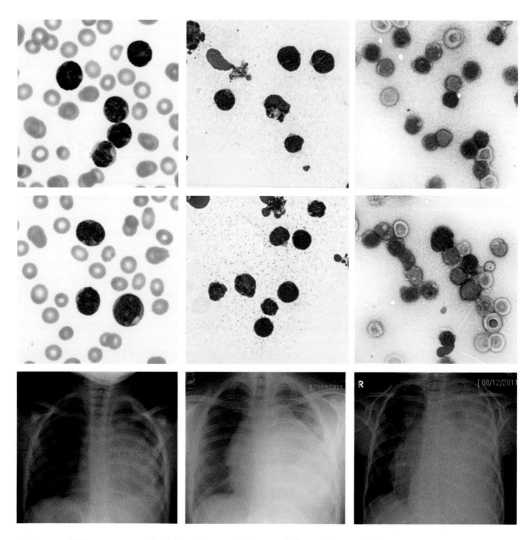

A 6-year-old boy presented with pallor and disrupted sleep due to night sweats. On examination, he appeared pale and unwell but no specific features were apparent. His full blood count showed Hb 88 g/l, WBC 63×10^9/l, neutrophils 1×10^9/l and platelets 32×10^9/l. His blood film showed pleomorphic blast cells with nucleoli, prominent nuclear clefts and basophilic cytoplasm (left images) (all microscopy images ×100 objective). The blasts had a CD45 weak, TdT+, cCD3+, CD7+, CD5+, CD2+, CD4/CD8+, CD3−, CD1a+ immunophenotype in keeping with a cortical T-lymphoblastic leukaemia. The chest X-ray (bottom left) showed a large mediastinal mass.

A second patient, a 22-year-old man, presented with rapidly increasing fatigue and dyspnoea when attempting his daily run. His full blood count showed Hb 157 g/l, WBC 5.2×10^9/l, neutrophils 2.6×10^9/l and platelets 192×10^9/l. A chest X-ray showed a large mediastinal mass (bottom centre) and echocardiography showed involvement of the pericardium with an effusion causing early cardiac tamponade so a pericardial fluid aspiration was undertaken. The cytospin showed large numbers of blast cells amongst cellular debris (centre microscopy images, facing page) and these had a CD45 weak, TdT+, cCD3+, CD7+, CD5+, CD2+, CD8+, CD3−, CD4−, CD1a+ immunophenotype. The bone marrow aspirate was normal so the diagnosis was cortical T-lymphoblastic lymphoma.

A third patient, an 8-year-old girl, presented with a persistent dry cough and dyspnoea. She had clinical features in keeping with a large left pleural effusion. This was confirmed on a chest X-ray, which also showed a large mediastinal mass (bottom right). The full blood count was normal. The mediastinal mass was not easily accessible to a percutaneous biopsy so the pleural effusion was partly drained. The fluid showed large numbers of blast cells but the morphological detail was difficult to define (microscopy images right, facing page). Nevertheless, flow cytometric studies were able to show the blasts had a CD45 weak, TdT+, CD7+, CD5+, CD2+, surface membrane CD3+, CD8−, CD4−, CD1a+ immunophenotype, in keeping with cortical T-lymphoblastic lymphoma. The bone marrow was not involved.

MCQ

Cortical T-lymphoblastic leukaemia/lymphoma:

1 Can have a normal blood count
2 Is associated with a better prognosis than other subtypes of T-lymphoblastic leukaemia/lymphoma
3 Is defined by expression of CD1a and CD3
4 Is now often classified as early T-cell precursor lymphoblastic leukaemia
5 Usually shows loss of expression of CD7

For answers and discussion, see page 206.

92 Trypanosomiasis

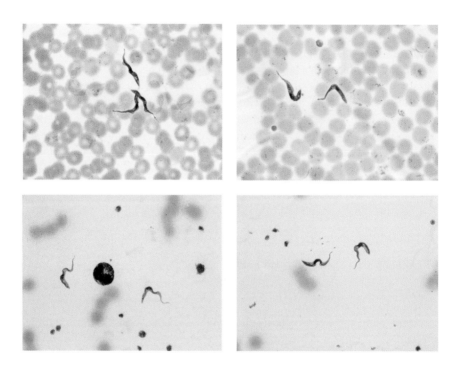

The images above (all images ×100 objective) are from two patients infected with *Trypanosoma brucei rhodesiense*. The top images are from a patient who was febrile following return from a safari in Serengeti National Park, Tanzania, while the bottom two images are from a patient who had recently returned from holidaying in Kenya. Note the graceful sinuous curves of the parasites, the undulating membrane, the flagellum and the presence of a central oval nucleus. The kinetoplast (most visible in the top left image) is very small. *Trypanosoma brucei rhodesiense* and *Trypanosoma brucei gambiense* cannot be distinguished on morphological grounds but their geographical distributions show little overlap. The former is found in Eastern and Southern Africa and the latter in Western and Central Africa with the two occurring in different areas of Uganda.

The images on the facing page are from two patients from South America who had travelled to the UK, both being infected by *Trypanosoma cruzi*. In the first patient (top images) the parasites are more compact with fewer curves than *Trypanosoma brucei* but the most striking difference between the two species is the presence of a large kinetoplast. In the second patient (bottom images) some of the parasites are more sinuous but again the prominent kinetoplast is apparent. Often *Trypanosoma cruzi* assumes a C or O shape (top right and bottom left).

Haematology: From the Image to the Diagnosis, First Edition. Mike Leach and Barbara J. Bain.
© 2022 John Wiley & Sons Ltd. Published 2022 by John Wiley & Sons Ltd.

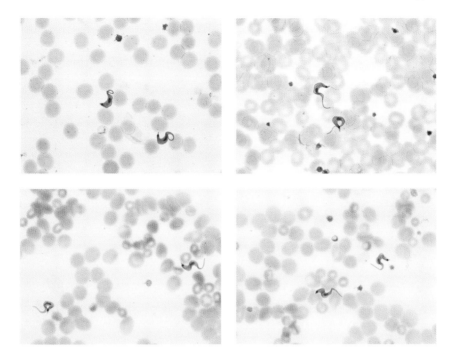

MCQ

Trypanosoma brucei infection:

1 Can cause disseminated intravascular coagulation
2 Causes eosinophilia
3 Is the cause of African sleeping sickness
4 Is transmitted by mosquitoes
5 Typically causes chronic cardiomyopathy

For answers and discussion, see page 206.

93 Acute myeloid leukaemia with myelodysplasia-related changes

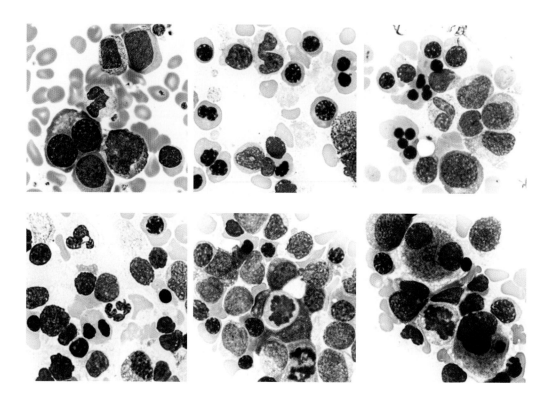

A 24-year-old woman underwent a laparoscopic cholecystectomy for gallstones. This was complicated by post-operative infection and an abscess developed requiring surgical drainage. The surgical team phoned for advice as her full blood count was abnormal, showing Hb 83 g/l, MCV 114 fl, WBC 1.8×10^9/l, neutrophils 0.9×10^9/l and platelets 81×10^9/l. On review of her records the FBC had been abnormal 6 months previously, showing a macrocytic anaemia and mild neutropenia. There were no laboratory records prior to this. Haematinic assays were normal. Her blood film showed hypogranular neutrophils and an occasional nucleated red cell. Her bone marrow aspirate was particulate and hypercellular, showing an excess of myeloblasts accounting for 38% of nucleated cells (all images ×100 objective). Notably, there was also trilineage dysplasia: note the prominent erythroid dysplasia with frequent binucleated forms, including a binucleated early erythroblast (top left); marked hypogranularity and abnormal nuclei in the myeloid series including an abnormal metamyelocyte and cell with a ring nucleus (top centre); and abnormal hypolobated megakaryocytes, some binucleated (bottom right). Flow cytometry showed the blasts to have a CD34+, CD117+, CD13+, CD33+, MPO+ immunophenotype; the karyotype was normal and no mutation of *NPM1* or *FLT3* was identified. A diagnosis of acute myeloid leukaemia with myelodysplasia-related changes (AML-MRC) was made.

For a diagnosis of AML-MRC at least one of three criteria must be met: AML with a preceding history of MDS or MDS/MPN; AML with more than 50% dysplastic cells in two or more cell lines; or AML with MDS-related cytogenetic abnormalities (complex cytogenetic abnormality, specified unbalanced abnormalities involving chromosome 5, 7, 11, 12, 13 or 17, and certain specified balanced abnormalities). There are also exclusion criteria to be met. Mutations in *ASXL1*, *U2AF1* and *TP53* are common. This patient satisfies the diagnostic criteria, both because of the bone marrow morphology and also on the basis of a likely preceding MDS phase. The condition is important to identify for a number of reasons. Firstly, it may have evolved from a prior MDS or MDS/MPN and it is important to look at retrospective laboratory records for evidence of such. Secondly, it carries a poor prognosis with inferior outcomes compared to many other AML subtypes; this diagnosis alone is an indication for allogeneic stem cell transplantation in first remission in patients of appropriate age and fitness. Thirdly, patients with this condition are eligible for treatment with CPX-351, a liposomal encapsulated formulation of daunorubicin with cytarabine in a synergistic 1:5 ratio. This formulation allows a longer duration of exposure and preferential uptake by leukaemic blasts, resulting in improved remission rates and potential for transplantation, compared with standard chemotherapy.

MCQ

The WHO category of acute myeloid leukaemia with myelodysplasia-related changes (AML-MRC) can be diagnosed in a patient with:

1 AML with complex cytogenetic abnormalities following previous treatment of Hodgkin lymphoma with combination chemotherapy
2 AML with erythroid and granulocytic dysplasia, monosomy 7 and del(5q)
3 AML with t(3;3)(q21.3;q26.2) with erythroid dysplasia, micromegakaryocytes and multinucleated megakaryocytes
4 AML with t(6;9)(p23;q34.1) with erythroid and granulocytic dysplasia, Auer rods and increased basophils
5 Pancytopenia with 15% bone marrow blast cells, some with Auer rods, with bilineage dysplasia

For answers and discussion, see page 206.

94 Blastic plasmacytoid dendritic cell neoplasm

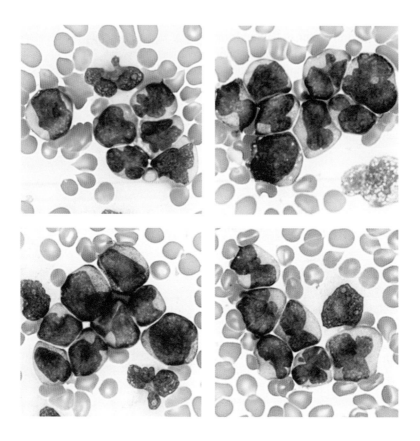

A 62 year-old man had been unwell for 2 weeks with fatigue, fever and bruising before presenting to the Accident and Emergency department. He collapsed in the waiting room. On examination he was obtunded with a right third nerve palsy. His brain CT showed an extensive intracerebral haemorrhage with intraventricular extension, midline shift and pressure on the brainstem. He died shortly afterwards. His full blood count showed Hb 128 g/l, WBC 189×10^9/l and platelets 96×10^9/l. His blood film showed a population of large cells with pale blue cytoplasm, fine chromatin and multiple nuclear clefts with some cells having distinct nucleoli (all images ×100 objective). Only a subset of cells showed fine cytoplasmic granulation (bottom left) and some showed vacuolation (top right). An acute monocytic leukaemia was suspected at the base hospital. Flow cytometry showed the large cells to express no lineage specific markers; surface CD45, CD33, HLA-DR and CD7 were all expressed. Only a subset of cells (approximately 25%) expressed CD15, whilst CD14, CD64 and CD11b were not expressed at all. This made a monocytic/monoblastic leukaemia much less likely as CD15, CD11b and CD64 are all consistently expressed in these leukaemias. Further immunophenotyping showed the cells to express CD4, CD56 and CD123. A leukaemic presentation of blastic plasmacytoid dendritic cell neoplasm (BPDCN) now seemed very likely. This is a rare neoplasm of plasmacytoid dendritic cell precursors; the mature forms are antigen-presenting cells that are normally located in the skin. This condition, which typically affects older males, often presents with skin infiltration appearing as focal thickening,

Haematology: From the Image to the Diagnosis, First Edition. Mike Leach and Barbara J. Bain.
© 2022 John Wiley & Sons Ltd. Published 2022 by John Wiley & Sons Ltd.

purplish discoloration or nodules; bone marrow involvement frequently follows. The liver, spleen, lymph nodes and CNS can all be involved. The neoplastic cells have a unique phenotype and typically express CD33, HLA-DR, CD4, CD56 and CD123 whilst lineage-specific markers are absent (Garnache-Ottou *et al.* 2019). The morphology of BPDCN is highly variable and there is no specific recurrent cytogenetic or molecular abnormality associated with it although various abnormalities of chromosomes 13, 12, 7, 9, 15, 5, 6 and 17 have been described. Although skin involvement is frequent, a fulminant systemic leukaemic presentation is also recognised, as in the patient described here. It is important to consider this diagnosis when the above constellation of features is apparent. Furthermore, there is no current consensus on optimal induction therapy, with a variety of AML, ALL and high-grade lymphoma-based therapies being reported with variable success (Garnache-Ottou *et al.* 2019). There is some agreement that once remission is achieved allogeneic stem cell transplantation offers the best long-term survival option.

Reference

Garnache-Ottou F, Vidal C, Biichlé F, Renosi F, Poret E, Pagadoy M *et al.* (2019) How should we diagnose and treat blastic plasmacytoid dendritic cell neoplasm patients? *Blood Adv*, **3**, 4238–4251.

MCQ

Blastic plasmacytoid dendritic cell neoplasm:

1 Can be associated with myelodysplastic features
2 Can have cytoplasmic tails and vacuolation among the cytological features
3 Is likely to be derived from a lymphoid stem cell
4 Often has complex karyotypic abnormalities
5 Usually shows expression of CD34 and TdT

For answers and discussion, see page 206.

95 Inherited macrothrombocytopenias

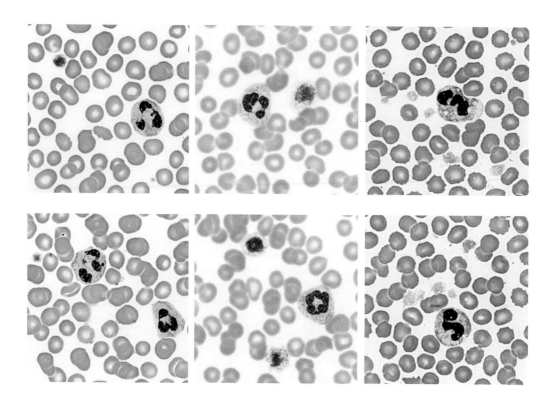

A 35-year-old woman was found to have a moderate thrombocytopenia after attending her GP with menorrhagia. The full blood count showed Hb 140 g/l, WBC 7.2×10^9/l and platelets 65×10^9/l. The blood film showed a true thrombocytopenia. The majority, but not all, of the neutrophils showed focal cytoplasmic blue blush inclusions which were often located near the periphery of the cell (left images) (all images ×100 objective). These are Döhle-like bodies typically seen in the May–Hegglin anomaly, an autosomal dominant inherited condition associated with macrothrombocytopenia. May–Hegglin anomaly is the most common variant of a family of macrothrombocytopenic conditions caused by mutation in the *MYH9* (non-muscle myosin heavy chain type IIa) gene. It is associated with a variable degree of thrombocytopenia and a mild bleeding tendency as platelet function is normal. The Döhle-like inclusions result from clusters of ribosomes arranged along myosin heavy chain filaments.

A second patient, a 35-year-old Iranian woman, was found to have a severe thrombocytopenia at a pre-operative assessment prior to removal of metal splints at the site of a previous ankle fracture. The automated impedance-based full blood count showed Hb 121 g/l, WBC 8.5×10^9/l and platelets 4×10^9/l. An automated optical platelet count was 40×10^9/l. Two sisters were also known to have thrombocytopenia, but surprisingly none gave a significant bleeding history. The blood film showed a true thrombocytopenia with very large platelets; the neutrophil morphology was normal (centre images). Platelet aggregation studies failed, likely due to the severity of thrombocytopenia but platelet CD42b expression was significantly reduced when assessed using flow cytometry.

Haematology: From the Image to the Diagnosis, First Edition. Mike Leach and Barbara J. Bain.
© 2022 John Wiley & Sons Ltd. Published 2022 by John Wiley & Sons Ltd.

Genetic analysis showed homozygosity for a c.182A>G mutation in exon 3 of the *GP9* gene consistent with a diagnosis of Bernard–Soulier syndrome. This is an autosomal recessive inherited disorder characterised by macrothrombocytopenia and deficiency of platelet glycoprotein Ib, which results in abnormal binding of the glycoprotein Ib-IX-V complex to von Willebrand factor and a moderate bleeding disorder.

A third patient, a 60-year-old man with a long history of easy bruising and epistaxis, was referred for investigation of thrombocytopenia. His full blood count showed Hb 139 g/l, WBC 4.1 $\times 10^9$/l and platelets 76 $\times 10^9$/l. The blood film showed a true thrombocytopenia but the platelets were large, with loss of normal granularity; the neutrophil morphology was normal (right images, facing page). These features are suggestive of grey platelet syndrome and investigations are on-going. Grey platelet syndrome is a rare autosomal recessive inherited disorder caused by mutations in the *NBEAL2* gene, resulting in depletion or absence of platelet alpha granules and a mild to moderate bleeding tendency. The thrombocytopenia can be progressive and there is a tendency to develop myelofibrosis and splenomegaly (Gunay-Aygun *et al.* 2010). An interesting curiosity, not yet explained, is that serum vitamin B12 levels tend to be high.

Reference

Gunay-Aygun M, Zivony-Elboum Y, Gumruk F, Geiger D, Cetin M, Khayat M *et al.* (2010) Gray platelet syndrome; natural history of a large patient cohort and locus assignment to chromosome 3p. *Blood*, **116**, 4990–5001.

MCQ

In inherited thrombocytopenias:

1 Grey platelets result from a reduction of alpha granules
2 Macrothrombocytopenia is anticipated in the Wiskott–Aldrich syndrome
3 *MYH9*-related disorders can be reliably detected by a search for Döhle-like inclusions in leucocytes
4 Platelets are of normal size when thrombocytopenia represents the presentation of Fanconi anaemia or dyskeratosis congenita
5 Platelet size may be underestimated by automated instruments

For answers and discussion, see page 206.

96   Persistent polyclonal B-cell lymphocytosis

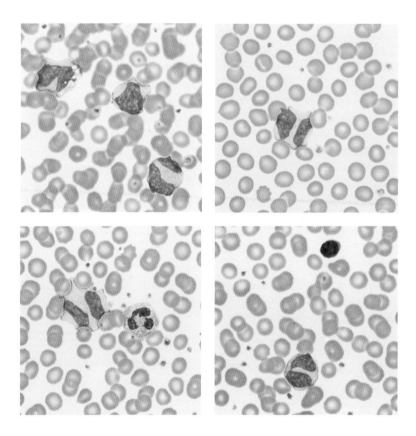

A 32-year-old woman was referred for investigation of lymphocytosis. She complained of headache, aches and pains, weight loss, fatigue, night sweats and itch. She had a 1 cm lymph node in the right axilla and a 2 cm node in the left axilla. Her FBC showed WBC $11.4 \times 10^9/l$, lymphocyte count $6.3 \times 10^9/l$, Hb 135 g/l and platelet count $340 \times 10^9/l$. An automated full blood count showed an increase in large unstained (peroxidase-negative) cells as well as in lymphocytes. Her blood film showed pleomorphic lymphocytes (top left) including binucleated forms (top images and bottom left) (all images ×100 objective). There were also lymphocytes with two distinct nuclear lobes joined by a thin filament. The abnormal lymphocytes had peripheral cytoplasmic basophilia. A provisional diagnosis of persistent polyclonal B-cell lymphocytosis was made. This was confirmed on immunophenotyping, which showed a CD19+, CD5+, CD79b+, FMC7+, CD20+, CD23+, CD22+ population with equal proportions of surface kappa and lambda.

Haematology: From the Image to the Diagnosis, First Edition. Mike Leach and Barbara J. Bain.
© 2022 John Wiley & Sons Ltd. Published 2022 by John Wiley & Sons Ltd.

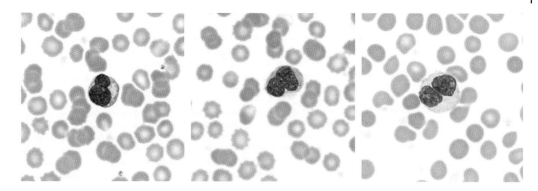

The images above are from a second patient with a mild lymphocytosis. Her full blood count showed Hb 128 g/l, WBC 13.28 × 10^9/l, lymphocytes 6.42 × 10^9/l, neutrophils 5.9 × 10^9/l and platelets 260 × 10^9/l. Note again the prominent bilobed nuclei. Immunophenotyping studies showed a polyclonal B-cell proliferation: CD19+, CD20+, CD79b+, CD22+, FMC7+, CD5−, CD10−, CD23−, surface kappa 48%, and surface lambda 47%.

MCQ

Persistent polyclonal B-cell lymphocytosis:

1 Can evolve into chronic lymphocytic leukaemia
2 Can have acquired chromosomal abnormalities
3 Can involve the bone marrow
4 Characteristically occurs in elderly male cigarette smokers
5 Shows an increase of polyclonal IgM

For answers and discussion, see page 206.

97 Acute myeloid leukaemia with t(6;9)(p23;q34.1)

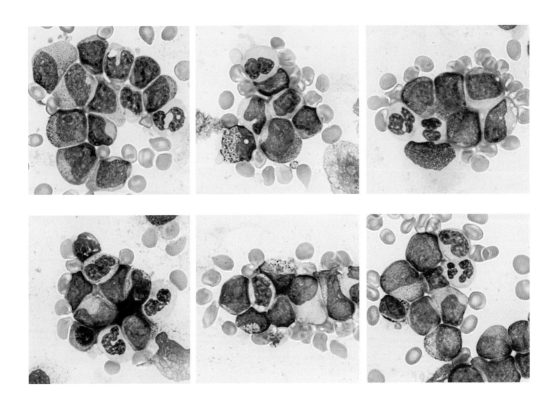

A 16-year-old boy presented with pallor and widespread bruising. His full blood count showed Hb 77 g/l, WBC 70 × 10^9/l, neutrophils 1.0 × 10^9/l and platelets 36 × 10^9/l. The blood film showed prominent blast cells and a small number of dysplastic neutrophils. His bone marrow aspirate was particulate and hypercellular with large numbers of myeloblasts showing prominent nucleoli and cytoplasmic granulation but without Auer rods (all images ×100 objective). In addition, there was trilineage dysplasia with marked neutrophil abnormalities with frequent hypogranularity and abnormal nuclear segmentation. Furthermore, hypogranular basophils and basophil myelocytes were prominent (top centre and bottom images). The myeloblasts had a CD34+, CD117+, CD13+, CD33+, HLA-DR+, MPO+ immunophenotype. The karyotype was t(6;9)(p23;q34.1), *NPM1* was wild type but a *FLT3* internal tandem duplication (ITD) was present. He was treated with two lines of induction chemotherapy but failed to achieve remission. Remission was subsequently successfully induced using the novel combination of venetoclax and gilteritinib (a FLT3 inhibitor). This treatment combination was extremely well tolerated and generated good recovery of the peripheral blood counts. His remission was consolidated using allogeneic stem cell transplantation. Post-transplant, the patient remains well and in remission and on the basis of recent approvals will continue gilteritinib maintenance therapy for a period of 2 years.

Haematology: From the Image to the Diagnosis, First Edition. Mike Leach and Barbara J. Bain.
© 2022 John Wiley & Sons Ltd. Published 2022 by John Wiley & Sons Ltd.

MCQ

Acute myeloid leukaemia with t(6;9)(p23;q34.1):

1 Can be therapy-related
2 Can occur *de novo* or follow MDS
3 Generally has a good prognosis
4 Often has *FLT3*-ITD
5 Often shows basophilic differentiation

For answers and discussion, see page 206.

98 B-cell prolymphocytic leukaemia

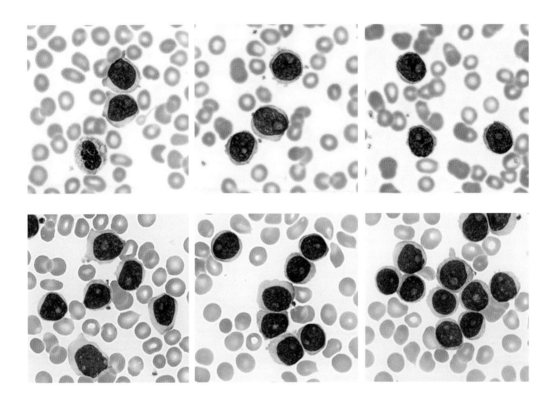

A 71-year-old woman had a full blood count done after a positive bowel screening test; it showed Hb 98 g/l, MCV 91 fl, WBC 63.8 × 10^9/l, neutrophils 2.3 × 10^9/l and platelets 130 × 10^9/l. Serum ferritin was normal. A small benign polyp was found on colonoscopy and excised. There was no lymphadenopathy but her spleen tip was just palpable. Her blood film showed large numbers of medium to large lymphoid cells with round or oval nuclei with condensed chromatin and a prominent, often single, nucleolus and a moderate amount of pale blue cytoplasm (top images) (all images ×100 objective). These cells had a CD19+, CD20+, FMC7+, CD79b+, HLA-DR+, surface kappa-restricted immunophenotype. The morphological features are typical of B-cell prolymphocytic leukaemia (B-PLL) whilst the flow cytometry merely identified a CD5–, pan-B phenotype, mature B-cell neoplasm. A t(8;14)(q24;q32) translocation was identified in 71% of cells. Deletion of chromosome 17p was not detected. She was treated with six cycles of bendamustine and rituximab and achieved a complete response which has been sustained 3 years later.

A second patient, a 91-year-old man, presented with abdominal pain and distension due to massive splenomegaly. His full blood count showed Hb 105 g/l, WBC 203.7 × 10^9/l, neutrophils 4.9 × 10^9/l and platelets 24 × 10^9/l. The blood film showed very similar features to the first case (bottom images) and the flow cytometry findings were identical. FISH studies identified deletion of one copy of *TP53* (17p13) in 89% of nuclei. These findings are also indicative of B-PLL. The loss of *TP53* gene function predicts chemotherapy refractoriness so he was given a trial of single-agent

Haematology: From the Image to the Diagnosis, First Edition. Mike Leach and Barbara J. Bain.
© 2022 John Wiley & Sons Ltd. Published 2022 by John Wiley & Sons Ltd.

rituximab therapy. Two years later, this has been remarkably effective with improvement in abdominal symptoms and correction of the leucocytosis, anaemia and thrombocytopenia.

There is no immunophenotype that is specific to B-PLL but the morphology of the cells is remarkably consistent; note the striking similarity of the morphology in the two cases above (compare with Theme 21). A careful morphological assessment in the context of an appropriate clinical presentation should suggest this diagnosis. Targeted molecular investigations should then further support the diagnosis and guide appropriate therapy.

MCQ

B-cell prolymphocytic leukaemia (B-PLL):

1 Can evolve from chronic lymphocytic leukaemia
2 If associated with t(8;14)(q24;q32), is likely to actually be Burkitt lymphoma
3 If associated with t(11;14)(q13;q32), is likely to actually be mantle cell lymphoma
4 Shows nuclear expression of cyclin D1
5 Usually shows weak or absent CD200 expression

For answers and discussion, see page 206.

99   Various red cell enzyme disorders

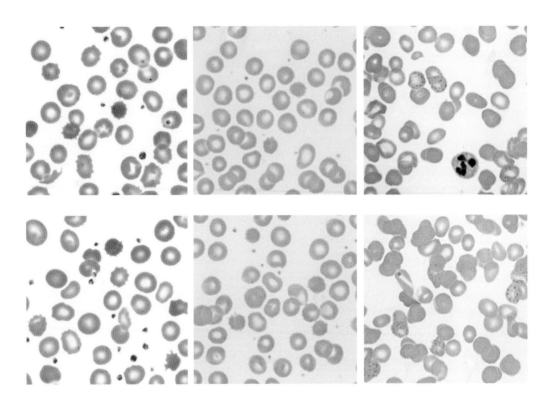

A 40-year-old man was referred by his GP for ongoing follow-up of a chronic haemolytic disorder, said to be due to hereditary spherocytosis, for which he had undergone splenectomy in another health board at the age of 3 years. His full blood count showed Hb 94 g/l, MCV 117 fl, WBC 5.6 × 10⁹/l and platelets 645 × 10⁹/l. A blood specimen was sent to our laboratory for eosin-5-maleimide (EMA) binding studies. His blood film (left images) (all images ×100 objective) showed post-splenectomy features (Howell–Jolly bodies and acanthocytes) and polychromasia but in addition echinocytes were present. Spherocytes were not present. These features are suggestive of pyruvate kinase (PK) deficiency and the clinical presentation requiring splenectomy at an early age is in keeping with this diagnosis. Red cell EMA binding was normal and a subsequent PK assay showed a level of 3.7 u/g Hb (NR 6.2–14.2). PK deficiency is an autosomal recessive disorder characterised by a moderate to severe chronic haemolytic anaemia which in most cases requires management with splenectomy (Grace and Barcellini 2020). It is the commonest of the non-G6PD enzymopathies and the presence of echinocytes, although they are not specific, should alert the morphologist to this possible diagnosis. *Echinus* is a genus of sea urchin and in Greek means 'hedgehog-like'.

The centre images are from the blood film of a second patient, a 10-year-old boy with a chronic haemolytic anaemia, myopathy and a neurodegenerative illness. They also show prominent echinocytes and polychromasia. He had a diagnosis of triose phosphate isomerase deficiency, another autosomal recessively inherited enzyme disorder, which carries a very poor prognosis.

Haematology: From the Image to the Diagnosis, First Edition. Mike Leach and Barbara J. Bain.
© 2022 John Wiley & Sons Ltd. Published 2022 by John Wiley & Sons Ltd.

Echinocytosis is a recognised feature of this deficiency but nevertheless it is so rare that it is unlikely to be suspected from the blood film.

The right images, facing page, are from a third patient, a 15-year-old female with a lifelong history of chronic haemolytic anaemia requiring transfusion from an early age. Her blood film shows prominent coarse basophilic stippling and polychromasia whilst the red cell morphology was otherwise unremarkable. Note the high frequency of the stippled cells and the coarseness of the stippling. In this context the blood film suggests a diagnosis of pyrimidine 5′ nucleotidase deficiency and this was subsequently confirmed on enzyme assay; both parents had borderline low levels but were asymptomatic heterozygotes. This is another autosomal recessively inherited condition. The blood film is a key component of the investigation and in this patient triggered the specific enzyme assay that confirmed the diagnosis.

The red blood cell requires three essential metabolic pathways in order to support its function in oxygen binding, transport and delivery to tissues. Glycolysis generates energy for maintaining cell structure and function, antioxidant pathways protect cells from extraneous damage and endogenous oxidants and nucleotide metabolism maintains purine and pyrimidine structure. Inherited enzymopathies are recognised in all these essential pathways; some have consequences only for red cell survival but others have, in addition, serious systemic consequences inducing skeletal and cardiac muscle disease, metabolic acidosis, recurrent infection and neurodegeneration. There is an increasing trend, with the evolution of genetic sequencing in the evaluation of red cell disorders, for the early utilisation of such technology at the expense of the simpler long learned tools at our disposal. We absolutely welcome the new technology but it is not infallible and can only be properly interpreted in the light of the other existing clinical and laboratory data.

Reference

Grace RF and Barcellini W (2020) Management of pyruvate kinase deficiency in children and adults. *Blood*, **136**, 1241–1249.

MCQ

Basophilic stippling:

1 Is characteristic of heavy metal poisoning
2 Is often seen in β thalassaemia heterozygosity
3 Leads to a positive Perls stain
4 Represents aggregates of ribosomes
5 Represents ectopically sited DNA

For answers and discussion, see page 206.

100   Sea-blue histiocytosis in multiple myeloma

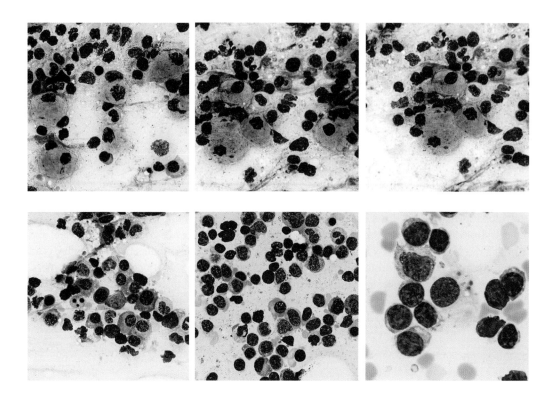

An 82-year-old woman was referred to the Renal department with a recent rapid decline in kidney function with urea 32.3 mmol/l and creatinine 300 μmol/l. She was noted to have a 40 g/l IgM kappa paraprotein, markedly elevated serum free kappa light chains, 3500 u/l, and Bence Jones proteinuria. There was no lymphadenopathy or splenomegaly.

Her full blood count showed Hb 97 g/l, WBC 13.5×10^9/l, neutrophils 10.5×10^9/l and platelets 626×10^9/l. The bone marrow aspirate was hypercellular. The initial most striking finding was of large numbers of sea-blue histiocytes (top images ×50 objective). On further examination an abnormal population including plasma cells was also apparent. This abnormal population included mature plasma cells, lymphoplasmacytoid lymphocytes and small lymphocytes (bottom images ×50, except right image ×100). Flow cytometry studies showed these cells to express CD138, CD38, CD20 and CD56, whilst CD45 and CD19 were negative. This confirms the diagnosis as IgM multiple myeloma and excludes a lymphoplasmacytic lymphoma (CD45+, CD19+, CD20+, CD79b+, CD38+/−). Cytogenetic studies showed t(11;14)(q13;q32). IgM myeloma differs in characteristics from class-switched myeloma. The t(11;14) translocation is much more often observed and is associated with cyclin D1 expression (Feyler *et al.* 2008, Castillo *et al.* 2017). Data are conflicting with regard to CD20 expression, which was reported in one of nine patients in one series (Feyler *et al.* 2008), in 10 of 15 in a second (Schuster *et al.* 2010) and in 15 of 26 in another (Castillo *et al.* 2017). When present in myeloma, the translocation of *CCND1* to the IGH locus is typically associated with CD20 expression and lymphoplasmacytic morphology (Heereema-McKenney *et al.* 2010).

It is clearly important to recognise this morphological variant of multiple myeloma, particularly as the bone marrow aspirate plasma cell quantitation by morphology is key to the diagnosis; in this setting it is likely that the neoplastic cells will be underestimated if the cells with lymphoplasmacytic and lymphocytic morphology are overlooked. Sea-blue histiocytes are also important to recognise as they frequently coexist with a number of bone marrow disorders.

References

Castillo JJ, Jurczyszyn A, Brozova L, Crusoe E, Czepiel J, Davila J *et al.* (2017) IgM myeloma: A multicenter retrospective study of 134 patients. *Am J Hematol*, **92**, 746–751.

Feyler S, O'Connor SJ, Rawstron AC, Subash C, Ross FM, Pratt G *et al.* (2008) IgM myeloma: a rare entity characterized by a CD20-CD56-CD117- immunophenotype and the t(11;14). *Br J Haematol*, **140**, 547–551.

Heereema-McKenney A, Waldron J, Hughes S, Zhan F, Sawyer J, Barlogie B and Shaugnessy JD (2010) Clinical, immunophenotypic and genetic characterisation of small lymphocyte-like plasma cell myeloma. A potential mimic of mature B-cell lymphoma. *Am J Clin Pathol*, **133**, 256–270.

Schuster SR, Rajkumar SV, Dispenzieri A, Morice W, Aspitia AM, Ansell S *et al.* (2010) IgM multiple myeloma: Disease definition, prognosis, and differentiation from Waldenstrom's macroglobulinemia. *Am J Hematol*, **85**, 853–855.

MCQ

Sea-blue histiocytes in the bone marrow can be a feature of:

1 Autoimmune thrombocytopenia
2 Chronic myeloid leukaemia
3 Gaucher disease
4 Niemann–Pick disease
5 Sickle cell anaemia

For answers and discussion, see page 206.

101   Enteropathy-associated T-cell lymphoma

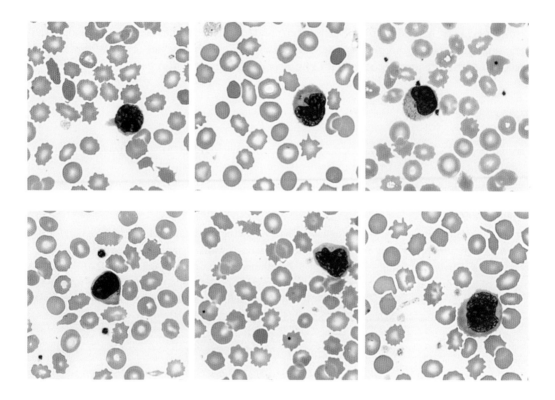

A 74-year-old woman with a long history of coeliac disease, compliant with a gluten-free diet, presented with anorexia and weight loss. Upper gastrointestinal endoscopy showed duodenal mucosal atrophy and biopsies showed increased intraepithelial T lymphocytes expressing CD3 but not CD4 or CD8. These findings were in keeping with type 2 refractory coeliac disease. A CT scan showed abnormal thickening of the ileum with adjacent mesenteric lymphadenopathy. During the period of investigation she developed a peripheral blood lymphocytosis. Her full blood count showed Hb 98 g/l, WBC 14.1×10^9/l, lymphocytes 8.5×10^9/l, neutrophils 4.5×10^9/l and platelets 318×10^9/l. Her blood film (all images ×100 objective) showed acanthocytes, target cells, irregular poikilocytes and Howell–Jolly bodies in keeping with hyposplenism. In addition, there was a population of medium to large pleomorphic lymphoid cells, with a mature chromatin pattern, occasional nucleoli and basophilic cytoplasm. Some cells showed fine azurophilic granules. Flow cytometry studies showed these cells to express cCD3, CD2 and CD7 with weak expression of CD103. CD4, CD8, CD5, CD56, CD57, CD30 and CD25 were not expressed. These findings indicate a clonal T-cell neoplasm and, in this clinical context, an enteropathy-associated T-cell lymphoma (EATL).

Enteropathy-associated T-cell lymphoma is a high-grade neoplasm arising from intraepithelial T cells that occurs in individuals with coeliac disease. It may arise from the enteropathy associated with poor dietary compliance or in those with type 2 refractory coeliac disease (independent of gluten avoidance). The tumour cells usually express CD3, CD7, CD103 and cytotoxic granule-associated proteins (TIA1, granzyme B and perforin). CD30 may be expressed in cases with large cell

Haematology: From the Image to the Diagnosis, First Edition. Mike Leach and Barbara J. Bain.
© 2022 John Wiley & Sons Ltd. Published 2022 by John Wiley & Sons Ltd.

morphology but CD56 is not usually expressed. The prevalence of this lymphoma, geographically, mirrors that of the underlying coeliac disease and in a significant proportion of cases the tumour develops in patients who were not aware of their gluten sensitivity. The small intestine is most frequently involved, but cases involving the stomach and colon have been described. The tumour spreads locally and to adjacent lymph nodes but involvement of bone marrow and blood is rare. This is an aggressive T-cell lymphoma which is difficult to treat. Furthermore, many patients are malnourished or have required surgery either to achieve a diagnosis, due to small bowel obstruction or as a result of tumour perforation and peritonitis.

A distinction should be made between EATL and MEITL (monomorphic epitheliotropic intestinal T-cell lymphoma). The latter is not associated with coeliac disease, has a worldwide distribution and has a characteristic immunophenotype with expression of CD3, CD8 and CD56. As the name suggests, the tumour cells show epitheliotropism and can spread diffusely through long lengths of small bowel mucosa. The prognosis is similarly poor.

MCQ

Haematological abnormalities in coeliac disease can result from:

1 Copper deficiency
2 Folic acid deficiency
3 Hyposplenism
4 Refractory iron deficiency anaemia
5 Vitamin B12 deficiency

For answers and discussion, see page 206.

Further discussion of the themes

1 Anaplastic large cell lymphoma with haemophagocytic syndrome

ALK-negative anaplastic large cell lymphoma:

1) Generally occurs at an older age than ALK-positive cases
2) Has a better prognosis than ALK-positive anaplastic large cell lymphoma
3) Has similar histological and immunophenotypic features to breast implant-associated anaplastic large cell lymphoma
4) Is usually associated with t(2;5)(p23.2-23.1;q35.1)
5) Usually presents with localised disease

Correct answers 1, 3

ALK-negative anaplastic large cell lymphoma typically occurs at an older age than ALK-positive cases and has a worse prognosis. Presentation is usually with stage III or IV disease. Although they are histologically indistinguishable, these are quite different conditions. It is ALK-positive cases that are associated with t(2;5), leading to formation of an *NPM1-ALK* fusion gene. Breast implant-associated cases are also histologically indistinguishable but are a quite distinct disease that usually remains localised and has a much better prognosis.

2 Bone marrow AL amyloidosis

Amyloid in tissue sections can be identified by positive staining with:

1) Congo red
2) Martius scarlet blue
3) Methenamine silver
4) Prussian blue
5) Sirius red

Correct answers 1, 5

Congo red and Sirius red both stain amyloid and, on examination by polarised light, there is apple-green birefringence. Martius scarlet blue stains collagen, methenamine silver stains fungi and Prussian blue stains haemosiderin.

Haematology: From the Image to the Diagnosis, First Edition. Mike Leach and Barbara J. Bain.
© 2022 John Wiley & Sons Ltd. Published 2022 by John Wiley & Sons Ltd.

> **3** Cup-like blast morphology in acute myeloid leukaemia

Acute myeloid leukaemia with mutated *NPM1* is typically associated with:

1) An abnormal karyotype
2) Cup-shaped nuclei
3) Cytoplasmic expression of NPM1
4) Expression of CD34
5) Poor prognosis

Correct answers 2, 3

The morphological findings are key in suspecting this subtype of AML; the cup-like nuclear morphology due to cytoplasmic organelle-rich invaginations into the nucleus is typical of *NPM1*-mutated AML, particularly when there is coexisting *FLT3*-ITD. In contrast to acute promyelocytic leukaemia (APL), in addition to the frequent cup-like forms, Auer rods are present but rarely multiple, the nuclei do not show bilobed or cleft forms and cytoplasmic granulation is not marked. Large, single, pseudo-Chédiak–Higashi granules may be present but giant granules are also occasionally seen in APL. A careful morphological assessment should help identify this entity, which can resemble other acute leukaemias, well before urgent FISH/cytogenetic/molecular results are available. The immunophenotype is a useful supplement to the morphology since CD34 is usually not expressed and HLA-DR is also negative in about a third of cases. The karyotype is abnormal in only about 15% of patients. NPM1 is normally expressed in the nucleolus but in this type of AML there is cytoplasmic expression. Prognosis is relatively good.

> **4** Neutrophil morphology

A botryoid ('grape-like') nucleus in a neutrophil can be a feature of:

1) Burns
2) Granulocyte colony-stimulating factor (G-CSF) therapy
3) Hyperthermia
4) Myelodysplastic syndrome
5) Sepsis

Correct answers 1, 3

A botryoid neutrophil nucleus is one that shows radial segmentation as a result of contraction of microfilaments radiating from the centriole, so that its shape resembles a bunch of grapes. It is a specific feature relating to exposure of cells to heat. It has been reported in patients suffering from burns, heat stroke and hyperthermia, the latter resulting, for example, from brainstem haemorrhage. The example that follows (×100 objective) is from a patient with hyperthermia resulting from cocaine abuse (Fumi *et al.* 2017). Methamphetamine abuse can also be causative.

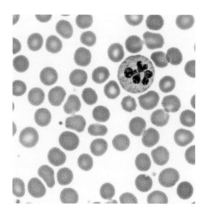

Reference

Fumi M, Pancione Y, Sale S, Rocco V and Bain BJ (2017) Botryoid nuclei resulting from cocaine abuse. *Am J Hematol*, **92**, 1260–1261.

---

5 Primary myelofibrosis

Molecular mechanisms underlying primary myelofibrosis include:

1) *BCR-ABL1*
2) *CALR* mutation
3) *JAK2* V617F
4) *JAK2* exon 12 mutation
5) *MPL* mutation

Correct answers 2, 3, 5

JAK2 V617F, as found in this patient, is seen in half or more of patients with primary myelofibrosis, *CALR* mutation in about 30% and *MPL* mutation in about 8%. The remaining 10–15% of patients are 'triple negative'; these patients have a less favourable prognosis with a higher risk of AML and a shortened overall survival (Tefferi *et al.* 2014). *JAK2* exon 12 mutations are found in a minority of patients with polycythaemia vera but not in primary myelofibrosis. Rarely, *BCR-ABL1* has been described as a second event in primary myelofibrosis but this is not a molecular mechanism underlying the condition.

Reference

Tefferi A, Lasho TL, Finke CM, Knudson RA, Ketterling R, Hanson CH *et al.* (2014) *CALR* vs *JAK2* vs *MPL*-mutated or triple negative myelofibrosis: clinical, cytogenetic and molecular comparisons. *Leukemia*, **28**, 1472–1477.

---

6 Sarcoidosis

Caseating granulomas can be a feature of:

1) Fungal infection
2) Granulomatous response to follicular lymphoma
3) Granulomatous response to multiple myeloma
4) Sarcoidosis
5) Tuberculosis

Correct answers 1, 5

Caseating granulomas can occur in tuberculosis and fungal infections whereas sarcoidosis is charac-terised by non-caseating granulomas. Non-caseating granulomas are also occasionally seen in the bone marrow as a response to multiple myeloma or infiltration by follicular lymphoma. 'Caseating' refers to the cheese-like consistency of necrotic tissue. Bone marrow granulomas are most often due to miliary tuberculosis, cytomegalovirus or Epstein–Barr virus infection, lymphoma or sarcoidosis (Eid *et al.* 1996). Rare causes include cholesterol embolism and a response to deposition of uric acid.

Reference

Eid A, Carion W and Nystrom JS (1996) *Differential diagnoses of bone marrow granuloma West J Med*, **164**, 510–515.

---

7 Visceral leishmaniasis

Leishmaniasis involving the bone marrow:

1) Can be complicated by a haemophagocytic syndrome
2) Can cause granuloma formation
3) Can lead to significant dyserythropoiesis
4) Is easily detected with Grocott's methenamine silver stain
5) Is often associated with increased plasma cells

Correct answers 1, 2, 3, 5

Leishmaniasis can have many haematological manifestations, among which are pancytopenia, haemophagocytosis and increased bone marrow plasma cells and lymphocytes. Dyserythropoiesis has sometimes led to misdiagnosis as a myelodysplastic syndrome (Kopterides *et al.* 2007). Misdiagnosis as lymphoma and malignant histiocytosis has also occurred. Occasionally organisms are identified in peripheral blood neutrophils. In the bone marrow they may be found in neutro-phils and myelocytes, as well as in macrophages (Bhatia *et al.* 2011). Grocott's methenamine silver stain identifies fungi but protozoan parasites do not stain.

References

Bhatia P, Haldar D, Varma N, Marwaha RK and Varma S (2011) A case series highlighting the relative frequencies of the common, uncommon and atypical/unusual hematological findings on bone marrow examination in cases of visceral leishmaniasis. *Mediterr J Hematol Infect Dis*, **3**, e2011035.

Kopterides P, Mourtzoukou EG, Skopelitis E, Tsavaris N and Falagas ME (2007) Aspects of the association between leishmaniasis and malignant disorders. *Trans R Soc Trop Med Hyg*, **101**, 1181–1189.

---

8 Gelatinous transformation of the bone marrow

Myxoid degeneration (gelatinous transformation) can be a feature of:

1) Acquired immune deficiency syndrome
2) Anorexia nervosa
3) Extreme exercise
4) Metastatic carcinoma
5) Morbid obesity

Correct answers 1, 2, 3, 4.

Gelatinous transformation is commonly associated with the anaemia and cytopenias seen in patients with eating disorders. It can also occur in malnutrition, chronic infection including the acquired immune deficiency syndrome (AIDS), metastatic malignancy and any chronic wasting condition. Curiously, it can also occur in fit individuals undergoing extreme exercise (Huffman *et al.* 2017).

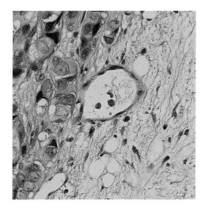

Occasionally, the primary pathology causing the malnourished state will also be apparent (above image, H&E ×50 objective) showing metastatic adenocarcinoma adjacent to gelatinous transformation.

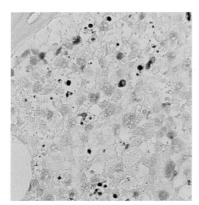 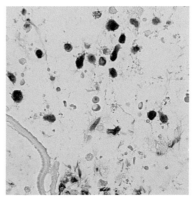

In contrast, the images on the facing page (H&E ×50) show bone marrow necrosis. This phenomenon usually has an infective or embolic cause or results from high-grade diseases growing rapidly or obliterating the marrow blood supply. The left image shows necrotic high-grade lymphoma whilst the right image shows necrotic normal marrow. Occasionally, gelatinous material is also apparent, in relation to fat cells, in a bone marrow aspirate.

Reference

Huffman BM, Wiisanen J, Shi M and Go RS (2017) Feeling run down: exercise-induced pancytopenia. *Br J Haematol*, **177**, 672.

9	Acanthocytic red cell disorders

Acanthocytes in a blood film can be the result of:

1) Anorexia nervosa
2) Liver failure
3) Splenectomy
4) Storage artefact
5) Transfusion of blood at the end of its shelf life

Correct answers 1, 2, 3

Red cell acanthocytic disorders represent a wide range of conditions, many having a defined genetic component with serious degeneration in a multitude of systems. A careful blood film analysis can be highly informative in a number of these syndromes and can provide a useful diagnostic pointer in patients with complex clinical presentations. A blood film in not only important in patients with abnormal full blood counts but can also be highly valuable in those with normal counts in selected clinical scenarios. Other causes of neurodegeneration with acanthocytosis include autosomal recessive neuroacanthocytosis due to mutation in *VPS13A*, autosomal dominant Huntington-like disease 2 due to *JPH3* mutation (some cases) and autosomal recessive pantothenate kinase-associated neurodegeneration due to *PANK2* mutation (some cases) (Bain and Bain 2013). A multidisciplinary approach to diagnosis is needed.

Acanthocytes are also seen in acquired disorders. Small numbers may be seen in anorexia nervosa and in starvation. Large numbers can be seen in haemolytic anaemia associated with liver failure, this sometimes being designated 'spur cell haemolytic anaemia' (Smith *et al.* 1964). Splenectomy is usually followed by the appearance of moderate numbers of acanthocytes but sometimes they are very numerous. However the cells that develop as a storage artefact are echinocytes rather than acanthocytes; in contrast to the acanthocyte, they have blunted projections that are regular in shape and evenly disposed over the surface of the erythrocyte. Small numbers of spiculated calls are also sometimes observed following blood transfusion; these are spheroechinocytes, resulting from adenosine triphosphate (ATP) depletion.

References

Bain BJ and Bain PG (2013) Choreo-acanthocytosis. *Am J Hematol*, **88**, 712.
Smith JA, Lonergan ET and Sterling K (1964) Spur-cell anemia: hemolytic anemia with red cells resembling acanthocytes in alcoholic cirrhosis. *N Engl J Med*, **271**, 396–398.

---

10 T-cell large granular lymphocytic leukaemia

T-cell large granular lymphocytic leukaemia:

1) Can lead to anaemia due to pure red cell aplasia or autoimmune haemolytic anaemia
2) Has specific diagnostic features on trephine biopsy
3) Shows an association with Felty syndrome
4) Shows an association with thymoma
5) Typically shows expression of CD3, CD8 and CD57.

Correct answers 1, 3, 5

T-cell large granular lymphocytic leukaemia (T-LGLL) is a fascinating condition with protean clinical manifestations including neutropenia due to maturation arrest, autoimmune thrombocytopenia and anaemia due to immune-mediated haemolysis or red cell aplasia. There is a strong association with Felty syndrome (rheumatoid arthritis with splenomegaly and neutropenia) and a less strong association with other autoimmune conditions, such as systemic lupus erythematosus. There is no association with thymoma. The lymphocytosis can be minor but it is important to consider the condition in patients with and without known rheumatological conditions. Trephine biopsy sections show variable, non-specific changes, which can include intrasinusoidal infiltration. No recurrent cytogenetic abnormality has been associated with this disorder. Flow cytometric studies can suggest a clonal T-cell disorder when multiple antigens are lost but confirmation of clonality ultimately needs gene sequencing. Typically there is the phenotype of a cytotoxic T cell with expression of CD3, CD8 and CD57. Patients with T-LGLL are more likely to have associated cytopenias when *STAT3* mutations (missense or insertion) are present; these are frequently located in the SH2 domain and lead to *STAT3* activation, which in turn prevents apoptosis (Koskela *et al.* 2012). The type of *STAT3* mutation can influence therapeutic management (Lamy *et al.* 2017). This condition should not escape the haematologist; it should always be in the differential diagnosis in patients with unexplained cytopenia.

References

Koskela HL, Eldfors S, Ellonen P, van Adrichem AJ, Kuusanmaki H, Andersson EI *et al.*
  (2012) Somatic STAT3 mutations in large granular lymphocytic leukemia. *N Engl J Med*, **366**,
  1905–1913.
Lamy T, Moignet A and Loughran TP (2017) LGL leukaemia: from pathogenesis to treatment. *Blood*,
  129, 1082–1094.

---

11 Pure erythroid leukaemia

Proerythroblasts in pure erythroid leukaemia often express:

1) CD34
2) CD61
3) CD117
4) E-cadherin (CD234)
5) Glycophorin A (CD235a)

Correct answers 3, 4, 5

Leukaemic proerythroblasts typically express CD36, CD71, CD117, E-cadherin and glycophorin A. They are usually CD34 negative. They do not express CD61, which is a marker of the megakaryocyte lineage. E-cadherin (detected on immunohistochemical staining) and glycophorin A are lineage specific. E-cadherin can be useful in detecting erythroid differentiation in very primitive cells that are not yet expressing glycophorin A (Caldwell *et al.* 2019, Bain and Leach 2021).

Flow cytometric immunophenotyping was diagnostic in this patient but this is not always so. The myeloblast population is small or absent, red cell lysis using ammonium chloride reduces the erythroid precursor population and modern acute leukaemia cytometry panels often include few erythroid-directed antibodies. The diagnosis relies heavily on morphological assessment. The images below, from this patient (×100 objective), emphasise the cytological features.

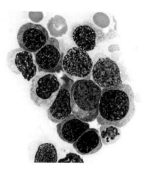 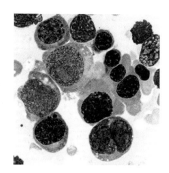

Note that the nuclei are often perfectly round and the chromatin pattern differs from that of a myeloblast – there is often a stippled or reticular pattern rather than the chromatin being diffuse. In some cells the Golgi zone stretches around the nuclear margin and cytoplasmic basophilia is notable. Note also the cytoplasmic vacuoles, which are generally indicative of the presence of glycogen. In resource-constrained settings, when appropriate immunophenotyping is not available, a periodic acid–Schiff stain to identify glycogen can still be used to support the diagnosis of erythroleukaemia.

References

Bain BJ and Leach M (2021) *Immunophenotyping for Haematologists: Principles and Practice*. Wiley Blackwell, Oxford.

Caldwell I, Ruskova A, Royle G, Liang J and Bain BJ (2019) Pure erythroid leukemia: The value of E-cadherin in making the diagnosis. *Am J Hematol*, **94**, 726–727.

12	Reactive mesothelial cells

Myeloid sarcoma:

1) Can be the first sign of relapse of acute myeloid leukaemia
2) Can have a green colour
3) Can be associated with t(8;21)(q22;q22.1)
4) Is common in acute promyelocytic leukaemia
5) Occurs only at a single site

Correct answers 1, 2, 3

Myeloid sarcoma refers to a solid mass of leukaemic cells at an extramedullary site (Aneja 2018). It can occur at presentation of AML or at relapse. It can occur at transformation of MDS and MDS/MPN and in therapy-related as well as *de novo* AML. When it is the presenting feature of AML, it can occur in the presence of bone marrow disease or as an isolated tumour with the bone marrow being normal. Myeloid sarcoma usually occurs at a single site but this is not always so; multiple tumours are present in less than 10% of cases (Pileri *et al.* 2017). In some cases the tumour is macroscopically green, as a result of the presence of myeloperoxidase, giving rise to the earlier designation of 'chloroma'. There is an association with t(8;21) but cases have also been reported with t(1;22), t(9;11), t(11;19), inv(16), *NPM1* mutation and biallelic *CEBPA* mutation, and also with other less specific chromosomal abnormalities such as trisomy 8, monosomy 7, del(5q) and del(7q). It has been reported but is very rare in acute promyelocytic leukaemia.

References

Aneja A (2018) Myeloid sarcoma pathology. *Medscape.* https://emedicine.medscape.com/article/1644141-overview

Pileri SA, Orazi A and Falini B (2017) Myeloid sarcoma. *In* Swerdlow SH, Campo E, Harris NL, Jaffe ES, Pileri S, Stein H and Thiele J (Eds) *WHO Classification of Tumours of Haematopoietic and Lymphoid Tissues*, revised 4th Edn. IARC Press, Lyon, pp. 167–168.

---

13 Plasmablastic myeloma

Plasmablastic myeloma:

1) Can represent disease evolution
2) Has a high proliferation index on Ki-67 staining
3) Has a worse prognosis than other cases of myeloma
4) Is associated with worse renal function than other cases of myeloma
5) Is associated with a higher serum calcium than other cases of myeloma

Correct answers 1, 2, 3, 5

Plasmablastic myeloma can occur *de novo* or represent disease evolution (Greipp *et al.* 1998, Lee *et al.* 2003). In a comparison with other cases, *de novo* plasmablastic myeloma is found to be a more aggressive disease with a high proliferation index and a worse prognosis (Greipp *et al.* 1998). In this large series of patients, an association was found with higher calcium levels but not with more renal impairment (Greipp *et al.* 1998). When plasmablastic myeloma represents transformation, there may be extramedullary disease.

References

Greipp PR, Leong T, Bennett JM, Gaillard JP, Klein B, Stewart JA *et al.* (1998) Plasmablastic morphology – an independent prognostic factor with clinical and laboratory correlates: Eastern Cooperative Oncology Group (ECOG) myeloma trial E9486 report by the ECOG Myeloma Laboratory Group. *Blood*, **91**, 2501–2507.

Lee CK, Ma ES, Shek TW, Lam CC, Au WY, Wan TS and Chan LC (2003) Plasmablastic transformation of multiple myeloma. *Hum Pathol*, **34**, 710–714.

---

14 Septicaemia

Neutrophil vacuolation can be a feature of:

1) Bacterial infection
2) Chédiak–Higashi syndrome
3) Ethanol toxicity
4) Neonatal necrotising enterocolitis
5) Neutral lipid storage disease

Correct answers 1, 3, 4, 5

Neutrophil abnormalities in sepsis include neutrophilia, toxic granulation, Döhle bodies, left shift and neutrophil vacuolation. Neutrophil vacuolation is particularly characteristic of bacterial infection and is so common in neonatal necrotising enterocolitis that, in its absence, the diagnosis is unlikely. Uncommonly it is observed as a feature of ethanol toxicity (Chetty-Raju *et al.* 2005). Chédiak–Higashi syndrome is not associated with vacuolation whereas it is a feature of a number of rare inherited lipid storage disorders (Markesbery *et al.* 1974, Chanarin *et al.* 1975, Lainey *et al.* 2008).

References

Chanarin I, Patel A, Slavin G, Wills EJ, Andrews TM and Stewart G (1975) Neutral-lipid storage disease: a new disorder of lipid metabolism. *BMJ*, **i**, 553–555.

Chetty-Raju N, Cook R and Erber W (2005) Vacuolated neutrophils in ethanol toxicity. *Br J Haematol*, **127**, 478.

Lainey E, Ogier H and Fenneteau O (2008) Vacuolation of neutrophils and acanthocytosis in a child with medium chain acyl-CoA dehydrogenase deficiency. *Br J Haematol*, **140**, 595.

Markesbery WR, McQuillen MP, Procopis PG, Harrison AR and Engel AG (1974) Muscle carnitine deficiency: association with lipid myopathy, vacuolar neuropathy, and vacuolated leukocytes. *Arch Neurol*, **31**, 320–324.

---

15 An unstable haemoglobin and a myeloproliferative neoplasm

Unstable haemoglobins:

1) Affect only the α or β globin chain
2) Can be associated with the presence of two variant haemoglobins as well as haemoglobin A
3) Can be detected by instability on heating or exposure to isopropanol
4) Have normal oxygen affinity
5) When clinically manifest, usually indicate homozygosity

Correct answers 2, 3

Unstable haemoglobins can result from mutation in an α, β, γ or δ globin gene. Because of the low percentage of haemoglobin A_2, δ globin gene mutations leading to instability of haemoglobin A_2 are of no clinical significance. Curiously, several patients have been described with two unstable haemoglobins, together with haemoglobin A. This potentially confusing observation results not from three β genes in the genome but from post-translational modification of an unstable haemoglobin. Detection requires a heat or isopropanol instability test, since there is not necessarily any abnormality on electrophoresis or high-performance liquid chromatography. Oxygen affinity can be abnormal, either increased or decreased. Most unstable haemoglobins cause clinical and haematological abnormalities in heterozygotes. Homozygosity is very rare.

---

16 Sickle cell anaemia in crisis

Causes of worsening anaemia that would be likely in a 30-year-old African or Afro-Caribbean woman with sickle cell anaemia include:

1) Folic acid deficiency
2) Haemolytic crisis
3) Parvovirus B19 infection
4) Splenic infarction
5) Splenic sequestration

Correct answers 1, 2

Worsening anaemia in a child with sickle cell anaemia can be due to splenic sequestration or parvovirus B19 infection but these would not be expected in an adult of African ancestry. Splenic sequestration beyond childhood is only likely in a patient with sickle cell anaemia associated with the Arab-Indian haplotype, when the higher haemoglobin F level can preserve the spleen from the recurrent infarction that leads to atrophy and fibrosis. Splenic infarction does not cause anaemia. Folic acid deficiency can lead to megaloblastic anaemia if a patient with sickle cell disease fails to take supplementary folic acid. In this patient haemolysis associated with malaria is the likely cause of the Hb being lower than otherwise expected. In other circumstances, a rapid fall in Hb following blood transfusion can be indicative of a transfusion reaction or hyperhaemolysis, in which recipient as well as donor cells are destroyed.

The blood film can be useful in suggesting some of the causes of worsening anaemia. Absence of polychromasia (and a low reticulocyte count) can indicate parvovirus B19 infection. Folic acid deficiency may show hypersegmented neutrophils and macrocytes.

---

17 Acute myeloid leukaemia with t(8;21)(q22;q22.1)

Acute myeloid leukaemia with t(8;21)(q22;q22.1); *RUNX1-RUNX1T1*:

1) Can be diagnosed despite blast cells being less than 20% in blood and bone marrow
2) May have an increase in bone marrow eosinophils and precursors
3) Often shows trilineage dysplasia
4) Should be classified as mixed phenotype acute leukaemia when there is expression of CD19, CD79a and PAX5
5) Shows an association with systemic mastocytosis with a *KIT* D816V mutation

Correct answers 1, 2, 5

This type of AML can be recognised despite not having 20% or more blast cells in the peripheral blood or bone marrow. Eosinophils are often increased in the bone marrow and occasionally there is significant peripheral blood eosinophilia. Dysplasia is largely confined to the granulocyte lineage, where it can be prominent. In addition to nuclear abnormalities, neutrophils may show uniform salmon-pink cytoplasm, Auer rods and, occasionally, giant (pseudo-Chédiak–Higashi) granules. There is an association with systemic mastocytosis (Bernd *et al.* 2004). The B-lineage markers, CD19 and PAX5, are often aberrantly expressed and sometimes also CD79a; however this does not lead to classification as mixed phenotype acute leukaemia (Arber *et al.* 2017).

References

Arber DA, Brunning RD, Le Beau MM, Falini B, Vardiman JW, Porwit A *et al.* (2017) Acute myeloid leukaemia (AML) with recurrent genetic abnormalities. *In* Swerdlow SH, Campo E, Harris NL, Jaffe ES, Pileri S, Stein H and Thiele J (Eds) *WHO Classification of Tumours of Haematopoietic and Lymphoid Tissues*, revised 4th Edn. IARC Press, Lyon, pp. 130−149.

Bernd H-W, Sotlar K, Lorenzen J, Osieka R, Fabry U, Valent P and Horny H-P (2004) Acute myeloid leukaemia with t(8;21) associated with "occult" mastocytosis. Report of an unusual case and review of the literature. *J Clin Pathol*, **57**, 324–328.

---

18   Chronic neutrophilic leukaemia

Increased neutrophil granulation ('toxic' granulation) is a usual feature of:

1) Chronic myeloid leukaemia, *BCR-ABL1*-positive
2) Chronic neutrophilic leukaemia
3) G-CSF (filgrastim) therapy
4) Leukaemoid reaction to multiple myeloma
5) Sepsis

Correct answers 2, 3, 4, 5

In patients with sepsis, toxic granulation is due to increased granulocyte colony-stimulating factor (G-CSF) synthesis whereas in a leukaemoid reaction to multiple myeloma and monoclonal gammopathy of undetermined significance it is due to production of G-CSF by neoplastic plasma cells (Bain and Ahmad 2015). Other tumours can similarly secrete G-CSF leading to neutrophilia with toxic granulation. In chronic neutrophilic leukaemia, toxic granulation is due to mutation in the gene that encodes the receptor for G-CSF, leading either to both constitutive overexpression of the receptor and ligand hypersensitivity or to cells becoming ligand independent (Maxson *et al.* 2013). *BCR-ABL1*-positive chronic myeloid leukaemia does not have any abnormality of neutrophil granulation. In chronic neutrophilic leukaemia there can also be neutrophil vacuolation and Döhle bodies. It is important to be aware that these abnormalities can be present in myeloid neoplasms as well as in reactive neutrophilia.

References

Bain BJ and Ahmad S (2015) Chronic neutrophilic leukaemia and plasma cell-related neutrophilic leukaemoid reactions. *Br J Haematol*, **171**, 400−410.

Maxson JE, Gotlib J, Pollyea DA, Fleischman AG, Agarwal A, Eide CA *et al.* (2013) Oncogenic CSF3R mutations in chronic neutrophilic leukemia and atypical CML. *New Engl J Med*, **368**, 1781–1790.

19 Essential thrombocythaemia

Essential thrombocythaemia:

1) Causes itch in a minority of patients
2) Is associated with *JAK2* V617F in more than half of patients
3) Is most often an incidental diagnosis in an asymptomatic patient
4) Is Ph+, *BCR-ABL1*+ in only a minority of patients
5) Typically has small platelets

Correct answers 1, 2, 3

Essential thrombocythaemia (ET) is now most often an incidental diagnosis. When there are clinical manifestations they can include headache, dizziness, visual disturbance, paraesthesia, peripheral vascular insufficiency, bleeding and thrombosis. Itch is present in a minority of patients. The *JAK2* V617F mutation is found in about two thirds of patients, *CALR* mutation in about a quarter and *MPL* mutation in 5–10%. The presence of *BCR-ABL1* excludes the diagnosis. Small platelets can be a feature of reactive thrombocytosis whereas in ET there is platelet anisocytosis with some large and giant platelets and sometimes some hypogranular platelets.

20 Hairy cell leukaemia

Hairy cell leukaemia:

1) Can be distinguished from chronic lymphocytic leukaemia on the basis of CD200 expression
2) Is associated with a *BRAF* V600E mutation in the majority of patients
3) Is best distinguished from hairy cell leukaemia variant by expression of CD25, CD123 and CD200
4) Requires assessment of tartrate-resistant acid phosphatase (TRAP) activity for a firm diagnosis
5) Usually has collagen fibrosis

Correct answers 2, 3

Hairy cell leukaemia typically shows expression of several markers that are otherwise uncommon in B-cell neoplasms, specifically CD11c (strongly expressed), CD25, CD103, CD123 and CD200. Of these, the most useful in making a distinction from hairy cell variant leukaemia are CD25, CD123 and CD200, which are usually negative in hairy cell leukaemia variant. CD200 expression is uncommon in other B-cell neoplasms but is expressed in chronic lymphocytic leukaemia so is of no use for making this distinction. CD10 can be expressed in HCL, as in the case presented here. Assessment of TRAP is not required unless appropriate immunophenotyping is unavailable. The discovery that the majority of patients have a *BRAF* V600E mutation has been very important for diagnosis since a monoclonal antibody that detects expression of the aberrant protein is now available. Reticulin fibrosis is common but collagen fibrosis is quite unusual.

21 Mantle cell lymphoma in leukaemic phase

Mantle cell lymphoma:

1) Can result from translocations involving *CCND1*, *CCND2* or *CCND3*
2) Is derived from marginal zone lymphocytes

3) Is the most common pathology underlying multiple lymphomatous polyposis
4) May show SOX11 expression on immunohistochemistry
5) Usually expresses CD200

Correct answers 1, 3, 4

Mantle cell lymphoma is usually associated with t(11;14)(q13;q32), which dysregulates the *CCND1* gene by proximity to the IGH locus, leading to expression of cyclin D1, the protein encoded by this gene. In a small minority of cases there is a variant translocation that leads to dysregulation of either *CCND2* or *CCND3*. Detection of SOX11 expression can be useful to confirm the diagnosis in cases that do not express cyclin D1 but expression is less likely in the leukaemic non-nodal subtype of the disease. This lymphoma originates within the mantle zone, which surrounds lymphoid follicles and is internal to the marginal zone. There is usually no expression of CD200, which is one of the many immunophenotypic features that permit a distinction from chronic lymphocytic leukaemia. Some cases present as multiple lymphomatous polyposis, with this being the lymphoma that most often underlies this diagnosis.

22	Infantile osteopetrosis

Infantile osteopetrosis can be associated with:

1) Autosomal recessive or dominant inheritance
2) Decreased osteoclasts
3) Fragile bones
4) Responsiveness to vitamin D that renders transplantation unnecessary
5) Increased osteoclasts

Correct answers 1, 2, 3, 5

Osteopetrosis, also known as marble bone disease, is a genetically heterogeneous group of disorders, which can be either autosomal recessive or autosomal dominant (Mazzolari *et al.* 2009, Blank 2017, Online Mendelian Inheritance in Man 2021). The infantile form is autosomal recessive and at least five genes have been implicated. Autosomal dominant cases are milder and occur later in life, with at least three genes being implicated. There is also an X-linked form of the disease. In infantile osteopetrosis, the blood film can be leucoerythroblastic and extramedullary haemopoiesis can lead to hepatosplenomegaly.

   Osteopetrosis results from decreased osteoclast function. Osteoclast numbers can be reduced, normal or increased. Paradoxically, although bones are dense and bone mass is increased, abnormal fragility can lead to pathological fractures. Vitamin D can lead to a short-term response but is not a definitive form of treatment for infantile cases.

References

Blank R (2017) Osteopetrosis. https://emedicine.medscape.com/article/123968
Mazzolari E, Forino C, Razza A, Porta F, Villa A and Notarangelo LD (2009) A single-center experience in 20 patients with infantile malignant osteopetrosis. *Am J Hematol*, **84**, 473–479.
Online Mendelian Inheritance in Man. https://www.omim.org/ (accessed January 2021).

23 Reactive eosinophilia

Reactive eosinophilia can occur in:

1) Acute lymphoblastic leukaemia
2) Acute myeloid leukaemia associated with inv(16)
3) Babesiosis
4) Filariasis
5) Strongyloidiasis

Correct answers 1, 4, 5

Reactive eosinophilia can occur in acute lymphoblastic leukaemia but in acute myeloid leukaemia associated with inv(16) the eosinophils are clonal and neoplastic. Other haematological neoplasms that can be associated with reactive eosinophilia include Hodgkin lymphoma, non-Hodgkin lymphoma and Sézary syndrome. Eosinophilia is a feature of filariasis and strongyloidiasis and many other parasitic infections but not of babesiosis.

Although the cytological features of eosinophils are not particularly helpful in making a diagnosis, careful examination of the blood film may provide convincing evidence of an underlying diagnosis with the observation of blast cells, lymphoma cells, Sézary cells, mast cells or filaria (Butt *et al.* 2017). When a drug reaction is causative there can also be reactive lymphocytes.

Reference

Butt NM, Lambert J, Ali S, Beer PA, Cross NC, Duncombe A *et al.*; British Committee for Standards in Haematology (2017) Guideline for the investigation and management of eosinophilia. *Br J Haematol*, **176**, 553–572.

24 Stomatocytic red cell disorders

Stomatocytosis can be a feature of:

1) Alcoholic excess and alcoholic liver disease
2) Hereditary xerocytosis
3) Hydroxycarbamide therapy
4) Triose phosphate isomerase deficiency
5) Zieve syndrome

Correct answers 1, 2, 3

Stomatocytes are characteristic of a number of inherited conditions but are more commonly seen as an acquired phenomenon, being associated with alcohol excess, with chronic liver disease, particularly due to alcohol, and with hydroxycarbamide, chlorpromazine and vinca alkaloid therapy (Ohsaka *et al.* 1989); they have even been reported in long distance runners immediately after the race (Reinhart and Chien 1985). They can also develop artefactually in normal individuals if blood films are poorly dried. In alcoholic liver disease and during hydroxycarbamide therapy there is both macrocytosis and stomatocytosis. Zieve syndrome is also associated with liver disease but in this case the typical cell associated with a haemolytic anaemia is an irregularly contracted cell.

Among the relevant inherited conditions, the overhydrated variant of hereditary stomatocytosis, as exemplified by the third patient, is associated with numerous stomatocytes.

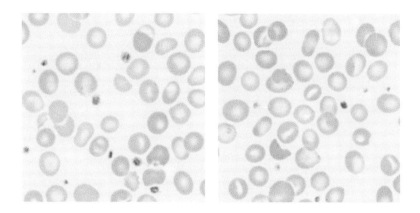

The dehydrated variant of hereditary stomatocytosis, also known as hereditary xerocytosis (images above ×100 objective), also has stomatocytes but they are much less numerous and there are also echinocytes, hypochromia, haemoglobin puddling and irregularly contracted cells. Hereditary spherocytosis due to protein 4.2 deficiency can have spherostomatocytes as well as typical spherocytes so that the differential diagnosis with hereditary xerocytosis can be difficult. Splenectomy is contraindicated in both variants of hereditary stomatocytosis so correct diagnosis is important (Andolfo *et al.* 2018). The diagnosis of Southeast Asian ovalocytosis is not, however, problematical, since the blood film is very distinctive. Diagnosis of this condition can be important in a pregnant woman since there is dominant inheritance and significant anaemia can occur in neonates. Hereditary phytosterolaemia, as exemplified by the second patient, is an example of stomatocytosis that is not due to an intrinsic red cell disorder but to a disorder of lipid metabolism. Red cell enzyme deficiencies are not associated with stomatocytosis.

References

Andolfo I, Russo R, Gambale A and Iolascon A (2018) Hereditary stomatocytosis: An underdiagnosed condition. *Am J Hematol*, **93**, 107–121.

Ohsaka A, Kano Y, Sakamoto S, Kanzaki A, Hashimoto M, Yawata Y and Miura Y (1989) A transient hemolytic reaction and stomatocytosis following vinca alkaloid administration. *Nihon Ketsueki Gakkai Zasshi*, **52**, 7–17.

Reinhart WH and Chien S (1985) Stomatocytic transformation of red blood cells after marathon running. *Am J Hematol*, **19**, 201–204.

25 Reactive lymphocytosis due to viral infection

Infectious mononucleosis due to the Epstein–Barr virus:

1) Can be associated with pure red cell aplasia
2) Can be complicated by haemophagocytic lymphohistiocytosis
3) Can be followed by aplastic anaemia

4) Is associated with a subsequent increased incidence of Hodgkin lymphoma
5) Predisposes to B-lineage acute lymphoblastic leukaemia

Correct answers 1, 2, 3, 4

Pure red cell aplasia, aplastic anaemia and haemophagocytic lymphohistiocytosis are all recognised, albeit uncommon or rare, complications of infectious mononucleosis (Grishaber *et al.* 1988, Xu *et al.* 2013). Primary EBV infection is associated with an increased incidence of Hodgkin lymphoma thereafter but there is no association with acute lymphoblastic leukaemia.

References

Grishaber JE, McClain KL, Mahoney DH and Fernbach DJ (1988) Successful outcome of severe aplastic anemia following Epstein–Barr virus infection. *Am J Hematol*, **28**, 273–275.
Xu L-H, Fang J-P, Weng W-J, Huang K, Guo H-X, Liu Y and Zhang J-H (2013) Pure red cell aplasia associated with cytomegalovirus and Epstein-Barr virus infection in seven cases of Chinese children. *Hematology*, **18**, 56–59.

> **26** Therapy-related acute myeloid leukaemia with eosinophilia

Therapy-related acute leukaemia:

1) Can be associated with 5q−, monosomy 5, 7q− and monosomy 7
2) Can be lymphoblastic or myeloid
3) Has an equally poor prognosis, regardless of the causative agent, the blast percentage or any cytogenetic abnormalities present
4) Has identical characteristics whether it follows alkylating agents or topoisomerase II inhibitors
5) Increases in incidence with the age of exposure to the causative agent

Correct answers 1, 2, 5

Abnormalities of chromosome 5 and chromosome 7 are commonly present. Complex karyotypes, often including del(3p), del(11q), del(13q), del(20q) and loss of the short arm or the whole chromosome 17, are common. More than 90% of cases show a cytogenetic abnormality. Mutations in *TP53* are common. The leukaemia can be lymphoblastic or myeloid, the former being associated particularly with t(9;22)(q34.1;q11.2) (Block *et al.* 2002) or with rearrangements of *KMT2A*. Cases that follow topoisomerase II inhibitors can have balanced chromosomal translocations including t(8;21)(q22;q22.1) and inv(16)(p13.1q22); they have a shorter latent period and a better prognosis than cases following alkylating agents. The blast percentage is not of major prognostic significance with even therapy-related myeloid neoplasms classified as myelodysplastic syndrome rather than as acute leukaemia generally having a poor prognosis. Interestingly, cases following alkylating agents increase in incidence with increasing age.

Reference

Block A-MW, Carroll AJ, Hagemeijer A, Michaux L, van Lom K, Olney HJ and Baer MR (2002) Rare recurring balanced chromosome abnormalities in therapy-related myelodysplastic syndromes and acute leukemia: report from an International Workshop. *Genes Chromosomes Cancer*, **33**, 401–412.

27   Red cell fragmentation syndromes

Microangiopathic haemolytic anaemia can result from:

1) A defective prosthetic cardiac valve
2) Haemolytic uraemic syndrome following *Escherichia coli* O157:H7 infection
3) Pregnancy-associated HELLP syndrome
4) Severe aortic or mitral valve disease
5) Thrombotic thrombocytopenic purpura

Correct answers 2, 3, 5

Microangiopathic haemolytic anaemia (MAHA) is an important haematological condition to recognise. Similar haematological changes can result from trauma to red cells in large blood vessels and can be seen with failing heart valves or as a result of a ventricular assist device, as seen in the third patient, but these are not designated MAHA. Red cell fragmentation resulting from microvascular disease and fibrin deposition has diverse aetiologies, including haemolytic uraemic syndrome, thrombotic thrombocytopenic purpura and the pregnancy-associated **H**aemolysis, **E**levated **L**iver enzymes, **L**ow **P**latelets (HELLP) syndrome. Some of the conditions that give rise to MAHA are life-threatening and require urgent intervention. A careful assessment of an underlying clinical trigger is therefore critical. Most cases result either from activation of coagulation (DIC), as a result of sepsis, disseminated carcinoma or acute promyelocytic leukaemia, or from multifocal small vessel platelet aggregation typically seen in thrombotic thrombocytopenic purpura and haemolytic uraemic syndrome. The blood film assessment can be very important in highlighting a potential diagnosis to other clinical specialties.

28   NK/T-cell lymphoma in leukaemic phase

Extranodal NK/T-cell lymphoma, nasal type:

1) Does not involve lymph nodes
2) Is angiocentric
3) Is strongly associated with EBV
4) Is usually cCD3 negative on flow cytometry
5) Occurs only in Chinese and other Asian populations

Correct answers 2, 3, 4

Although this lymphoma is primarily extranodal, secondary lymph node involvement can occur. Typically, the lesions are angiocentric with vascular damage and necrosis and sometimes ulceration of overlying mucous membrane. There is a very strong association with EBV, which is present in clonal form in the lymphoma cells. Although flow cytometry showed cytoplasmic expression of CD3 in this patient, this is variable in practice and depends on the target CD3 epitope of the diagnostic antibody. About 90% of cases are of NK lineage and only 10% of T lineage. Immunohistochemistry, however, often shows cCD3 expression as the antibody used detects CD3ε, which is expressed by NK cells. This lymphoma is most often seen in China, Korea and Japan but is not confined to these populations. It occurs also in Mexico, in Central and South America, in some Pacific islands and sporadically in other countries.

---

29 Myelodysplastic syndrome with del(5q)

The WHO category of myelodysplastic syndrome with isolated del(5q):

1) By definition, cannot have any other cytogenetic abnormality
2) By definition, can have thrombocytopenia but not thrombocytosis
3) Can benefit from lenalidomide therapy
4) Has a poor prognosis
5) Is more common in females

Correct answers 3, 5

Counterintuitively, the WHO category designated 'myelodysplastic syndrome with isolated del(5q)' can have another single cytogenetic abnormality as long as this is not monosomy 7 or del(7q). The definition was changed between the 2008 and 2016 WHO classifications but without a change of name (Hasserjian *et al.* 2017). The reason for the change was that the relatively good prognosis is not altered by an extra cytogenetic abnormality other than those of chromosome 7. Thrombocytosis is also compatible with this diagnosis, being seen in a third or more of patients. It should be noted that the cytologically abnormal megakaryocytes in this condition are small but they are not 'micro'; micromegakaryocytes are similar in size to a promyelocyte and are associated with a worse prognosis. The 5q– megakaryocyte is correctly described as 'non-lobated' not 'monolobated' since the nucleus has no lobes.

  The pathogenetic mechanism is likely to be haploinsufficiency for one or more of the genes that are found in the commonly deleted segment. The interstitial deletion is generally detectable on standard cytogenetic analysis or, if this fails, on FISH. Rarely the deletion is cryptic (Medlock *et al.* 2017) so observation of the typical cytological abnormalities should lead to further investigation if the expected abnormality is not detected on cytogenetic or FISH analysis.

This diagnosis is important because of the responsiveness to lenalidomide, which can lead to a cytogenetic as well as haematological response.

References

Hasserjian RP, Le Beau MM, List AF, Bennett JM, Brunning RD and Thiele J (2017) Myelodysplastic syndrome with isolated del(5q). *In* Swerdlow SH, Campo E, Harris NL, Jaffe ES, Pileri S, Stein H and Thiele J (Eds) *WHO Classification of Tumours of Haematopoietic and Lymphoid Tissues*, revised 4th Edn. IARC Press, Lyon, pp. 115–116.

Medlock R, Barrans S, Cargo C and Kelly R (2017) Cryptic 5q deletion in a patient with myelodysplastic syndrome. *Br J Haematol*, **177**, 347.

---

30 Classical Hodgkin lymphoma

Classical Hodgkin lymphoma:

1) Has the Epstein–Barr virus (EBV) as an aetiological factor in a significant proportion of cases
2) Is a neoplasm of uncertain lineage
3) Is increased in frequency in patients carrying the human immunodeficiency virus (HIV)

4) Is more common in children and adolescents in developing countries than in developed countries

5) When the bone marrow is infiltrated, can usually be diagnosed by the presence of Reed–Sternberg cells and mononuclear Hodgkin cells in a bone marrow aspirate

Correct answers 1, 3, 4

Despite obvious bone marrow involvement by Hodgkin lymphoma it is rarely possible to identify the neoplastic cells in the bone marrow aspirate since associated fibrosis makes aspiration of the neoplastic cells difficult. The images below are from a patient with confirmed bone marrow involvement by Hodgkin lymphoma. Remarkably, both Reed–Sternberg and mononuclear Hodgkin cells are clearly visible in the aspirate (×100 objective). When encountered it is important to consider this diagnosis and recognise these cells for what they are and what they represent.

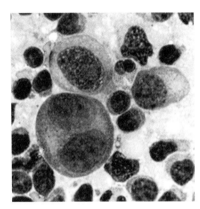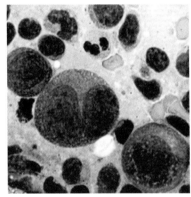

Known factors contributing to the aetiology of classical Hodgkin lymphoma include HIV and EBV infection. EBV has a directly oncogenic role whereas HIV infection is relevant because of the resultant immune deficiency. The proportion of cases where EBV has an aetiological role varies between developed and developing countries with a higher proportion of such cases being seen in developing countries. This accounts for the higher proportion of cases in children and adolescents in developing countries where this viral infection tends to occur at a younger age. The neoplastic cells in classical Hodgkin lymphoma are known to be B cells, although crippling mutations in various genes lead to failure to express many normal B-cell antigens. Expression of PAX5, as in this patient, provides evidence of their B-cell nature. A minority of cases also express CD20, usually weakly, whilst CD79a expression is usually weak or absent. The occasional transformation of follicular lymphoma to classical Hodgkin lymphoma provides indirect evidence of the B-cell nature of the latter.

---

31 Cryoglobulinaemia

Type II cryoglobulinaemia:

1) Can be a feature of hepatitis C infection
2) Can occur in Sjögren syndrome
3) Has no monoclonal component

4) Is occasionally a feature of a lymphoproliferative disorder
5) Is typically found in multiple myeloma

Correct answers 1, 2, 4

Cryoglobulinaemia was first described by Wintrobe and Buell, as long ago as 1933, in a patient with myeloma (Wintrobe and Buell 1933) with the term 'cryoglobulin' being first used in 1947 (Lerner and Watson 1947).

Type II cryoglobulinaemia, by definition, has a monoclonal component. This monoclonal component has rheumatoid factor activity and complexes polyclonal immunoglobulin. Type II cryoglobulinaemia is often a feature of hepatitis C infection and sometimes of Sjögren syndrome or other autoimmune disease. Less often it is the result of a lymphoproliferative disorder (Bryce *et al.* 2006, Mogabgab *et al.* 2016). It is type I rather than type II cryoglobulinaemia that is typically found in multiple myeloma and lymphoplasmacytic lymphoma. Autoimmune diseases can also be also associated with type III cryoglobulinaemia.

References

Bryce AH, Kyle RA, Dispenzieri A and Gertz MA (2006) Natural history and therapy of 66 patients with mixed cryoglobulinaemia. *Am J Hematol*, **81**, 511–518.

Lerner A and Watson C (1947) Studies of cryoglobulins: unusual purpura associated with the presence of a high concentration of cryoglobulin (cold precipitable serum globulin). *Am J Med Sci*, **214**, 410–415.

Mogabgab ON, Osman NY, Wei K, Batal I and Loscalzo J (2016) Clinical problem-solving. A complementary affair. *N Engl J Med*, **374**, 74–81.

Wintrobe M and Buell M (1933) Hyperproteinemia associated with multiple myeloma, with report of case in which extraordinary hyperproteinemia was associated with thrombosis of retinal veins and symptoms suggesting Raynaud's disease. *Bull Johns Hopkins Hosp*, **52**, 156–165.

32 Congenital dyserythropoietic anaemia

Congenital dyserythropoietic anaemia type I is characterised by:

1) A positive acid lysis test
2) Frequent splenomegaly and gallstones
3) Giant erythroblasts with multiple nuclei
4) Internuclear chromatin bridges
5) Responsiveness to interferon

Correct answers 2, 4, 5

Congenital dyserythropoietic anaemia (CDA) represents a rare constellation of inherited red cell disorders, which are assigned to three main categories based on morphological and genetic characteristics: types I, II and III. It is impossible to discuss this condition without identifying the important scientific contribution to the understanding of all forms of CDA from our late haematology colleague Sunitha Wickramasinghe. His publications on this subject are too numerous to cover here but this review is notable (Wickramasinghe and Wood 2005).

Congenital dyserythropoietic anaemia type I, is characterised by ineffective erythropoiesis, intramedullary death of erythroid precursors and multiple morphological abnormalities of erythroblasts (Roy and Babbs 2019). Internuclear chromatin bridges (in a minority of erythroblasts) are among the characteristic abnormalities in CDA type I, whereas giant multinucleated erythroblasts are a feature of CDA type III. A positive acid lysis test characterises CDA type II. Minor skeletal abnormalities such as syndactyly are seen in some type I patients but the bony exostoses in this patient are likely unrelated. Gallstones are found in more than half of adult patients. The spleen is often palpable and imaging shows that splenomegaly is usual. CDA type I typically presents with a macrocytic anaemia of variable severity with iron loading, with Hb ranging from 70 g/l to normal in different families. In fact, the relative preservation of the Hb levels in this patient had initially somewhat diverted the investigating team from this possible diagnosis. Misdiagnosis of CDA is not rare, with wrong diagnoses including membrane defects, enzyme defects and myelodysplastic syndromes. A correct diagnosis is important because of responsiveness of type I to alpha interferon and the need to manage iron overload.

The images below (×100 objective) show CDA type II, also known as Hempas — **H**ereditary **E**rythroid **M**ultinuclearity with **P**ositive **A**cidified **S**erum test. Morphologically it is characterised by bi- and multinuclearity and erythroblasts with lobulated nuclei.

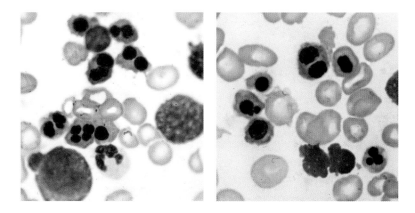

CDA type III (images below ×100) has the most distinctive cytology with giant erythroblasts, which can have a single nucleus or be multinucleated.

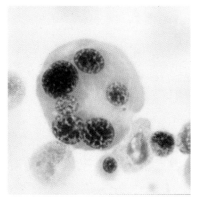
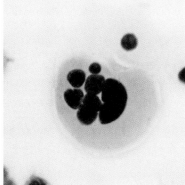

References

Roy NBA and Babbs C (2019) The pathogenesis, diagnosis and management of congenital dyserythropoiesis type I. *Br J Haematol*, **185**, 436–449.

Wickramasinghe SN and Wood WG (2005) Advances in the understanding of the congenital dyserythropoietic anaemias. *Br J Haematol*, **131**, 431–446.

---

33   Acute monoblastic leukaemia with t(9;11)(p21.3;q23.3)

Acute monoblastic/monocytic leukaemia associated with t(9;11)(p21.3;q23.3):

1) Can occur following therapy with topoisomerase II-interactive drugs
2) Is more likely than acute myeloblastic leukaemia to have infiltration of gums, skin and other extramedullary sites
3) Not infrequently expresses CD4, CD11b, CD14, CD64 and strong HLA-DR
4) Often has blast cells that do not express CD34 or myeloperoxidase
5) Should be confirmed by non-specific esterase staining

Correct answers 1, 2, 3, 4

Acute leukaemia with t(9;11) can follow therapy with topoisomerase II-interactive drugs and is then classified as a therapy-related myeloid neoplasm rather than being assigned to the WHO category acute myeloid leukaemia with t(9;11)(p21.3;q23.3); *KMT2A-MLLT3*.

Monoblastic leukaemia, including cases with this translocation, has a predilection for extramedullary sites with involvement of gingivae, skin (leukaemia cutis), soft tissues, lymph nodes and the CNS not infrequently being reported either at diagnosis or relapse. CNS localisation presents a serious therapeutic challenge needing both intrathecal and CNS-penetrating systemic cytotoxic drugs and furthermore it frequently heralds systemic relapse of the leukaemia.

The blast cells express markers characteristic of immature cells of the monocyte lineage but may fail to express CD34 and MPO. Non-specific esterase is strongly positive but is not necessary for diagnosis, except in a resource-constrained environment.

---

34   Chronic myeloid leukaemia presenting with myeloid sarcoma

---

The peripheral blood in *BCR-ABL1*-positive chronic myeloid leukaemia (CML):

1) Can show occasional nucleated red blood cells and megakaryocyte nuclei
2) Characteristically shows a double peak of myelocytes and neutrophils
3) Has monocytes increased in proportion to the increase in neutrophils
4) Often shows hypogranular neutrophils
5) Rarely shows thrombocytosis without leucocytosis

Correct answers 1, 2, 5

The peripheral blood differential count in CML typically shows a double peak of myelocytes and segmented neutrophils, with fewer promyelocytes than myelocytes and fewer blast cells than promyelocytes (Spiers *et al.* 1977). Basophilia is almost invariably present with eosinophilia being present in about 90% of cases. Neutrophils are normally granulated. Nucleated red blood cells and megakaryocyte nuclei may be seen. The monocyte count is increased but, except in the rare cases with a variant breakpoint and a p190 BCR-ABL1 protein, monocytes are NOT increased in proportion to neutrophils. Thrombocytosis without leucocytosis is found in about 1% of patients (Savage *et al.* 1997).

References

Savage DG, Szydlo RM and Goldman JM (1997) Clinical features at diagnosis in 430 patients with chronic myeloid leukaemia seen at a referral centre over a 16-year period. *Br J Haematol*, **96**, 111–116.

Spiers ASD, Bain BJ and Turner JE (1977) The peripheral blood in chronic granulocytic leukaemia. *Scand J Haematol*, **18**, 25–38.

---

35   Glucose-6-phosphate dehydrogenase deficiency

Heinz bodies:

1) Are removed by the spleen
2) Are specific for defects of the pentose shunt
3) Can be detected during acute haemolytic episodes in G6PD deficiency
4) Can sometimes be identified on an MGG-stained blood film
5) Represent denatured haemoglobin

Correct answers 1, 3, 4, 5

Heinz bodies are precipitates of denatured haemoglobin resulting from oxidant damage. They are removed from circulating red cells by splenic macrophages, resulting in formation of a 'bite cell' or keratocyte. They can be detected by supravital staining with methylene violet. However, they can often also be detected in an MGG-stained film, either protruding from a cell or as an inclusion within the otherwise empty cytoplasm of a ghost or hemighost cell (Bain 2008).

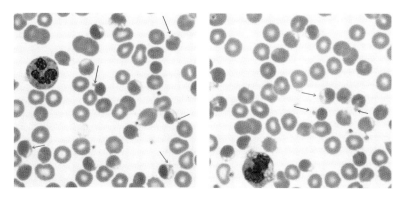

The images above (×100 objective), from a heterozygous woman who suffered haemolysis after eating fava beans, show irregularly contracted cells and hemighosts. However, in addition they show Heinz bodies protruding from erythrocytes (red arrows) and Heinz bodies within the otherwise empty cytoplasm of hemighosts (green arrows). Although characteristic of haemolysis resulting from defects in the pentose shunt, the presence of Heinz bodies can also reflect the presence of an unstable haemoglobin or can result from exposure to a strongly oxidant drug or chemical in a patient with normal red cell enzymes.

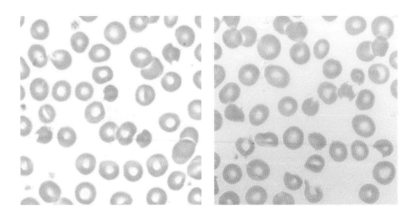

The images above (×100) are from a patient with a skin disorder and mild anaemia on dapsone therapy. Note the prominent bite cells and the irregularly contracted cells. However, the full spectrum of features seen in acute oxidative haemolysis in the context of G6PD deficiency are not present here. Drug-induced oxidant haemolysis is sometimes overinterpreted as indicative of G6PD deficiency. The clinical history is important, with consideration of the ethnic origin, the gender and any exposure to oxidant substances, including industrial chemicals and recreational agents.

References

Bain BJ (2008) Sudden onset of jaundice in a Sardinian man. *Am J Hematol*, **83**, 810.

---

36 Leukaemic presentation of hepatosplenic γδ T-cell lymphoma

---

Hepatosplenic T-cell lymphoma:

1) Consistently expresses γδ T-cell receptor
2) Has a good prognosis
3) Has a strong association with isochromosome 7q
4) Not infrequently arises in the setting of chronic immune suppression
5) Rarely involves the bone marrow

Correct answers 3, 4

Hepatosplenic T-cell lymphoma is a rare T-cell neoplasm, often presenting with infiltration of these organs, absent lymphadenopathy and a karyotype typically showing isochromosome 7q. The prognosis is poor. The majority of cases express γδ T-cell receptor (TCR) but in a minority there is expression of αβ TCR with or without γδ TCR. This is recognised as an immunosuppression-related lymphoma in around a fifth of cases, both following transplantation and associated with immuno-suppressive treatment of inflammatory bowel disease. The bone marrow is often involved, with intrasinusoidal infiltration being typical. A leukaemic presentation is very unusual with this mostly being recognised at disease relapse.

It is important to recognise this entity and differentiate it from acute lymphoblastic leukaemia as the treatment algorithm is very different. As noted here, the subtle but unusual order of antigen acquisition for T-ALL and the clinical presentation led to a consideration of the confirmed diagnosis.

---

37 Myelodysplastic syndromes

Hypogranularity of neutrophils can be a feature of:

1) Chédiak–Higashi syndrome
2) Human immunodeficiency virus (HIV) infection
3) Inherited specific granule deficiency
4) Myelokathexis
5) Therapy-related acute myeloid leukaemia

Correct answers 2, 3, 5

Rarely, hypogranularity of neutrophils is congenital, as in specific granule deficiency (previously known as lactoferrin deficiency) (McIlwaine *et al*. 2013) and in several rare congenital neutrope-nias. In Chédiak–Higashi syndrome, granules are large and have abnormal staining characteris-tics, whilst myelokathexis has hypersegmentation but normal granularity. HIV infection can cause a variety of dysplastic features, among which is variable neutrophil hypogranularity (Bain 1997). Hypogranularity can be a feature not only of MDS and myelodysplasia-related AML but also of therapy-related AML, which often has dysplastic features.

Neutrophil hypogranularity, due to a reduction of specific granules, is a strong pointer to MDS or a related myeloid neoplasm but it is necessary to be aware of other potential causes.

References

Bain BJ (1997) The haematological features of HIV infection. *Br J Haematol*, **99**, 1–8.
McIlwaine L, Parker A, Sandilands G, Gallipoli P and Leach M (2013) Neutrophil-specific granule deficiency. *Br J Haematol*, **160**, 735.

---

38 Pelger–Huët anomaly

The pseudo-Pelger–Huët anomaly can be a feature of:

1) Azathioprine therapy
2) Mycophenolate mofetil therapy
3) Myelodysplastic syndromes

4) Sodium valproate therapy
5) Therapy-related acute myeloid leukaemia

Correct answers 2, 3, 4, 5

An acquired (pseudo-)Pelger–Huët anomaly is often seen in MDS and in myelodysplasia-related and therapy-related AML and is of adverse prognostic significance. It is distinguished from the inherited anomaly by being present in a lower proportion of cells and often being accompanied by neutrophil hypogranularity and other dysplastic features. A pseudo-Pelger anomaly can also be caused by a number of immunosuppressive drugs, including mycophenolate mofetil and tacrolimus (Banerjee *et al.* 2000, Wang *et al.* 2011), but not azathioprine. Other drugs that can be causative include sodium valproate, palbociclib, taxols (paclitaxel and docetaxil) and ganciclovir (Banerjee *et al.* 2000, Wang *et al.* 2011). A clue to a drug-induced pseudo-Pelger anomaly is that sometimes there are also detached nuclear fragments.

References

Banerjee R, Halil O, Bain BJ, Cummins D and Banner NR (2000) Neutrophil dysplasia caused by mycophenolate mofetil. *Transplantation*, **70**, 1608–1610.
Wang E, Boswell E, Siddiqi I, Lu CM, Sebastian S, Rehder C and Huang Q (2011) Pseudo-Pelger–Huët anomaly induced by medications: a clinicopathologic study in comparison with myelodysplastic syndrome-related pseudo-Pelger–Huët anomaly. *Am J Clin Pathol*, **135**, 291–303.

---

39 Russell bodies in lymphoplasmacytic lymphoma

Recognised features when neoplastic cells show plasmacytic differentiation include:

1) Auer rods
2) Cytoplasmic crystals
3) Dutcher bodies
4) Flame cells
5) Mott cells

Correct answers 2, 3, 4, 5

Cells showing plasmacytic differentiation do not contain Auer rods, which by definition are myeloperoxidase positive. However, Auer rod-like inclusions are one of two types of crystalline inclusion that can occur with plasmacytic differentiation; they are composed of lysosomal enzymes and are azurophilic (Hütter *et al.* 2009). The other type of crystal is composed of immunoglobulin and is colourless. Immunoglobulin can also form globular inclusions as in Dutcher bodies (Dutcher and Fahey 1959) and Russell bodies (Russell 1890). It is of interest that when William Russell first described the eponymous inclusions in an address to the Pathological Society of London on 2 December 1890 and to the Medico-Chirurgical Society of Edinburgh the next day, he did not recognise that the inclusions were in plasma cells and thought that he had discovered the organism that caused cancer (Russell 1890). A Mott cell, also sometimes called a morular cell, has multiple small Russell bodies in its cytoplasm; it is named for Frederick Walker Mott, who described it in the brains of monkeys with trypanosomiasis (Mott 1905). Although these immunoglobulin inclusions are indicative of plasmacytic differentiation, none of them is specific for neoplasia. Flame cells have been associated particularly with IgA-secreting plasma cells.

Some Historical Names

William Russell, Scottish pathologist and physician (1852–1940)
Thomas F. Dutcher, American pathologist (1923–1999)
Frederick Walker Mott, British physician and pathologist (1853–1926)

References

Dutcher TF and Fahey JL (1959) The histopathology of the macroglobulinemia of Waldenström. *J Natl Cancer Inst*, **22**, 887–917.

Hütter G, Nowak D, Blau IW and Thiel E (2009) Auer rod like intracytoplasmic inclusions in multiple myeloma: A case report and review of literature. *Int J Lab Hematol*, **31**, 236–240.

Mott FW (1905) Observations on the brains of men and animals infected with various forms of trypanosomes. Preliminary note. *Proc Roy Soc London*, **76**, 235–242. https://doi.org/10.1098/rspb.1905.0016

Russell W (1890) An address on a characteristic organism of cancer. *BMJ*, **ii**, 1358–1360. https://www.ncbi.nlm.nih.gov/pmc/articles/PMC2208600/pdf/brmedj04652-0016.pdf

40	T-cell prolymphocytic leukaemia

T-cell prolymphocytic leukaemia:

1) Can respond to alemtuzumab, directed at CD52
2) Is aetiologically related to a retroviral infection
3) Is unusual among mature T-cell neoplasms in that both CD4 and CD8 may be expressed
4) Responds well to combination chemotherapy
5) Should be suspected if there is expression of CD7 by a mature T-cell neoplasm

Correct answers 1, 3, 5

T-cell prolymphocytic leukaemia is a rare mature T-cell neoplasm, typically presenting with a high leucocyte count, lymphadenopathy and hepatosplenomegaly. A significant proportion of patients show leukaemic skin infiltration and this can be quite unpleasant and disfiguring. The morphological characteristics are variable between cases, as shown here, where the spectrum of features is captured. The cells typically show a mature pan-T phenotype without antigen loss and are uniformly positive for CD26; the majority of cases express CD4 and not CD8, but CD4−CD8+ and CD4+CD8+ cases also occur. The expression of CD7 is diagnostically very useful since such expression is uncommon in neoplasms of mature T cells. The most frequent chromosomal abnormalities involve chromosome 14 with inversions or translocations involving breakpoints at 14q11.2 and 14q32.1. Abnormalities of chromosome 8, del(12p), del(22q) and amplification of 5p also occur and FISH and molecular studies may show deletions or missense mutations in the *ATM* gene at 11q22.3. There is no aetiological link to retroviral infection. The disease is aggressive and refractory to standard chemotherapy. Current approaches using alemtuzumab and purine analogues can achieve remissions in younger patients who can tolerate such therapy.

---

41 Myeloid maturation arrest

Maturation arrest in the granulocytic series can be a feature of:

1) Acute promyelocytic leukaemia
2) Copper deficiency
3) Drug-induced agranulocytosis
4) Myelokathexis
5) Some types of congenital neutropenia

Correct answers 1, 2, 3, 5

Maturation arrest at the promyelocyte stage is seen in acute promyelocytic leukaemia and drug-induced agranulocytosis. Some but not all congenital neutropenias show this feature; it has been reported, for example, in hyperimmunoglobulin M syndrome, Barth syndrome and with *SRP54* mutation. In myelokathexis, neutrophil morphology is abnormal but full myeloid maturation is seen. Arrest at the myelocyte stage has been described in copper deficiency. The patient described below illustrates another potential cause of myeloid maturation arrest.

A 55-year-old woman with rheumatoid arthritis (RA) developed neutropenia on methotrexate therapy, which failed to resolve on stopping the medication. Her marrow aspirate images below (×100 objective) show no maturation beyond the myelocyte stage. The neutropenia resolved with 3 days of granulocyte colony-stimulating factor (G-CSF) therapy. Patients with RA are prone to neutropenia due to myeloid maturation arrest either from effects of medication, as a component of Felty syndrome or in relation to coexistent large granular lymphocytic leukaemia (see Theme 10).

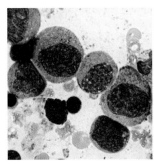 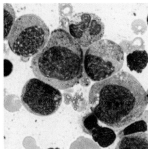 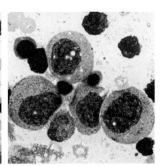

---

42 MDS/MPN with ring sideroblasts and thrombocytosis

Myelodysplastic/myeloproliferative neoplasm with ring sideroblasts and thrombocytosis (MDS/MPN-RS-T) is defined in the WHO classification by:

1) A platelet count of at least $450 \times 10^9/l$
2) At least 5% ring sideroblasts in the bone marrow if an *SF3B1* mutation is present
3) At least 15% ring sideroblasts in the bone marrow
4) Less than 20% bone marrow blast cells
5) No previous exposure to leukaemogenic drugs

Correct answers 1, 3, 5

Myelodysplastic/myeloproliferative neoplasm with ring sideroblasts and thrombocytosis is a disease of the elderly and anaemia is virtually always present. It is defined in the 2016 WHO classification as a condition characterised by the presence of thrombocytosis with ring sideroblasts being at least 15% of erythroblasts, with dyserythropoiesis and with less than 1% blast cells in the peripheral blood and less than 5% in the bone marrow (Orazi *et al.* 2017). This is now a well-defined entity with both dysplastic (ring sideroblasts) and proliferative (thrombocytosis) components, with the latter being driven by mutations in *JAK2* or, less often, *CALR* or *MPL*. By definition, the condition is *BCR-ABL1* negative. There is no consistent cytogenetic abnormality but mutations in *SF3B1* are frequent and the absence of such should cause one to question the diagnosis; a significant minority of patients have a mutation in *TET2*, *ASXL* or *DNMT2A* (Meggendorfer *et al.* 2018, Palomo *et al.* 2020). In the presence of an *SF3B1* mutation, 5% ring sideroblasts is sufficient for a diagnosis of myelodysplastic syndrome with ring sideroblasts but a diagnosis of MDS/MPN-RS-T requires the higher threshold. Therapy-related cases are categorised separately. Prognostic information is currently limited but empirically this condition carries a number of favourable features and therefore has an anticipated low risk of progression to AML. The ultimate dilemma is deciding on the relative merits of managing the proliferative and dysplastic elements as cytoreductive therapy, akin to that used in the management of essential thrombocythaemia, can often worsen the anaemia.

References

Meggendorfer M, Jeromin S. Haferlach C, Kern W and Haferlach T (2018) The mutational landscape of 18 investigated genes clearly separates four subtypes of myelodysplastic/myeloproliferative neoplasms. *Haematologica*, **103**, e192–e195.

Orazi A, Hasserjian RP, Cazzola M, Thiele J and Malcovati L (2017) Myelodysplastic/myeloproliferative neoplasm with ring sideroblasts and thrombocytosis (MDS/MPN-RS-T). *In* Swerdlow SH, Campo E, Harris NL, Jaffe ES, Pileri S, Stein H and Thiele J (Eds) *WHO Classification of Tumours of Haematopoietic and Lymphoid Tissues*, revised 4th Edn. IARC Press, Lyon, pp. 93–94.

Palomo L, Meggendorfer M, Hutter S, Twardziok S, Ademà V, Fuhrmann I *et al.* (2020) Molecular landscape and clonal architecture of adult myelodysplastic/myeloproliferative neoplasms. *Blood*, **136**, 1851–1862.

---

43   Acute myeloid leukaemia with inv(16)(p13.1q22)

AML with inv(16)(p13.1q22):

1) Can be therapy-related
2) Generally has a good prognosis
3) Has a *RUNX1-RUNX1T1* fusion gene that is demonstrable on FISH analysis
4) Has identical features to AML with t(16;16)(p13.1;q22)
5) Is often complicated by disseminated intravascular coagulation

Correct answers 1, 2, 4

Acute myeloid leukaemia with inv(16)(p13.1q22) and with t(16;16)(p13.1;q22) probably have identical features, although in one series of patients the prognosis was less good in those with t(16;16)

(Weisser *et al.* 2005). They can occur as a therapy-related AML following treatment with topoi-somerase inhibitors, with more than 10% of cases being therapy-related and classified as such in the WHO classification (Schoch *et al.* 2003, Weisser *et al.* 2005). The prognosis is generally good but is worse in the therapy-related cases. The fusion gene is *CBFB-MYH11*, *RUNX1-RUNX1T1* being associated with t(8;21). Disseminated intravascular coagulation is not a feature.

References

Schoch C, Schnittger S, Kern W, Dugas M, Hiddemann W and Haferlach T (2003) Acute myeloid leukemia with recurring chromosome abnormalities as defined by the WHO-classification: incidence of subgroups, additional genetic abnormalities, FAB subtypes and age distribution in an unselected series of 1,897 patients with acute myeloid leukemia. *Haematologica*, **88**, 351–352.

Weisser M, Schnittger S, Kern W, Hiddemann W, Haferlach T and Schoch C (2005) Prognostic factors in CBFB-MYH11 positive AML: trisomy 21, age, and t(16;16) are associated with inferior outcome. *Blood*, **106**, 146a.

---

44 Babesiosis

Babesiosis:

1) Can be transmitted by blood transfusion
2) Can cause leucopenia, neutropenia and thrombocytopenia
3) Has a similar distribution to malaria
4) Is more likely to be severe in hyposplenic patients
5) Is transmitted by mosquitoes

Correct answers 1, 2, 4

Babesia microti occurs in north-eastern and upper mid-western United States, where it is transmitted from rodents to humans by an *Ixodes* tick bite. The disease is usually only moderately severe unless the patient is hyposplenic, immune deficient or elderly. *Babesia divergens* occurs in cattle in Europe, including the United Kingdom and the Republic of Ireland, and is transmitted to humans by a tick bite. Severe disease is seen in hyposplenic patients. The first UK case was reported from Scotland in 1979 in a patient who had had a splenectomy and was immunosuppressed as a result of treatment of ongoing Hodgkin lymphoma (Entrican *et al.* 1979). Although most cases described in Europe have been severe, patients with normal immunity and a functioning spleen can have mild or asymptomatic disease; serological surveys suggest that this might actually be quite common.

As well as tick bite, transmission can be by blood transfusion (Leiby 2006) or transplacentally. In addition to haemolytic anaemia, leucopenia, neutropenia, thrombocytopenia, lymphopenia and atypical lymphocytes, when the disease is severe, there can be pancytopenia, haemophagocytic syndrome and disseminated intravascular coagulation. The disease distribution differs from that of malaria, being worldwide but with most reports being from temperate zones where incidence often varies according to season (Cunha 2018, Homer *et al.* 2000).

Babesia can also be recognised in a thick film and pyriform forms may be apparent (facing page, Field stain ×100 objective, Babesia divergens) but importantly, a thin film is likely to be needed to make a definite distinction from *Plasmodium falciparum*.

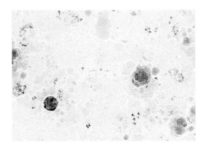

References

Cunha BA (2018) Babesiosis. *Medscape.* https://emedicine.medscape.com/article/212605-overview

Entrican JH, Williams H, Cook IA, Lancaster WM, Clark JC, Joyner LP and Lewis D (1979) Babesiosis in man: a case from Scotland. *Br Med J*, **2**, 474.

Homer MJ, Aguilar-Delfin I, Telford SR, Krause PJ and Persing DH (2000) Babesiosis. *Clin Microbiol Rev*, **13**, 451–469.

Leiby DA (2006) Babesiosis and blood transfusion: flying under the radar. *Vox Sang*, **90**, 157–165.

45	Haemoglobin E disorders

Haemoglobin E:

1) Can be regarded as a thalassaemic haemoglobinopathy
2) Can cause a mild sickling disorder when co-inherited with haemoglobin S
3) In heterozygotes, constitutes about 50% of haemoglobin
4) Is a high-affinity haemoglobin
5) Is of no significance in heterozygotes

Correct answers 1, 2

Haemoglobin E can be regarded as a thalassaemic haemoglobinopathy since the variant β chain is synthesised at a reduced rate. For this reason, in heterozygotes it usually constitutes only about 25% of total haemoglobin and is usually associated with red cell indices that resemble those of β thalassaemia trait. Oxygen affinity is normal. Although the heterozygous state is of little clinical significance it can cause diagnostic confusion and it is of considerable genetic significance. The detection of haemoglobin E trait is thus important in antenatal screening programmes. Worldwide, compound heterozygous states with β thalassaemia are a major cause of β thalassaemia intermedia and major (Bain 2020). The presence of α chain inclusions (particularly evident in splenectomised patients) illustrated the considerable chain imbalance that occurs. These inclusions cause damage to developing erythroblasts, leading to dyserythropoiesis and ineffective erythropoiesis.

Reference

Bain BJ (2020) *Haemoglobinopathy Diagnosis*, 3rd Edn. Wiley Blackwell, Oxford, pp. 275–290.

46 Juvenile myelomonocytic leukaemia

Recognised features of juvenile myelomonocytic leukaemia (JMML) include:

1) Frequent complex chromosomal abnormalities
2) Increased haemoglobin F
3) Reduced erythrocyte carbonic anhydrase
4) Reduced haemoglobin A_2
5) Right shifted oxygen dissociation curve

Correct answers 2, 3, 4

Juvenile myelomonocytic leukaemia (JMML) often shows reversion to features of fetal erythropoiesis. Specifically, the haemoglobin F percentage, glucose-6-phosphate dehydrogenase activity and the expression of the i antigen are increased whilst the haemoglobin A_2 percentage, red cell carbonic anhydrase activity and the expression of the I antigen are reduced. The oxygen dissociation curve is left shifted when haemoglobin F is high, rather than right shifted. Cytogenetic analysis is usually normal.

47 Non-haemopoietic tumours

Bone marrow infiltration by a non-haemopoietic tumour:

1) Can show cohesive masses of cells in both the aspirate and trephine biopsy sections
2) Can show moulding of cells by adjacent cells
3) Is often associated with fibrosis and osteosclerosis
4) Is strongly suggested if cells show expression of CD10
5) May show increased osteoblasts and osteoclasts in a bone marrow aspirate

Correct answers 1, 2, 3, 5

The haematologist will encounter metastatic non-haemopoietic tumour, through examination of either the bone marrow or tissue fluid specimens. The clinical history is often important in this regard but not infrequently the metastatic presentation is the primary reason for the health care encounter. One should suspect a non-haemopoietic tumour morphologically when the cells encountered are not easily recognisable, when the tumour cells form clumps, when aspirate particles are scarce and abnormal cells infrequent and when there are signet ring cells (indicative of adenocarcinoma) or moulding of cells by adjacent cells (suggestive of small cell lung carcinoma). Non-haemopoietic tumours frequently generate marrow fibrosis and interfere with marrow aspiration. Bone marrow necrosis, osteolysis and new bone formation can also be seen and bone cells may be seen in increased numbers in the aspirate. The suspicion needs to be supported by analysis of suspect cells using flow cytometry supported by immunohistochemistry. The latter is often more informative as a larger range of antigen specificities can be studied. Non-haemopoietic tumours frequently show expression of non-lineage-specific antigens which are associated with, but are not diagnostic of, primary haematological disorders, examples being CD56, CD33, CD117, CD10 and CD15. In these circumstances it is important to look for antigens indicating lineage specificity such as cCD3 (T lineage), CD79a and CD19 (B lineage) and MPO (myeloid lineage). CD10 expression is not strongly suggestive of a non-haemopoietic tumour since, although renal cell carcinoma is usually positive, expression is also seen in ALL, Burkitt lymphoma and follicular lymphoma. Finally, the ultimate histopathological diagnosis will be made using a large panel of antibodies alongside directed genetic and molecular studies to support the diagnosis, inform prognosis and guide selection of available targeted therapies.

The bone marrow trephine biopsy sections below (H&E ×100 objective) are from a patient with hypercalcaemia due to metastatic breast carcinoma. The marrow is clearly heavily involved by carcinoma and no residual haemopoietic tissue is evident. Hypercalcaemia in metastatic carcinoma can result from direct osteoclast activation, through ectopic parathyroid hormone secretion or through direct resorption of bone by the tumour; the latter mechanism seems to be the mechanism in this case.

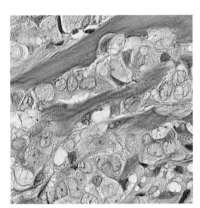
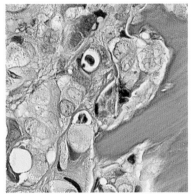

48   Richter transformation of chronic lymphocytic leukaemia

Richter syndrome:

1) Can usually be effectively managed with chemoimmunotherapy appropriate for a large cell lymphoma
2) Consistently involves the peripheral blood and bone marrow
3) Describes the development of a large B-cell lymphoma in a patient with chronic lymphocytic leukaemia
4) Has no known aetiological factors
5) Usually represents transformation of a clonal B cell

Correct answers 3, 5

The term Richter syndrome describes the development of a high-grade B-cell lymphoma in a patient with CLL. Strictly speaking, the term 'Richter transformation' should be reserved for the majority of cases in which this represents transformation of a clonal B cell, but often the detailed investigation to know if this is the case is not available. Richter transformation of CLL is a devastating development for any patient. It is a high-grade B-cell neoplasm, usually developing in involved nodal sites, showing rapid growth, high proliferation fraction, high serum LDH and acute clinical decline. The peripheral blood and bone marrow may show only CLL. Typically, it proves highly refractory to R-CHOP type therapy as *TP53* mutations are common. Effective management is difficult but prognosis is somewhat better in cases that do not originate in a clonal B cell. Cases that have a different clonal origin have immunosuppression and Epstein–Barr virus (EBV) infection as aetiological factors. EBV can also have an aetiological role when the origin is from a clonal B cell. The new biological therapies for CLL, notably Bruton's kinase inhibitors such as ibrutinib and *BCL2* inhibitors such as venetoclax, have revolutionised CLL therapy but Richter transformation still remains a relatively frequent cause of loss of disease control.

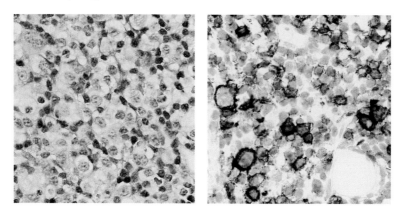

The bone marrow trephine section images above are from another CLL patient with Richter transformation. Note the mixture of large nucleolated cells interspersed with CLL cells (left image, H&E ×100) and the different intensity of CD20 expression by the two populations (right image, immunoperoxidase for CD20 ×100).

---

49 Sickle cell–haemoglobin C disease

In comparison with sickle cell anaemia, sickle cell–haemoglobin C disease has:

1) A higher haematocrit
2) A higher incidence of retinal disease and bone marrow necrosis
3) A lower oxygen affinity
4) Less evidence of hyposplenism
5) Shorter red cell survival

Correct answers 1, 2, 4

Haemoglobin C has a higher oxygen affinity than haemoglobin S, hence the higher Hb and haematocrit in the compound heterozygous state in comparison with sickle cell anaemia (Bain 2020). Red cell survival is longer so that gallstones are less frequent. Hyposplenism is less and splenic sequestration and splenic infarction can thus occur beyond infancy. Retinitis proliferans and vitreous haemorrhages are more common and correlate with a higher Hb. Bone marrow necrosis and embolism of necrotic bone marrow to the lungs are more common. Life expectancy is longer.

Reference

Bain BJ (2020) *Haemoglobinopathy Diagnosis,* 3rd Edn. Wiley Blackwell, Oxford.

---

50   T cell/histiocyte-rich B-cell lymphoma

T cell/histiocyte-rich B-cell lymphoma (THRBCL):

1) Can occur *de novo* or evolve from nodular lymphocyte predominant Hodgkin lymphoma
2) Is one of the more common type of large B-cell lymphoma
3) Often presents with advanced stage disease
4) Usually expresses CD15 and CD30
5) Usually harbours the Epstein–Barr virus

Correct answers 1, 3

T cell/histiocyte-rich B-cell lymphoma is an infrequent subtype of diffuse large B-cell lymphoma accounting for less than 10% of cases. It typically affects middle-aged males presenting with B symptoms, advanced-stage disease and bone marrow involvement. The neoplastic cells do not usually express CD15 or CD30, whereas both of these antigens are usually expressed in classical Hodgkin lymphoma; in nodular lymphocyte predominant Hodgkin lymphoma (NLPHL) there is not usually any expression of either (see Theme 83). The diagnosis can be elusive and even when affected tissue is examined it is important not to misinterpret it as a T-cell neoplasm, classical Hodgkin lymphoma or NLPHL. The latter, also being a B-cell neoplasm with a T-cell infiltrate, can mimic THRBCL. The main differences between the two are summarised in the table below.

Nodular lymphocyte predominant Hodgkin lymphoma	T cell/histiocyte-rich B-cell lymphoma
Low-volume nodes	Large nodes
Non-axial nodes	Widespread nodal and extranodal disease
Often stage 1 or 2	Often stage 4
No B symptoms	B symptoms common
No splenic involvement	Splenic involvement common
Normal FBC	Frequent cytopenias
Bone marrow involvement rare	Bone marrow involvement common
CD20+ LP cells	CD20+ DLBCL cells
CD4+ T-cell rosettes	CD8+ T-cell reaction

Finally, and to complicate matters further, NLPHL can transform to a THRBCL so every aspect of the clinical and laboratory presentation needs to be considered. A simple rule of thumb is that if a patient with an apparent NLPHL appears sick with B symptoms and, in particular, has focal splenic infiltrates, evolution to THRBCL should be considered. This lymphoma is not related to EBV.

---

51   Miliary tuberculosis

Tuberculosis:

1) Can be complicated by haemophagocytic lymphohistiocytosis
2) Can be excluded if there are tissue granulomas but the Ziehl–Neelsen stain is negative

3) Can cause anaemia of chronic disease
4) Can cause bone marrow necrosis
5) Is often associated with more numerous bacteria in bone marrow lesions than are found in atypical mycobacterial infection

Correct answers 1, 3, 4

There are numerous and variable potential haematological effects of tuberculosis, including neutrophilia, neutropenia, monocytosis, monocytopenia, lymphopenia, thrombocytosis, thrombocytopenia, anaemia of chronic disease, increased bone marrow macrophages and iron stores, haemophagocytic lymphohistiocytosis, bone marrow necrosis and bone marrow granulomas, sometimes with caseation. Staining for the bacilli is insensitive so that a negative result does not exclude this infection. Organisms are generally much more numerous in atypical mycobacterial infection.

---

52 Pure red cell aplasia

Chronic red cell aplasia can be a feature of:

1) ABO-incompatible allogeneic stem cell transplantation
2) Autologous stem cell transplantation
3) Development of an anti-erythropoietin antibody
4) Parvovirus infection in an immunodeficient patient
5) Systemic lupus erythematosus

Correct answers 1, 3, 4, 5

Chronic acquired red cell aplasia is a rare condition which has been associated with low-grade lymphomas, large granular lymphocytic leukaemia, solid tumours, autoimmune disorders, drugs and infection. Among the drugs that can be causative are epoetin and darbepoetin, the mechanism being development of an anti-erythropoietin antibody. Red cell aplasia can also complicate ABO-incompatible allogeneic stem cell transplantation. Thymoma has long been known to be associated with myasthenia gravis and red cell aplasia; the tumour (which is frequently benign) can impair normal T-lymphocyte development and lead to relative deficiency of CD8+ regulatory T cells, resulting in loss of self-tolerance. Removal of the tumour leads to resolution of the aplasia in some but not all cases, possibly due to persistence of T-cell imbalance. In this case, the introduction of ciclosporin, which blocks T-cell signalling and expansion, appeared effective in permitting recovery of erythropoiesis.

---

53 Lymphoblastic transformation of follicular lymphoma

Follicular lymphoma can transform into:

1) B lymphoblastic leukaemia/lymphoma
2) Burkitt lymphoma
3) Diffuse large B-cell lymphoma
4) Lymphoma with features intermediate between Burkitt lymphoma and diffuse large cell lymphoma
5) Mantle cell lymphoma

Correct answers 1, 2, 3, 4

Lymphoblastic transformation of follicular lymphoma is a rare but well-documented phenomenon that carries a poor prognosis (Young *et al.* 2008, Jaffe *et al.* 2017). More typically, transformation is to a diffuse large B-cell lymphoma (DLBCL) but it can also be to Burkitt lymphoma or a lymphoma with features intermediate between Burkitt lymphoma and DLBCL (Jaffe *et al.* 2017). The findings here indicate lymphoblastic transformation with a change in clinical symptoms, blood and bone marrow morphology and immunophenotype together with features of bone marrow failure. Importantly, the original genetic signature is present in the transformed cells but there will be additional genetic events. A *MYC* translocation may be found not only in cases with transformation to Burkitt lymphoma but also in lymphoblastic transformation. In transformation to DLBCL, a mature phenotype will normally be preserved, very similar to that seen at diagnosis. The patient was commenced on a lymphoblastic leukaemia type regimen but the disease proved refractory to treatment.

References

Jaffe AS, Harris NL, Swerdlow SH, Ott G, Nathwani BN, de Jong G *et al.* (2017) Follicular lymphoma. *In* Swerdlow SH, Campo E, Harris NL, Jaffe ES, Pileri SA, Stein H and Thiele J (Eds) *World Health Organization Classification of Tumours of Haematopoietic and Lymphoid Tissues*, revised 4th Edn. IARC Press, Lyon, pp. 266–273.

Young KH, Xie Q, Zhou G, Eickhoff JC, Sanger WG, Aoun P and Chan WC (2008) Transformation of follicular lymphoma to precursor B-cell lymphoblastic lymphoma with c-*myc* gene rearrangement as a critical event. *Am J Clin Pathol*, **129**, 157–166.

54 Primary hyperparathyroidism

The histological changes of hyperparathyroidism can be seen in the bone marrow as a result of:

1) Chronic renal insufficiency
2) Osteopetrosis
3) Osteosclerosis
4) Paget disease
5) Parathyroid adenoma

Correct answers 1, 5

The bone marrow changes of hyperparathyroidism can be seen in both primary and secondary hyperparathyroidism. The changes of osteopetrosis (see Theme 22), osteosclerosis and Paget disease are different. Primary hyperparathyroidism usually results from a parathyroid adenoma; much less often it is due to parathyroid hyperplasia or a carcinoma of the parathyroid. Secondary hyperparathyroidism usually results from chronic renal insufficiency.

55 Gamma heavy chain disease

Gamma heavy chain disease:

1) Almost always involves the bone marrow
2) Can involve Waldeyer's ring

3) Histologically does not differ from multiple myeloma
4) Shows an association with autoimmune disease
5) Usually involves liver, spleen and lymph nodes

Correct answers 2, 4, 5

Gamma heavy chain disease is a rare B-lineage lymphoproliferative disorder, which can resemble a lymphoplasmacytic or marginal zone B-cell lymphoma (either splenic or mucosa-associated lymphoid tissue) and thus generally differs histologically from multiple myeloma. Clinicopathological features can include lymphadenopathy, splenomegaly, hepatomegaly and involvement of the gastrointestinal tract and Waldeyer's ring. The bone marrow is involved in 30–60% of cases. The condition is characterised by the production of truncated gamma heavy chains that are unable to associate with light chains to form an intact IgG molecule. It shows female predominance, an association with autoimmune disease, systemic upset (anorexia, fever, weight loss) and recurrent infections (Bieliauskas *et al.* 2014). The serological assessment is important in that the free gamma heavy chains may not initially be identified and quantified unless specific gamma immunofixation studies are performed.

Flame cells, as seen in this patient, are plasma cells with cytoplasm staining red/purple with an MGG stain and sometimes having irregular cytoplasmic projections. They are thought to result from excess accumulation of glycoproteins; they are normally associated with IgA myeloma but can be seen in other plasma cell neoplasms including gamma heavy chain disease (further images below ×100). The flame cell (below right) also shows blue cytoplasmic precipitates, which may represent free gamma chains.

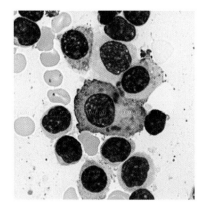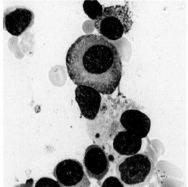

It is also interesting that in this case the pulmonary nodules were due to AL amyloid deposition; there was mild excess of serum free kappa chains and a low concentration IgG kappa paraprotein. This suggests that a small subset of neoplastic cells produced gamma heavy chains that were still able to combine with kappa light chains. Interestingly, nodular pulmonary amyloidosis can be derived from a combination of both heavy and light chains (Grogg *et al.* 2013), which we suspect in this case. We attempted to stain the lung biopsy for gamma heavy chain but no residual tissue was available from the block. Gamma heavy chain disease likely represents a spectrum of disorders, the nature of which we are only just beginning to understand.

References

Bieliauskas S, Tubbs RR, Bacon CM, Eshoa C, Foucar K, Gibson SE *et al.* (2014) Gamma heavy-chain disease: defining the spectrum of associated lymphoproliferative disorders through analysis of 13 cases. *Am J Surg Pathol*, **36**, 534–543.

Grogg KL, Aubry MC, Vrana JA, Theis JD and Dogan A (2013) Nodular pulmonary amyloidosis is characterised by local immunoglobulin deposition and is frequently associated with an indolent B-cell lymphoproliferative disorder. *Am J Surg Pathol*, **37**, 406–412.

---

56 Acute promyelocytic leukaemia with t(15;17)(q24.1;q21.2)

Acute promyelocytic leukaemia:

1) Always has abnormal promyelocytes in the peripheral blood film when a careful search is done
2) Can be complicated by thrombosis
3) Can be reliably diagnosed when a case of acute myeloid leukaemia does not express CD34 or HLA-DR
4) Is more common in the elderly
5) Morphologically, can simulate acute megakaryoblastic leukaemia

Correct answers 2, 5

Acute promyelocytic leukaemia has three morphological variants: (i) hypergranular, (ii) microgranular/hypogranular (this case) and (iii) hyperbasophilic. The hyperbasophilic variant can have not only basophilic cytoplasm but also cytoplasmic blebs so that acute megakaryoblastic leukaemia is simulated. In the hypergranular variant the WBC can be low or normal and sometimes no leukaemic cells are found in the peripheral blood, despite a diligent search. Although CD34 and HLA-DR negativity is typical, this is also true of a significant proportion of cases of AML with *NPM1* mutation; the immunophenotype is thus important for offering rapid support for the morphological diagnosis but cannot be relied on in isolation. Unlike many subtypes on AML, APL has a lower prevalence in the elderly. Paradoxically, although bleeding is characteristic, a significant minority of patients suffer thrombotic events.

---

57 AA amyloidosis

Recognised causes of AA amyloidosis include:

1) Crohn's disease
2) Familial amyloidosis due to mutation in the transthyretin gene (*TTR*)
3) Familial Mediterranean fever
4) Osteomyelitis
5) Plasma cell myeloma

Correct answers 1, 3, 4

AA amyloidosis is seen in patients with chronic infective and inflammatory disorders and should be distinguished from AL amyloidosis seen in patients with clonal lymphoproliferative and plasma cell disorders, and from various type of familial amyloidosis in which the protein that gives rise to the amyloid differs (Picken 2020, Vaxman and Gertz 2020). The clinical consequences can be similar and major organs such as the heart and kidney are frequently affected. AA amyloid is derived from the serum amyloid A protein, which is closely related to C-reactive protein. It is an acute phase reactant synthesised by the liver and is frequently elevated in serum over long periods in patients with these inflammatory diseases. One of us (ML) remembers this principle well from many years ago: during examination for a distinction in medicine in final MB ChB, I was asked to examine a female patient who was breathless at rest and who had finger clubbing and bibasal coarse crepitations on chest auscultation. I was asked for a working diagnosis and suggested bronchiectasis. The renal physician examiner enquired what I might find on urine dipstick analysis and what the mechanism might be. I offered proteinuria due to renal AA amyloidosis and I can remember his grin to this day.

References

Picken MM (2020) The pathology of amyloidosis in classification: a review. *Acta Haematol*, **143**, 322–334.

Vaxman J and Gertz M (2020) When to suspect a diagnosis of amyloidosis. *Acta Haematol*, **143**, 304–311.

---

58 Acquired sideroblastic anaemia

Sideroblastic erythropoiesis is a feature of:

1) *ALAS2* mutation
2) Copper deficiency
3) GATA1 deficiency
4) Pearson syndrome
5) Zinc deficiency

Correct answers 1, 2, 4

In the WHO classification, sideroblastic erythropoiesis is, by definition, a feature of certain myelodysplastic and myelodysplastic/myeloproliferative neoplasms, specifically MDS with ring sideroblasts and either single-lineage or multilineage dysplasia and myelodysplastic/myeloproliferative neoplasm with ring sideroblasts and thrombocytosis. In all of these there is a strong association with a somatic *SF3B1* mutation. This mutation can also be seen in other myeloid neoplasms. Acquired sideroblastic erythropoiesis is a feature of copper deficiency (Mangles *et al.* 2007), including copper deficiency resulting from zinc excess (Ramadurai *et al.* 1993), and can be caused by drugs, such as isoniazid (Piso *et al.* 2011). It is important to be aware of these associations to avoid misdiagnosis as MDS (Mangles *et al.* 2007). There are many causes of congenital sideroblastic anaemia but all are rare. The most common is *ALAS2* mutation but a mitochondrial gene mutation can also be responsible, as in Pearson syndrome. *GATA1* mutation is associated with microcytosis but this is due to β thalassaemia rather than sideroblastic erythropoiesis.

It should be noted that microcytosis, as observed in this patient, is uncommon when sideroblastic erythropoiesis is a feature of MDS. More frequently the hypochromic microcytic cells are a smaller proportion and the MCV is characteristically increased. Elliptocytes associated with hypochromic microcytic anaemia are usually a feature of iron deficiency ('pencil cells') but it should be noted that small numbers can also be seen in thalassaemia trait and both congenital and acquired sideroblastic anaemias.

We advise that an iron stain is done on the first bone marrow aspirate of all patients. However, it is also possible to suspect sideroblastic erythropoiesis when dysplastic features are not excessive and there is poor haemoglobinisation of a proportion of late erythroblasts.

References

Mangles SE, Abdalla SH, Gabriel CM and Bain B (2007) Case Report 37: Neutropenia and macrocytosis in a middle-aged man. *Leuk Lymphoma*, **48**, 1846−1848.

Piso RJ, Kriz K and Desax MC (2011) Severe isoniazid related sideroblastic anemia. *Hematol Rep*, **3**, e2.

Ramadurai J, Shapiro C, Kozloff M and Telfer M (1993) Zinc abuse and sideroblastic anemia. *Am J Hematol*, **42**, 227−228.

---

59 Diffuse large B-cell lymphoma

Diffuse large B-cell lymphoma:

1) Can be a feature of the acquired immune deficiency syndrome (AIDS)
2) Can result from Epstein–Barr virus or human herpes virus 8 infection
3) Can result from immune suppression following transplantation
4) Consistently shows a germinal centre immunophenotype
5) Is the most frequently observed non-Hodgkin lymphoma

Correct answers 1, 2, 3, 5

Diffuse large B-cell lymphoma is the most frequent non-Hodgkin lymphoma we encounter. A significant proportion of cases result from immune deficiency, either inherited, virus-induced (AIDS) or iatrogenic (including following transplantation). Both the Epstein–Barr virus and human herpes virus 8 are recognised aetiological factors. Some cases have a germinal centre immunophenotype but others, including 'activated B-cell like', do not.

DLBCL can involve any tissue and frequently therefore can be a challenge in diagnosis and ultimately in treatment. Intravascular B-cell lymphoma can be particularly difficult to identify as patients typically present with vascular occlusive symptoms but without lymphadenopathy or foci of abnormal tissue on detailed imaging. The serum LDH is often elevated; together with the above features this can be a clue to the diagnosis. The bone marrow images that follow are from a patient who presented with acute systemic decline, confusion and night sweats. Note the giant lymphoma cells in the aspirate (left image ×100 objective), in the marrow sinusoids (centre image, H&E ×50) with strong expression of CD20 (right image, immunoperoxidase ×50).

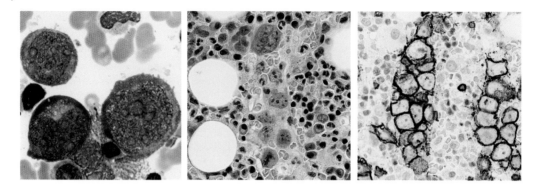

The intensity of the treatment approach in DLBCL has to take account of all elements of the disease including clinical stage, histology and cell-of-origin (and possible evolution from low-grade disease or related to immunosuppressive therapy), International Prognostic Score, CNS relapse risk and molecular characteristics, particularly focusing on those with dual or triple translocations involving *MYC*, *BCL2* and *BCL6*. These latter cases show aggressive clinical behaviour, frequent extranodal disease and poorer outcomes with standard R-CHOP chemotherapy. Diffuse large B-cell lymphoma is a collective term encompassing many different mature B-cell neoplasms. As many affected patients can be cured with appropriate therapy, an increased understanding of the biology of the disease and effective therapeutic risk stratification is certainly needed.

60	Hickman line infection

Recognised complications of indwelling central venous lines include:

1) Bacterial infection
2) Cardiac arrhythmia
3) Fungal infection
4) Pneumothorax
5) Venous thrombosis

Correct answers 1, 2, 3, 4, 5

Infection in central venous lines is most often bacterial infection, particularly by *Staphylococcus aureus* or *Staphylococcus epidermidis*, but fungal colonisation, for example with *Candida* species, has also been reported, and may be recognised in a blood film (Arnold *et al.* 1999). Some Gram-negative bacteria such as *E. coli*, *Klebsiella* spp. and *Stenotrophomonas* spp. are serious pathogens in venous access device-related infection and when implicated, because of their propensity for causing septic shock, the line will often require removal. Bacteria can colonise the fibrinous sheath that often forms within the catheter lumen; showers of bacteria can be released when the line is accessed and flushed. It is common in neutropenic sepsis to not identify the causative organism and patients are often treated empirically. This case is unusual in that large numbers of bacteria must have been displaced from the line so that they were subsequently visible in the blood film and within cells. It is fortunate that the organism responsible was a relatively low-grade pathogen; such a heavy bacteraemia from a more virulent pathogen could have led to more serious consequences in a neutropenic patient.

Reference

Arnold JA, Jowzi Z and Bain BJ (1999) Images in haematology: *Candida glabrata* in a blood film. *Br J Haematol*, **104**, 1.

---

61 Monocytes and their precursors

Promonocytes:

1) Can be distinguished from monoblasts by their lack of expression of CD34
2) Can be present in acute myeloid leukaemia with t(9;11) and *KMT2A* rearrangement
3) Can be readily differentiated from monocytes on immunophenotyping
4) Often express CD11b, CD11c, CD14 and CD64
5) Sometimes show chromatin condensation

Correct answers 2, 4

Promonocytes cannot be distinguished reliably from monoblasts on the basis of CD34 negativity since monoblasts can also be CD34 negative. They often have a phenotype very similar to that of immature or mature monocytes: CD13+, CD33+, HLA-DR+, CD11b+, CD11c+, CD14+, CD64+ and CD15+ with CD34 and CD117 not being expressed. This is one situation, therefore, where immunophenotyping cannot be relied upon for assessing promonocytic blast equivalents. AML with t(9;11) often shows monocytic differentiation. Promonocytes do not show any chromatin condensation; this is a crucial feature in distinguishing them from immature monocytes. A good morphological assessment with differential leucocyte count is therefore essential for accurate disease classification.

---

62 Paroxysmal cold haemoglobinuria

Paroxysmal cold haemoglobinuria:

1) Can be caused by syphilis
2) Is associated with intravascular haemolysis
3) Is caused by an antibody directed at the P antigen
4) Is caused by an IgG antibody so that IgG is usually detected when a direct antiglobulin tests is done
5) Occurs most often in children

Correct answers 1, 2, 3, 5

At the beginning of the twentieth century paroxysmal cold haemoglobinuria (PCH) was often the result of syphilis. The condition was first described by Julius Donath and Karl Landsteiner in 1904 in cases of congenital and tertiary syphilis. In that instance haemolysis was episodic, hence the designation 'paroxysmal'. PCH is now generally seen following a viral infection (including measles, mumps, chickenpox, cytomegalovirus, Epstein–Barr virus, parvovirus B19 and respiratory syncytial virus) but also sometimes following bacterial infection or immunisation. The antibody, directed at the red cell P antigen, binds complement at a low temperature leading to intravascular haemolysis and subsequent haemoglobinuria on rewarming. The red cells of the great majority of individuals express the P antigen and thus they are susceptible to PCH. The IgG antibody elutes from the red cell membrane on rewarming so that when a direct antiglobulin test is done only complement is detected.

63 Transient abnormal myelopoiesis

Transient abnormal myelopoiesis of Down syndrome:

1) Can occur in mosaic Down syndrome
2) Generally requires chemotherapy to lower the white cell count
3) Is associated with a *GATA1* mutation
4) On cytogenetic analysis, shows only trisomy 21
5) Represents a leukaemoid reaction

Correct answers 1, 3

Transient abnormal myelopoiesis is a clonal neoplastic condition (Roberts *et al.* 2013, Tunstall *et al.* 2018) seen in Down syndrome and it can occur in mosaic forms of the condition. Typically it shows spontaneous resolution. In all cases there is a *GATA1* mutation in addition to trisomy 21. Some patients with TAM also have an additional acquired cytogenetic abnormality, which disappears when the condition remits. Chemotherapy is not usually necessary. When TAM is followed by acute myeloid leukaemia during infancy the same *GATA1* mutation is present.

References

Roberts I, Alford K, Hall G, Juban G, Richmond H, Norton A *et al.*; Oxford-Imperial Down Syndrome Cohort Study Group (2013) GATA1-mutant clones are frequent and often unsuspected in babies with Down syndrome: identification of a population at risk of leukemia. *Blood*, **122**, 3908–3917.
Tunstall O, Bhatnagar N, James B, Norton A, O'Marcaigh AS, Watts T *et al.*; British Society for Haematology (2018) Guidelines for the investigation and management of transient leukaemia of Down syndrome. *Br J Haematol*, **182**, 200–211.

64 Systemic lupus erythematosus

Haematological manifestations of systemic lupus erythematosus (SLE) include:

1) Autoimmune neutropenia
2) Autoimmune thrombocytopenia ('ITP')
3) Cold haemagglutinin disease
4) Evans syndrome
5) Pure red cell aplasia

Correct answers 1, 2, 4, 5

The haematological complications of SLE include: (i) autoimmune manifestations such as antiphospholipid syndrome, warm autoimmune haemolytic anaemia, neutropenia, thrombocytopenia and bone marrow hypoplasias (including red cell aplasia, agranulocytosis and aplastic anaemia); (ii) reactive bone marrow changes sometimes associated with dysplastic features including sideroblastic erythropoiesis; and (iii) in some cases bone marrow fibrosis (shown below, left and centre, H&E and reticulin stains ×50 objective) (Jiminez-Balderas *et al.* 1994, Costallat *et al.* 2012, Chalayer *et al.* 2017). Furthermore, some patients show other peripheral blood abnormalities that can be a clue to the diagnosis. In the peripheral blood images from a third patient (below right ×100) note the fluffy very weakly basophilic precipitates due to cryofibrinogenaemia. Rarely, LE cells are observed in a bone marrow aspirate (Abdulsalam *et al.* 2012).

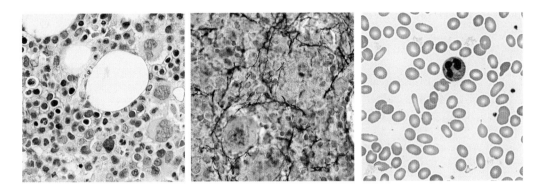

This range of abnormalities together indicate that reduced bone marrow function and blood cell survival can be consequences of this disease (Chalayer *et al.* 2017). The challenging question in this patient with severe marrow aplasia is how this should best be managed. She commenced high-dose corticosteroid therapy, with an improvement in joint symptoms but the severe cytopenias initially persisted. At 8 weeks, however, on prednisolone 50 mg daily, an improvement was noted: Hb 94 g/l, WBC 3.7×10^9/l, neutrophils 2.6×10^9/l and platelets 61×10^9/l. The plan is to introduce hydroxychloroquine and slowly taper the steroid dosing.

References

Abdulsalam AH, Sabeeh N, Hatim A and Bain BJ (2012) Diagnosis of systemic lupus erythematosus from a bone marrow aspirate. *Am J Hematol*, **87**, 620.

Chalayer E, Costedoat-Chalumeau N, Beyne-Rauzy O, Ninet J, Durupt S, Tebib J *et al.* (2017) Bone marrow involvement in systemic lupus erythematosus. *QJM*, **110**, 701–711.

Costallat GL, Appenzeller S and Costallat LT (2012) Evans syndrome and systemic lupus erythematosus: clinical presentation and outcome. *Joint Bone Spine*, **79**, 362–364.

Jiminez-Balderas FJ, Morales-Polanco MR and Guttierez L (1994) Acute sideroblastic anemia in active systemic lupus erythematosus. *Lupus*, **3**, 157–159.

---

65   Granular blast cells in acute lymphoblastic leukaemia

Rearrangement of *KMT2A*:

1) Can be associated with lineage switch at relapse, from acute lymphoblastic leukaemia (ALL) to acute monoblastic leukaemia (AMoL) or mixed phenotype acute leukaemia (MPAL)

2) Can be therapy-related
3) Generally has a good prognosis
4) In ALL, is usually associated with a common ALL immunophenotype
5) Is occasionally found in congenital ALL

Correct answers 1, 2, 5

The *KMT2A* gene located at 11q23.3 (previously known as *MLL* – mixed lineage leukaemia) is an important oncogene implicated in the pathogenesis of AML, MPAL and both B- and, occasionally, T-ALL. Therapy-related cases are recognised following use of topoisomerase II-interactive drugs. This is a promiscuous gene, fusion genes with more than 100 partners having been reported. Genes involved include *AFF1* at 4q21.3-22.1 (B-ALL), *MLLT1* at 19p13.3 (T-ALL) and *MLLT3* at 9p21.3 (AML). Congenital cases of B-ALL have been recognised. The immunophenotype of B-lineage cases is usually that of pro-B ALL, not common ALL; in addition, co-expression of myeloid antigens, CD15 and CD65, can be present. The prognostic significance is determined in part by the translocation partner but is generally poor. The t(4;11) translocation identified in this case carries a poor prognosis and allogeneic transplantation is normally indicated in first complete remission.

---

66 Chronic myelomonocytic leukaemia

Chronic myelomonocytic leukaemia:

1) By definition, in the WHO classification, cannot be therapy-related
2) Can have an associated proliferation of plasmacytoid dendritic cells
3) Has an abnormal karyotype in 20–40% of patients
4) Is associated with an increase in haemoglobin F
5) Shows *BCR-ABL1* in a minority of patients

Correct answers 1, 2, 3

In the WHO classification, therapy-related cases are excluded from this diagnostic category. Rare cases of chronic myeloid leukaemia with a p190 *BCR-ABL1* protein can simulate CMML (Parilla and Venkataraman 2017) but, by definition, such cases are also excluded. There can be proliferation of clonally-related plasmacytoid dendritic cells (Patnaik and Tefferi 2020) and there can similarly be an association with clonally-related Erdheim–Chester disease (Goyal *et al.* 2019). The karyotype is abnormal in 20–40% of cases. It is juvenile myelomonocytic leukaemia that is associated with increased haemoglobin F, not CMML.

References

Goyal G, Liu Y, Ravindran A, Al-Kali A, Go RS, Patnaik MM and Rech KL on behalf of the Mayo Clinic Histiocytosis Working Group (2019) Concomitant Erdheim-Chester disease and chronic myelomonocytic leukaemia: genomic insights into a common clonal origin. *Br J Haematol*, **187**, e51–e54.
Parilla M and Venkataraman G (2017) The thin line between CML and CMML. *Blood*, **129**, 2456.
Patnaik MM and Tefferi A (2020) Chronic myelomonocytic leukemia: 2020 update on diagnosis, risk stratification and management. *Am J Hematol*, **95**, 97–115.

67 Burkitt lymphoma/leukaemia

Burkitt lymphoma/leukaemia:

1) Can involve the breasts and ovaries
2) Has a proliferation fraction approaching 100%
3) Is consistently associated with t(8;14)(q24;q32)
4) Is of marginal zone origin
5) Occurs in endemic, sporadic and immunodeficiency-related forms

Correct answers 1, 2, 5

Burkitt lymphoma occurs in endemic, sporadic and immunodeficiency-related forms. The endemic form, linked to the co-occurrence of holoendemic malaria and Epstein–Barr virus infection, occurs in sub-Saharan Africa and Papua New Guinea and is particularly characterised by tumours originating in the mandible, maxilla or orbital bones. EBV is a significant aetiological factor also in a proportion of patients with the non-endemic forms. Immunodeficiency-related cases are seen particularly in HIV-infected individuals but also following solid organ transplantation. Breast and ovaries can be involved with the former being seen particularly at puberty and during pregnancy and lactation. The proliferation fraction (Ki-67 expression) approaches 100%, this being a haematological neoplasm with a remarkable rate of tumour growth. Burkitt lymphoma is usually associated with t(8;14)(q24;q32) but not invariably; *MYC* can also be dysregulated by proximity to one of the immunoglobulin light chain loci. The origin is not in the marginal zone but in the germinal centre, with expression of CD10 and BCL6 being indicative.

68 Gaucher disease

Gaucher disease:

1) Can cause osteolytic bone lesions
2) Is associated with an increased incidence of multiple myeloma and lymphoplasmacytic lymphoma
3) Is associated with increased serum ferritin, indicative of iron overload
4) Has a high prevalence in Ashkenazi Jews
5) Requires a biopsy for diagnosis

Correct answers 1, 2, 4

Gaucher disease was first described by the French physician, Philippe Gaucher, in a doctoral thesis in 1882. Clinicopathological features that may lead to referral of a patient with undiagnosed Gaucher disease to a haematologist include splenomegaly, bleeding and bruising, anaemia, thrombocytopenia, pancytopenia and lytic bone lesions. The incidence of monoclonal gammopathy of undetermined significance, multiple myeloma and lymphoplasmacytic lymphoma is increased, probably as a result of chronic antigen stimulation and dysregulation of inflammatory cytokines (Thomas *et al.* 2014, Weinreb *et al.* 2018). Although serum ferritin measurements are increased, there is no iron overload (Morgan *et al.* 1983); this is a reminder that what is assayed as 'serum ferritin' is actually apoferritin. The carrier rate of the mutant gene is as high as one in 12 among Ashkenazi Jews (Thomas *et al.* 2014). Disease occurs in homozygotes. Although Gaucher disease is not infrequently diagnosed following bone marrow examination, neither this nor any other biopsy is necessary if the diagnosis is suspected. Non-invasive diagnosis is possible by DNA analysis or by assay of glucocerebrosidase in peripheral blood leucocytes (Thomas *et al.* 2014).

The haematologist needs to distinguish Gaucher disease from conditions associated with pseudo-Gaucher cells. Since specific treatment is now available, diagnosis is important.

References

Morgan MA, Hoffbrand AV, Laulicht M, Luck W and Knowles S (1983) Serum ferritin concentration in Gaucher's disease. *Br Med J (Clin Res Ed)*, **286**, 1864.

Thomas AS, Mehta A and Hughes DA (2014) Gaucher disease: haematological presentations and complications. *Br J Haematol*, **165**, 427–440.

Weinreb NJ, Mistry PK, Rosenbloom BE and Dhodapkar MV (2018) MGUS, lymphoplasmacytic malignancies, and Gaucher disease: the significance of the clinical association. *Blood*, **131**, 2500–2501.

---

69   Myelodysplastic syndrome with haemophagocytosis

In the myelodysplastic syndromes an adverse prognosis is associated with:

1) A complex karyotype
2) Del(5q)
3) Del(20q)
4) Monosomy 7
5) −Y

Correct answers 1, 4

An adverse prognosis in MDS is associated with a complex karyotype (more than three abnormalities), monosomy 7, del(7q) and monosomy 5. Certain specific chromosomal rearrangements are also adverse, specifically *KMT2A* rearrangements, t(6;9)(p23;q34.1) and 3q21.3q26.2 abnormalities. A good prognosis is associated with a normal karyotype, del(5q), del(12p), del(20q) and −Y. Trisomy 8 has an intermediate prognostic significance. Only 50% of patients with a diagnosis of MDS show a cytogenetic abnormality but a much higher proportion show gene mutations. Similar to the pattern seen with certain cytogenetic abnormalities, specific gene mutations are associated with morphological abnormalities in MDS. For example, *SF3B1* mutations are common in patients with ring sideroblasts and mutations in *TP53*, *ASXL1*, *RUNX1* and *SRSF2* are all associated with marked granulocyte dysplasia (Della Porta *et al.* 2015). Finally, dysplasia in multiple lineages is associated with an adverse outcome in MDS (Della Porta *et al.* 2015) though this may be confounded by presence of one or more poor-risk gene mutations noted above.

Reference

Della Porta MG, Travaglino E, Boveri E, Ponzoni M, Malcovati L, Papaemmanull E *et al.* (2015) Minimal morphological criteria for defining bone marrow dysplasia: a basis for clinical implementation of WHO classification of myelodysplastic syndromes. *Leukemia*, **29**, 66–75.

> **70** Primary oxalosis

Haematological features of oxalosis can include:

1) A leucoerythroblastic blood film
2) Oxalate crystals, osteoblasts, osteoclasts and multinucleated giant cells in bone marrow aspirates
3) Pancytopenia
4) Susceptibility to myeloid neoplasms
5) Thrombocytopenia

Correct answers 1, 2, 3, 5

Haematological features of oxalosis can include anaemia, thrombocytopenia, pancytopenia and a leucoerythroblastic blood film. There is no susceptibility to neoplasia. The anaemia is multifactorial, attributable to renal failure, hypersplenism and bone marrow fibrosis. When bone marrow can be aspirated, the aspirate can contain refractile oxalate crystals, increased macrophages, osteoblasts and osteoclasts and multinucleated giant cells (Sharma *et al.* 2018). The haematological features of oxalosis become more prominent in patients who are sustained on haemodialysis. In this setting, iron overload has also occurred.

Reference

Sharma S, Rao RN, Pani KC and Paul P (2018) Bone marrow oxalosis: An unusual cause of cytopenia in end-stage renal disease; report of two cases. *Ind J Pathol Microbiol*, **61**, 268–270.

> **71** Acute myeloid leukaemia with inv(3)(q21.3q26.2)

The inv(3)(q21.3q26.2) and t(3;3)(q21.3;q26.2) cytogenetic abnormalities:

1) Are associated with an appreciably better prognosis in MDS than in AML
2) Can occur in myeloid blast crisis of *BCR-ABL1*-positive chronic myeloid leukaemia
3) Can occur in therapy-related AML
4) Lead to formation of a fusion gene that is responsible for leukaemogenesis
5) Permit a diagnosis of MDS in a cytopenic patient without significant dysplasia.

Correct answers 2, 3, 5

These cytogenetic abnormalities occur in *de novo* and therapy-related AML, in MDS and in blast transformation of chronic myeloid leukaemia. Even cases classified as MDS have a poor prognosis. In the 2016 WHO classification, the presence of inv(3) or t(3;3) in a cytopenic patient is sufficient for a diagnosis of MDS, even in the absence of significant dysplasia. The mechanism of leukaemogenesis is dysregulation of *MECOM*, rather than formation of a fusion gene. *GATA2* haploinsufficiency also appears to contribute to this process.

---

72 Autoimmune haemolytic anaemia

Warm autoimmune haemolytic anaemia:

1) Can result from inherited immunodeficiency
2) Causes only extravascular haemolysis
3) Has a recognised association with levodopa therapy
4) Is more common in women than men
5) Is sometimes a complication of allogeneic haemopoietic stem cell transplantation

Correct answers 1, 3, 4, 5

In children and young adults, particularly those who are refractory to therapy, an underlying inherited immunodeficiency with autoimmunity and lymphoproliferation should be considered. These result from germline mutations in a number of genes including *CTLA4*, *LRBA*, *PIK3CD*, *PIK3R1* and *STAT3* gain of function (GOF). *STAT3* mutations can lead to loss of function, implicated in hyperimmunoglobulin E syndrome, or Job syndrome, whereas GOF mutations are associated with immune cytopenias (anaemia, neutropenia, thrombocytopenia), multiorgan autoimmunity (lung, skin, liver, thyroid, pancreas), lymphoproliferation, increased numbers of CD4/CD8 double-negative T cells and hypogammaglobulinaemia (Milner *et al.* 2015). The latter leads to reduction in numbers of T regulatory cells which are important in self-tolerance. The condition shows incomplete penetrance and so may have only minor manifestations or appear to skip a generation completely. A recent 70-year-old patient with a *STAT3* GOF mutation was referred with isolated splenomegaly. Her grandson, aged 10 years, with the same mutation had a history of highly refractory AIHA. This had remitted completely after the introduction of sirolimus which targets the JAK-STAT pathway. Consideration of these conditions is important therefore not only in understanding pathogenesis but also in indicating potential therapeutic options.

Haemolysis in warm AIHA is largely extravascular but in severe cases there can be significant intravascular haemolysis with haemoglobinuria. Therapy with levodopa, and also mefenamic acid and procainamide, can lead to AIHA. Both idiopathic and secondary cases are more common in women. AIHA can follow allogeneic stem cell transplantation (donor antibodies against donor red cells) (O'Brien *et al.* 2004).

References

Milner JD, Vogel TP, Forbes L, Ma CA, Stray-Pedersen A, Niemela JE *et al.* (2015) Early-onset lymphoproliferation and autoimmunity caused by germline STAT3 gain-of-function mutations. *Blood*, **125**, 591–599.

O'Brien TA, Eastlund T, Peters C, Neglia JP, Defor T, Ramsay NKC and Baker KS (2004) Autoimmune haemolytic anaemia complicating haematopoietic cell transplantation in paediatric patients: high incidence and significant mortality in unrelated donor transplants for non-malignant disease. *Br J Haematol*, **127**, 67–75.

---

73 Chronic eosinophilic leukaemia with *FIP1L1-PDGFRA* fusion

---

The most appropriate treatment for the first patient described is:

1) Corticosteroids
2) Imatinib

3) Midostaurin
4) Ruxolitinib
5) Vemurafenib

Correct answer 2

The most appropriate treatment is imatinib or another related tyrosine kinase inhibitor. This can be preceded or accompanied by corticosteroids to reduce the eosinophil count and lessen the chance of cardiac damage. Ruxolitinib could be used for other myeloproliferative neoplasms, midostaurin for systemic mastocytosis and vemurafenib for hairy cell leukaemia or Erdheim–Chester disease with a *BRAF* V600E mutation. Note that although mast cells can be increased in association with *FIP1L1-PDGFRA*, this condition must be distinguished from systemic mastocytosis with a *KIT* mutation, for which the treatment is quite different. Although the eosinophil morphology is usually abnormal, this does not permit reliable differentiation from reactive eosinophilia (Goasguen *et al.* 2020).

The molecular lesion results from a cryptic interstitial deletion at 4q12. This can be detected using molecular analysis or by FISH to show deletion of the *CHIC2* gene, which is within the deleted segment (Chung *et al.* 2006, Bain *et al.* 2017). Cytogenetic analysis is almost always normal but the same disease features occasionally result from a translocation that leads to fusion of *PDGFRA* with another partner.

References

Bain BJ, Horny H-P, Arber DA, Tefferi A and Hasserjian RP (2017) Myeloid/lymphoid neoplasms with eosinophilia and rearrangements of *PDGFRA*, *PDGFRB*, *FGFR1*, or with *PCM1-JAK2*. *In* Swerdlow SH, Campo E, Harris NL, Jaffe ES, Pileri S, Stein H and Thiele J (Eds) *WHO Classification of Tumours of Haematopoietic and Lymphoid Tissues*, revised 4th Edn. IARC Press, Lyon, pp. 71–79.

Chung KF, Hew M, Score J, Jones AV, Reiter A, Cross NC and Bain BJ (2006) Cough and hypereosinophilia due to *FIP1L1-PDGFRA* fusion gene with tyrosine kinase activity. *Eur Respir J*, **27**, 230–232.

Goasguen JE, Bennett JM, Bain BJ, Brunning R, Zini G, Vallespi M-T *et al.*; International Working Group on Morphology of MDS (2020) The role of eosinophil morphology in distinguishing between reactive eosinophilia and eosinophilia as a feature of a myeloid neoplasm. *Br J Haematol*, **191**, 497–504.

---

74 Leukaemic phase of follicular lymphoma

Follicular lymphoma:

1) Can be detected reliably by bone marrow aspiration and immunophenotyping when the bone marrow is infiltrated
2) Consistently shows a translocation involving *BCL2*
3) Is cytologically difficult to distinguish from chronic lymphocytic leukaemia
4) Is of germinal centre origin, as shown by expression of CD19 and CD20
5) Typically shows paratrabecular infiltration in the bone marrow

Correct answer 5

Making a distinction between CLL and follicular lymphoma on the basis of cytology is generally not difficult. In follicular lymphoma, in addition to narrow nuclear clefts in some cells, the cells are often smaller, the cytoplasm is even scantier, the chromatin is more evenly condensed and smear cells are less common. Bone marrow infiltration can be missed on bone marrow aspiration because of focal involvement and increased reticulin deposition in an infiltrated area. A trephine biopsy, which typically shows paratrabecular infiltration, is therefore important if there is a need to know whether or not the marrow is infiltrated. The great majority of cases have a translocation involving *BCL2* and an immunoglobulin locus (heavy chain, kappa or lambda) but a translocation involving *BCL6* is an alternative mechanism of lymphomagenesis (Horsman *et al.* 2003). The germinal centre origin of follicular lymphoma is shown by expression of CD10 and strong BCL2, not by expression of CD19 and CD20, although it should be noted that circulating lymphoma cells do not always show CD10 expression.

Reference

Horsman DE, Okamoto I, Ludkovski O, Le N, Harder L, Gesk S *et al.* (2003) Follicular lymphoma lacking the t(14;18)(q32;q21): identification of two disease subtypes. *Br J Haematol*, **120**, 424–433.

75	Megaloblastic anaemia

Severe megaloblastic anaemia due to vitamin B12 or folate deficiency is characterised by:

1) Dysplastic haemopoiesis
2) Increased conjugated bilirubin
3) Increased macrophage iron
4) Increased reticulocyte count
5) Ineffective haemopoiesis

Correct answers 1, 3, 5.

Haemopoiesis is dysplastic, to the extent that misdiagnosis as a myelodysplastic syndrome has occurred. In addition to the asynchronous maturation of nucleus and cytoplasm that characterises megaloblastic erythropoiesis, erythroid precursors can show nuclear irregularity, detached nuclear fragments and binuclearity, sometimes with two nuclei in a cell having different characteristics. Partially megaloblastic erythropoiesis can be a feature of erythroleukaemia and MDS but the nuclear/cytoplasmic dyssynchrony is not universal and giant metamyelocytes are rarely seen. Haemopoiesis is ineffective, i.e. the bone marrow is hypercellular and yet the production of mature end cells is reduced as a result of intramedullary death of haemopoietic cells. Ineffective haemopoiesis leads to an increase in unconjugated bilirubin but not conjugated. The reticulocyte count is inappropriately low rather than raised. Macrophage iron is typically increased since iron that would previously have been in the haemoglobin of erythrocytes and late erythroblasts is now present in increased amounts in macrophages.

76	Reactive bone marrow and an abnormal PET scan

The erythrocyte sedimentation rate (ESR) is:

1) Consistently increased in multiple myeloma
2) Higher in women than in men and higher still in pregnancy

3) Important in the diagnosis of temporal arteritis
4) Increased by a high plasma fibrinogen
5) Increased in polycythaemia

Correct answers 2, 3, 4

The erythrocyte sedimentation rate was first described by the British surgeon John Hunter (1728–1793) in his posthumous work *A Treatise on the Blood, Inflammation, and Gun-Shot Wounds* (Madrenas *et al.* 2005). It is increased in anaemia and when there is an increase in high molecular weight plasma proteins such as fibrinogen, immunoglobulin, von Willebrand factor and α2 macroglobulin. It is reduced in polycythaemia. Although the ESR is usually increased in multiple myeloma, it may be normal in Bence Jones myeloma and non-secretory myeloma, any increase being due to anaemia. Giant cell arteritis is an inflammatory arteritis of unknown aetiology. It most often affects medium and small arteries including the temporal arteries but can also affect the aorta and other large vessels. An ESR of above 50 mm in 1 h suggests a diagnosis of giant cell arteritis rather than another type of vasculitis (Salvarani *et al.* 2008) and is important in facilitating the rapid diagnosis of temporal arteritis.

References

Madrenas J, Potter P and Cairns E (2005) Giving credit where credit is due: John Hunter and the discovery of erythrocyte sedimentation rate. *Lancet*, **366**, 2140–2141.
Salvarani C, Cantini F and Hunder GG (2008) Polymyalgia rheumatica and giant-cell arteritis. *Lancet*, **372**, 234–245.

---

77 Acute megakaryoblastic leukaemia

Characteristic cytogenetic abnormalities in acute megakaryoblastic leukaemia include:

1) t(1;22)(p13;q13.1)
2) t(3;3)(q21.3;q26.2)
3) t(8;21)(q22;q22.1)
4) t(9;11)(p21.3;a22)
5) t(9;22)(q34.1;q11.2)

Correct answer 1

Only t(1;22) is characteristic of acute megakaryoblastic leukaemia, being often seen in paediatric cases. Some cases of acute myeloid leukaemia with t(3;3) or inv(3) show expression of CD41 or CD61 and the presence of dysplastic megakaryocytes but the leukaemia is usually acute myeloblastic rather than acute megakaryoblastic. t(9;22) is present in megakaryoblastic transformation of chronic myeloid leukaemia but is not characteristic of acute megakaryoblastic leukaemia. t(8;21) and t(9;11) are not associated with this entity.

---

78 Erythrophagocytosis and haemophagocytosis

Diagnostic criteria for haemophagocytic lymphohistiocytosis include:

1) Haemophagocytosis in any organ
2) Increased erythrocyte sedimentation rate

3) Increased plasma fibrinogen
4) Increased serum ferritin
5) Increased serum triglycerides

Correct answers 1, 4, 5

Diagnostic criteria for haemophagocytic lymphohistiocytosis (HLH) include haemophagocytosis, increased ferritin and triglycerides, and low rather than increased fibrinogen (Lehmberg and Ehl 2013). The low fibrinogen can lead to a low ESR. Haemophagocytosis may be infrequent or even not detected in a bone marrow aspirate but the diagnosis can nevertheless be made if enough other criteria are met.

Erythrophagocytosis can be a feature of HLH, with other cells also being phagocytosed, or an isolated phenomenon. It can be a feature of neoplastic cells in certain subtypes of acute myeloid leukaemia or can result from activation of macrophages, when the alternative designation of 'macrophage activation syndrome' is often used. Erythrocyte abnormalities, including an abnormal red cell membrane and binding of immunoglobulin or complement to the membrane, can also be causative. The altered red cell membrane in various forms of sickle cell disease can lead to erythrophagocytosis and, interestingly, the bone marrow of the patient with HLH described also showed occasional examples of phagocytosis of sickled cells (image below ×100 objective). The intact macrophage depicted also contains a nucleated red blood cell. In addition, there is a crushed cell that contains a sickled cell and two morphologically normal erythrocytes.

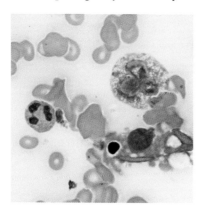

Reference

Lehmberg K and Ehl S (2013) Diagnostic evaluation of patients with suspected haemophagocytic lymphohistiocytosis. *Br J Haematol*, **160**, 275–287.

---

79 Hyposplenism

Hyposplenism is associated with an increased risk of:

1) Autoimmune haemolytic anaemia
2) Babesiosis
3) *Capnocytophaga canimorsus* infection
4) Pneumococcal infection
5) Thrombotic thrombocytopenic purpura

Correct answers 2, 3, 4

The finding of a hyposplenic state indicates that a patient has an increased susceptibility to overwhelming bacterial infection. Vaccinations for meningococcus, pneumococcus and *Haemophilus influenzae* type b should be given and, depending on the circumstances, prophylactic antibiotic therapy may also be advised (Davies *et al.* 2011). The patient should be warned of the risk of malaria, babesiosis (see Theme 44) and dog and cat bites (*Capnocytophaga canimorsus* and *Capnocytophaga cynodegmi* infection) and should be issued with a card to alert health professionals to the hyposplenic state.

Reference

Davies JM, Lewis MP, Wimperis J, Rafi I, Ladhani S and Bolton-Maggs PH (2011) Review of guidelines for the prevention and treatment of infection in patients with an absent or dysfunctional spleen: British Committee for Standards in Haematology. *Br J Haematol*, **155**, 308–317.

80 Acquired haemoglobin H disease

Features that favour acquired rather than inherited haemoglobin H disease include:

1) Dimorphic blood film
2) Dysplasia in non-erythroid lineages
3) Normal number of alpha genes
4) Occurrence in a female
5) Unusually high percentage of haemoglobin H

Correct answers 1, 2, 3, 5

The blood film in acquired haemoglobin H disease is often dimorphic whereas this is not so in the inherited condition. The images below show the blood films of two typical cases of inherited haemoglobin H disease. The left image is from an adult female with RBC 5.0×10^{12}/l, Hb 99 g/l, MCV 66 fl, MCH 20.1 pg and MCHC 300 g/l. The centre image is from an adult female with RBC 4.6×10^{12}/l, Hb 98 g/l, MCV 69 fl, MCH 21.3 pg and MCHC 309 g/l (both images ×100 objective). Both show hypochromia, microcytosis and poikilocytosis. The red cell indices are informative. Note that in contrast to the findings in β thalassaemia trait and in α thalassaemia trait when only one or two alpha genes are deleted, the MCHC is reduced. In contrast to iron deficiency, the RBC is normal. The right image is of HPLC on a Bio-Rad Variant II instrument showing, at the left, the very characteristic early double peak of haemoglobin H. Note also that haemoglobin A_2 is reduced.

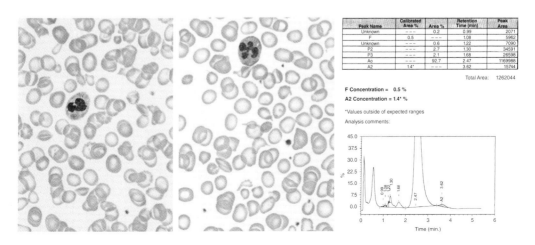

Peak Name	Calibrated Area %	Area %	Retention Time (min)	Peak Area
Unknown	---	0.2	0.99	2071
F	0.5	---	1.08	5962
Unknown	---	0.6	1.22	7090
P2	---	2.7	1.30	34591
P3	---	2.1	1.68	26598
Ao	---	92.7	2.47	1169988
A2	1.4*	---	3.62	15744

Total Area: 1262044

F Concentration = 0.5 %

A2 Concentration = 1.4* %

*Values outside of expected ranges

Analysis comments:

Acquired haemoglobin H disease is associated with a normal number of alpha genes, expression being down regulated. Rarely inherited haemoglobin H disease has a normal number of alpha genes when two of the four genes are mutated, as in $\alpha^{\text{TSaudi}}\alpha/\alpha^{\text{TSaudi}}\alpha$, but a normal number of alpha genes certainly favours the acquired condition (Bain 2020). The inherited condition occurs equally in males and females, whereas more than 90% of acquired cases have been in males so that the occurrence in a female does not favour the acquired condition. The percentage of haemoglobin H in the acquired condition is very variable, from a few percent to as high as 60–65%, whereas in the inherited condition the level is typically around 12–15%.

Reference

Bain BJ (2020) *Haemoglobinopathy Diagnosis*, 3rd Edn. Wiley Blackwell, Oxford, pp. 325–328.

81 Cystinosis

Factors that can contribute to anaemia in cystinosis include:

1) Bone marrow fibrosis
2) Haemolysis
3) Hypersplenism
4) Hyperthyroidism
5) Renal impairment

Correct answers 1, 3, 5

The major cause of anaemia in cystinosis is renal impairment (Elmonem *et al.* 2016). Replacement of haemopoietic marrow by cystine-containing macrophages, hypersplenism and in some cases bone marrow fibrosis can also contribute to anaemia and other cytopenias. Cystinosis can cause hypothyroidism, not hyperthyroidism. Bone marrow trephine biopsies can also occasionally show renal osteodystrophy or osteosclerosis.

Reference

Elmonem M, Veys KR, Soliman NA, van Dyck M, van den Heuvel LP and Levtchenko E (2016) Cystinosis: a review. *Orphanet J Rare Dis*, **11**, 47.

82 Familial platelet disorder with a predisposition to AML

The *RUNX1* gene is involved in:

1) Acute lymphoblastic leukaemia with t(12;21)(p13.2;q22.2)
2) Acute lymphoblastic, myeloid or mixed phenotype leukaemia with t(4;11)(q21;q23.3)
3) Acute myeloid leukaemia with inv(16)(p13.1q22)
4) Acute myeloid leukaemia with t(8;21)(q22;q22.1)
5) The grey platelet syndrome

Correct answers 1, 4

A variety of mutations in *RUNX1* have been described in familial platelet disorder with a predisposition to AML (FPD/AML); there can be a large intragenic deletion, a point mutation or a small deletion or insertion, leading to missense, nonsense or frame shift mutations (Sood *et al.* 2017). The *RUNX1* gene at 21q22.2 is also involved in ALL with t(12;21)(p13.2;q22.1), in which there is an *ETV6-RUNX1* fusion gene, and in AML with t(8;21)(q22;q22.1), in which there is a *RUNX1-RUNX1T1* fusion gene. AML can also be associated with somatic mutation of *RUNX1*, this being a provisional entity in the 2016 WHO classification. The *RUNX1* gene has no involvement in acute leukaemias with t(4;11) or inv(16). There can be a proportion of 'grey' platelets in FPD/AML due to reduction in alpha granules but the grey platelet syndrome is the result of an *NBEAL2* mutation. In addition to *RUNX1*, mutations in *ANKRD26* and *ETV6* are also responsible for platelet disorders with germline predisposition to myeloid neoplasms (Galera *et al.* 2019).

References

Galera P, Dulau-Florea A and Calvo KR (2019) Inherited thrombocytopenia and platelet disorders with germline predisposition to myeloid neoplasia. *Int J Lab Haematol*, **41** (Suppl 1), 131–141.

Sood R, Kamikubo Y and Liu P (2017) Role of RUNX1 in hematological malignancies. *Blood*, **129**, 2070–2082.

---

83   Nodular lymphocyte predominant Hodgkin lymphoma

Nodular lymphocyte predominant Hodgkin lymphoma:

1) Can relapse as diffuse large B-cell lymphoma
2) Differs from classical Hodgkin lymphoma in that the neoplastic cells have a more clearly B-lineage immunophenotype
3) Is often related to the Epstein–Barr virus
4) Shows an increased incidence in family members
5) Usually shows expression of CD15 and CD30

Correct answers 1, 2, 4

The neoplastic cells of nodular lymphocyte predominant Hodgkin lymphoma have a germinal centre B-cell immunophenotype: CD45+, CD20+, CD75+, CD79a+, PAX5+, OCT2+ and BCL6+ but they do not express CD10 or CD15 and only rarely express weak CD30. In contrast, the neoplastic cells of classical Hodgkin lymphoma less often express CD45 and B-cell markers and expression may be weaker, whereas they do express CD15 and CD30. Classical Hodgkin lymphoma is quite often related to the Epstein–Barr virus but this is true of only a small minority of cases of the lymphocyte predominant disease. Transformation to diffuse large B-cell lymphoma can occur. There is an increased incidence in family members (Saarinen *et al.* 2011, 2013).

It is important that this entity is distinguished from T cell/histiocyte-rich B-cell lymphoma (see Theme 50) and classical Hodgkin lymphoma (see Theme 30). A common feature to all three of these conditions is the relatively small number of neoplastic cells, which need to be identified within the reactive environment around them. The type of reaction encountered can also inform the diagnosis. It should be noted that bone marrow examination is not necessarily indicated in this condition but was done in the present patient because of the cytopenias.

References

Saarinen S, Vahteristo P, Launonen V, Franssila K, Kivirikko S, Lehtonen R *et al.* (2011) Analysis of *KLHDC8B* in familial nodular lymphocyte predominant Hodgkin lymphoma. *Br J Haematol*, **154**, 413–415.

Saarinen S, Pukkala E, Vahteristo P, Mäkinen MJ, Franssila K and Aaltonen LA (2013) High familial risk in nodular lymphocyte-predominant Hodgkin lymphoma. *J Clin Oncol*, **31**, 938–943.

---

84   Acute monocytic leukaemia with *NPM1* mutation

NPM1-mutated AML:

1) According to the WHO classification, can be therapy-related
2) Cannot be diagnosed if multilineage dysplasia is present
3) Is often associated with unbalanced chromosomal rearrangement
4) Shows aberrant cytoplasmic expression of NPM1
5) Shows a specific association with cup-shaped nuclei

Correct answer 4

By definition, *NPM1*-mutated AML occurs *de novo*, therapy-related cases with mutation of this gene not being included in this category in the WHO classification. Multilineage dysplasia is present in a significant proportion of cases and does not preclude the diagnosis. The great majority of cases have a normal karyotype. The NPM1 protein (nucleophosmin) is normally expressed in the nucleus, particularly the nucleolus; the cytoplasmic location when mutation is present can serve as a surrogate marker for this subtype of AML. There is a strong association with cup-shaped nuclei but the association is not specific.

---

85   Adult T-cell leukaemia/lymphoma

Human lymphotropic virus 1 (HTLV-1):

1) In carriers, is associated with a low percentage of atypical lymphocytes with lobulated nuclei
2) Is endemic in Japan and the Caribbean
3) Is not transmitted by breastfeeding so antenatal screening is not important
4) Is the cause of tropical spastic paraparesis
5) Leads to immunodeficiency

Correct answers 1, 2, 4, 5

Human lymphotropic virus 1 (HTLV-1), the causative agent of ATLL, is endemic in Japan, the Caribbean, several foci in South America (including northern Brazil, Colombia, Guyana), some areas of Africa (South Africa, Nigeria, Sierra Leone, Gambia, Central Africa), the Philippines, Papua New Guinea, Vanuatu, Romania, Taiwan, the Fujian province of China, in some areas of the Middle East including the Khorasan province of Iran, and in Inuit, Amerindians and Australian aboriginals (European Centre for Disease Prevention and Control 2015). HTLV-1 is the cause of tropical spastic paraparesis, now more often designated HTLV-1-associated myelopathy. Individuals who carry the virus can also develop neuropathy, uveitis, pneumonitis, polymyositis, thyroiditis, hepatitis, arthropathy, alveolitis (with T-cell infiltration), Sjögren syndrome and immune suppression. Transmission is transplacentally, by breastfeeding, by sexual intercourse and by blood transfusion. Blood donors in the United Kingdom are screened for HTLV-1 but as yet there is no screening of antenatal patients, whereas such screening is established practice in Japan.

The images below (×100 objective) are from a 41-year-old Afro-Caribbean woman with HTLV-1-associated myelopathy. Her FBC showed WBC 6.7×10^9/l, Hb 112 g/l, lymphocyte count 2.8×10^9/l and platelet count 92×10^9/l. The small lymphocyte with a lobulated nucleus seen in the left image is typical of the cells that are seen, in low numbers, in carriers of this virus. It is less usual to see larger, more pleomorphic cells as shown in the right image.

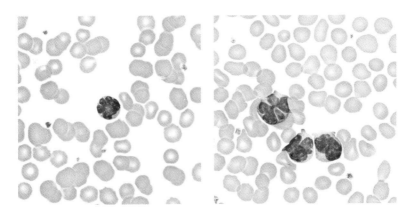

Reference

European Centre for Disease Prevention and Control (2015) Geographical distribution of areas with a high prevalence of HTLV-1 infection. https://ecdc.europa.eu/sites/portal/files/media/en/publications/Publications/geographical-distribution-areas-high-prevalence-HTLV1.pdf

---

86 Hereditary elliptocytosis and pyropoikilocytosis

Hereditary pyropoikilocytosis:

1) Can result from coinheritance in *cis* to a mutation that usually causes hereditary elliptocytosis and an α spectrin low expression allele, α spectrin[Lely]
2) In the neonatal period, can be confused with hereditary elliptocytosis
3) Is more severe in the neonatal period than later in life
4) Is uniformly associated with hereditary elliptocytosis in both parents
5) Shows reduced eosin-5-maleimide (EMA) binding

Correct answers 2, 3, 5

Hereditary pyropoikilocytosis (HPP) is genetically heterogeneous. Hereditary elliptocytosis may be apparent in one or both parents or neither. It is co-inheritance in *trans* to a mutation that usually causes hereditary elliptocytosis and α spectrin[Lely] that can lead to HPP; co-inheritance in *cis* actually ameliorates the phenotype of hereditary elliptocytosis. The condition can be more severe in the neonatal period, attributed to haemoglobin F binding 2,3-DPG less well than does haemoglobin A, with the free 2,3-DPG weakening spectrin–actin interactions. Hereditary elliptocytosis can similarly be more severe in the neonatal period, leading to the possibility of it being confused with HPP. EMA binding is best known as a test for hereditary spherocytosis but in fact it is also reduced in HPP.

---

87 Sézary syndrome

On immunophenotyping, Sézary cells show:

1) Consistent expression of CD7
2) Expression of CD3
3) Expression of CD4
4) No expression of CD26
5) Usually expression of CD8

Correct answers 2, 3, 4

Characteristically, immunophenotyping shows expression of CD3 and CD4. CD8 is not expressed and, as with many lymphomas of mature T cells, CD7 expression is often lost. There can be expression of CD2 and CD5. There is also expression of CD279 (PD-1). In contrast to activated T cells, there is no expression of CD26. A CD4+, CD7−, CD26− phenotype can thus be useful in making a distinction from an inflammatory erythroderma and in identifying low level disease in the blood. Sézary syndrome was previously regarded as a leukaemic form of mycosis fungoides but they are now considered to be separate entities, with Sézary syndrome being derived from a circulating central memory T cell and mycosis fungoides from a skin-resident memory T cell (Whittaker *et al.* 2017).

Reference

Whittaker SJ, Cerroni L and Willemze R (2017) Sézary syndrome. *In* Swerdlow SH, Campo E, Harris NL, Jaffe ES, Pileri S, Stein H and Thiele J (Eds) *WHO Classification of Tumours of Haematopoietic and Lymphoid Tissues*, revised 4th Edn. IARC Press, Lyon, pp. 390–391.

---

88 Spherocytic red cell disorders

Microspherocytes can be a feature of the blood film in:

1) Burns
2) Hereditary pyropoikilocytosis
3) Mechanical haemolytic anaemia
4) Pyrimidine 5′ nucleotidase deficiency
5) Thrombotic thrombocytopenic purpura

Correct answers 1, 2, 3, 5

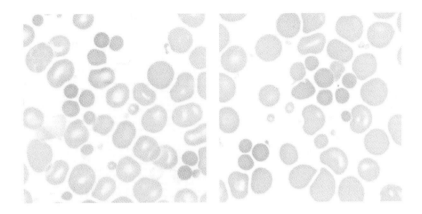

Microspherocytes are red cell fragments, hence the name spheroschistocyte is also sometimes used. They can be a feature of microangiopathic haemolytic anaemia, as in the haemolytic uraemic syndromes and thrombotic thrombocytopenic purpura. They can also result from fragmentation in large vessels or in relation to defective prosthetic valves within the heart in mechanical haemolytic anaemia. In the case of hereditary pyropoikilocytosis the red cell fragmentation is a result of the very abnormal red cell membrane (see also Theme 86). Unique features are seen in thermal burns. The images above (×100 objective) are from the blood film of a patient with severe burns. In this case, the microspherocytes are formed by budding off of part of the red cell, as can be seen bottom right in the left image. There can also be budding of red cell fragments that retain their disc shape and their central pallor, as is very evident in the right image, which shows three microdiscocytes. The history of burns is normally self-evident but for the morphologist the features are almost diagnostic and due to the extent of heat exposure necessary to cause them they certainly carry prognostic significance; similar features can be seen when a blood specimen has been accidentally heated before arrival in the laboratory. Interestingly, hereditary pyropoikilocytosis, in which microspherocytes are just one of several types of poikilocyte present, shows increased heat sensitivity *in vitro*, hence the name of the condition.

The spherocyte and the microspherocyte are therefore easily recognised morphological forms, with somewhat different diagnostic significance. As in all aspects of haematology, the true significance depends on a full evaluation of all clinical and laboratory information. The scenarios highlighted here offer examples of where the recognition of such cells can have important diagnostic and therapeutic implications.

---

89 Acute myeloid leukaemia and metastatic carcinoma

Bone marrow infiltration by prostatic cancer can be associated with:

1) Cytokeratin expression
2) Fibrosis
3) Haemophagocytic syndrome
4) Intravascular infiltration
5) Osteosclerosis

Correct answers 1, 2, 5

Infiltration of the bone marrow by prostatic carcinoma can have associated fibrosis and osteosclerosis with a leucoerythroblastic blood film. Haemophagocytosis and intravascular infiltration are not features. Cytokeratin is expressed but more specific markers are prostate-specific antigen and prostate-specific acid phosphatase. Identification of the primary site of a metastatic tumour is important for the choice of therapy.

---

90   Chédiak–Higashi syndrome

Abnormally large neutrophil granules can be a feature of:

1) Acute myeloid leukaemia
2) Chronic neutrophilic leukaemia
3) May–Hegglin anomaly
4) Mucopolysaccharidoses (Alder–Reilly anomaly)
5) Myelodysplastic syndrome

Correct answers 1, 4, 5

Giant neutrophil granules, designated pseudo-Chédiak–Higashi granules, are sometimes seen in acute myeloid leukaemia (Abdulsalam *et al.* 2011) (see also Theme 3). Rarely, similar granules are seen in myelodysplastic syndromes. Chronic neutrophilic leukaemia (see Theme 18) is characterised by strongly staining granules but these are of normal size. Various mucopolysaccharidoses can have large as well as strongly staining granules. The May–Hegglin anomaly (see Theme 95) and other MYH9-related disorders have abnormal cytoplasmic inclusions but granules are normal.

Reference

Abdulsalam AH, Sabeeh N and Bain BJ (2011) Pseudo-Chédiak–Higashi inclusions together with Auer rods in acute myeloid leukemia. *Am J Hematol*, **86**, 602.

---

91   Cortical T-lymphoblastic leukaemia/lymphoma

Cortical T-lymphoblastic leukaemia/lymphoma:

1) Can have a normal blood count
2) Is associated with a better prognosis than other subtypes of T lymphoblastic leukaemia/lymphoma
3) Is defined by expression of CD1a and CD3
4) Is now often classified as early T-cell precursor lymphoblastic leukaemia
5) Usually shows loss of expression of CD7

Correct answers 1, 2, 3

Cortical T-lymphoblastic lymphoma is thought to arise in a thymic T-cell precursor with secondary involvement of the bone marrow in T-lymphoblastic leukaemia. The leukaemic cells typically show a cCD3+, CD7+, CD5+, CD2+, CD1a+ immunophenotype with the expression of

CD1a by leukaemic cells of T lineage being the defining characteristic. Surface membrane CD3 may be positive or negative. CD7 expression is often lost in neoplasms of mature T cells (with the exception of T-prolymphocytic leukaemia) but is retained by leukaemic T lymphoblasts. Some cases show early differentiation toward CD4 or CD8 (second case), some show both CD4 and CD8 expression (first case) and some neither (third case). Cases expressing CD1a are not now reclassified as early T-cell precursor lymphoblastic leukaemia, although some cases once designated pro-T or pre-T ALL are reclassified. The thymic origin explains the mediastinal mass which is frequently present and which may influence early patient management in cases with superior vena cava obstruction or pericardial or pleural effusions. The thymic origin also explains why the blood count is sometimes normal, as exemplified by the second and third patients. The prognosis is generally better that that of other subtypes of T-lymphoblastic leukaemia/lymphoma (Schabath *et al.* 2003, Marks *et al.* 2009). As noted here, therapeutic fluid aspirations can also yield a rapid diagnosis when a mediastinal mass biopsy would be difficult or dangerous and when a general anaesthetic for a directly visualised biopsy is contraindicated. Note that despite the poorly preserved morphology in the latter two cases, flow cytometry was able to accurately identify the tumour cells and the early introduction of corticosteroids with chemotherapy was then possible.

References

Marks DI, Paietta EM, Moorman AV, Richards SM, Buck G, DeWald G *et al.* (2009) T-cell acute lymphoblastic leukemia in adults: clinical features, immunophenotype, cytogenetics, and outcome from the large randomized prospective trial (UKALLXII/ECOG2993). *Blood*, **114**, 5136–5145.
Schabath R, Ratei R and Ludwig W-D (2003) The prognostic significance of antigen expression in leukemia. *Best Pract Res Clin Haematol*, **16**, 613–628.

---

92 Trypanosomiasis

Trypanosoma brucei infection:

1) Can cause disseminated intravascular coagulation
2) Causes eosinophilia
3) Is the cause of African sleeping sickness
4) Is transmitted by mosquitoes
5) Typically causes chronic cardiomyopathy

Correct answers 1, 3

Trypanosoma brucei is the cause of African sleeping sickness, a serious condition that occurs in 36 countries in sub-Saharan Africa (Centers for Disease Control and Prevention 2020, World Health Organization 2020). This condition is more acute with *Trypanosoma brucei rhodesiense* infection (in East Africa) than with *Trypanosoma brucei gambiense* infection (in West and Central Africa). Typically there is fever, headache and malaise and, in West African cases, lymphadenopathy; the more severe East African cases can be complicated by disseminated intravascular coagulation. The disease progresses to meningoencephalitis, which is fatal if untreated. The incidence of trypanosomiasis has declined markedly in East Africa in recent decades.

Trypanosomes are not among the parasites that cause eosinophilia. They are transmitted by the tsetse fly, not by mosquitoes. It is *T. cruzi* infection (Chagas disease) that typically causes chronic cardiomyopathy, although cardiac damage can also occur with *T. brucei*.

Given the serious consequences of these diseases, the recognition of the parasites by the laboratory and diagnosis early in the course of the disease are of considerable importance. The organisms are motile and may be observed in a wet buffy coat preparation, as well as in stained blood films. For *Trypanosoma brucei gambiense*, which is now the cause of the great majority of cases, serological tests are also available.

References

Centers for Disease Control and Prevention (2020) Parasites – African trypanosomiasis (also known as sleeping sickness). https://www.cdc.gov/parasites/sleepingsickness/index.html

World Health Organization (2020) Trypanosomiasis, human African (sleeping sickness). https://www.who.int/news-room/fact-sheets/detail/trypanosomiasis-human-african-(sleeping-sickness)

---

93 Acute myeloid leukaemia with myelodysplasia-related changes

The WHO category of acute myeloid leukaemia with myelodysplasia-related changes (AML-MRC) can be diagnosed in a patient with:

1) AML with complex cytogenetic abnormalities following previous treatment of Hodgkin lymphoma with combination chemotherapy
2) AML with erythroid and granulocytic dysplasia, monosomy 7 and del(5q).
3) AML with t(3;3)(q21.3;q26.2) with erythroid dysplasia, micromegakaryocytes and multinucleated megakaryocytes
4) AML with t(6;9)(p23;q34.1) with erythroid and granulocytic dysplasia, Auer rods and increased basophils
5) Pancytopenia with 15% bone marrow blast cells, some with Auer rods, with bilineage dysplasia

Correct answer 2

It is important to note that AML with certain specified recurrent cytogenetic abnormalities, including t(6;9)(p23;q34.1) (see Theme 97), t(3;3)(q21.3;q26.2) and inv(3)(q21.3q26.2) (see Theme 71), often shows multilineage dysplasia but such cases are classified as acute myeloid leukaemia with recurrent genetic abnormalities. Similarly, cases that would otherwise meet the criteria for AML-MRC but with previous exposure to leukaemogenic drugs are categorised as therapy-related myeloid neoplasms. Importantly, these patients are also eligible for therapy with CPX-351. The existence of multilineage dysplasia, at the time of diagnosis of AML, needs to be interpreted in the light of all the available clinical and laboratory information, thus permitting a fully integrated report. The patient described in option 5 has a myelodysplastic syndrome with excess of blasts 2 rather than AML.

---

94 Blastic plasmacytoid dendritic cell neoplasm

Blastic plasmacytoid dendritic cell neoplasm:

1) Can be associated with myelodysplastic features
2) Can have cytoplasmic tails and vacuolation among the cytological features

3) Is likely to be derived from a lymphoid stem cell
4) Often has complex karyotypic abnormalities
5) Usually shows expression of CD34 and TdT

Correct answers 1, 2, 4

Blastic plasmacytoid dendritic cell neoplasm is derived from a myeloid rather than lymphoid stem cell. There can be associated myelodysplastic features and evolution to CMML and AML can occur. The presence of cytoplasmic tails, although not seen in this patient, can be a helpful diagnostic feature (Fernandes *et al.* 2018); this feature is more often observed in the bone marrow than in the blood (bone marrow image below, ×100 objective). CD34 is usually negative and TdT is not expressed whilst complex karyotypic abnormalities are common.

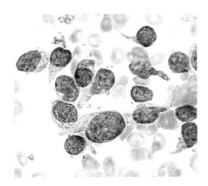

Reference

Fernandes F, Barreira R, Cortez J, Silveira M and Bain BJ (2018) The distinctive cytology and disease evolution of blastic plasmacytoid dendritic cell neoplasm. *Am J Hematol*, **93**, 1431–1432.

---

95 Inherited macrothrombocytopenias

In inherited thrombocytopenias:

1) Grey platelets result from a reduction of alpha granules
2) Macrothrombocytopenia is anticipated in the Wiskott–Aldrich syndrome
3) *MYH9*-related disorders can be reliably detected by a search for Döhle-like inclusions in leucocytes
4) Platelets are of normal size when thrombocytopenia represents the presentation of Fanconi anaemia or dyskeratosis congenita
5) Platelet size may be underestimated by automated instruments

Correct answers 1, 4, 5

It is essential to carefully assess the blood film in every patient presenting with thrombocytopenia. The latter needs to be confirmed because spuriously low counts can arise with EDTA-induced platelet clumping and from neutrophil satellitism and phagocytosis of platelets. When platelets are large, their numbers tend to be underestimated by automated analysers as they are misinterpreted as red cells in the impedance channel; an optical platelet count acquired from the reticulocyte channel will give a more accurate count. The platelet size may be similarly underestimated.

When large platelets are identified, particularly when the thrombocytopenia is longstanding and associated with a bleeding tendency, a number of inherited disorders need to be considered. It is important that the possibility is recognised and targeted investigations are undertaken using platelet aggregation, flow cytometry and genetic studies. This allows optimal management of the particular condition but should also prevent inappropriate therapy. The images below (×100 objective) are from a patient who was thought to have an immune thrombocytopenia but this appeared refractory to multiple lines of therapy; this resulted in a splenectomy. The post-splenectomy film showed macrothrombocytopenia and the neutrophils have clear Döhle-like inclusions, in keeping with the May–Hegglin anomaly. The presence of inclusions in neutrophils is an important clue to the diagnosis of MYH9-related disorders. However, it should be noted that sometimes these are not detectable in a blood film, even though they are detectable by immunofluorescence and are apparent on ultrastructural examination (Sun *et al.* 2013, Balduini and Pecci 2020). Inherited thrombocytopenia is often associated with large platelets but when the cause is a bone marrow failure syndrome they are of normal size and in the Wiskott–Aldrich syndrome they are small.

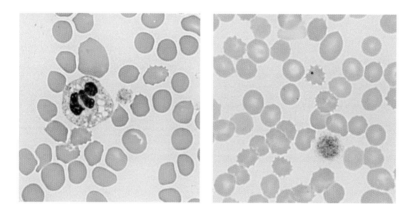

References

Balduini CL and Pecci A (2020) Inherited thrombocytopenias. *In* Invernizzi R (Ed) *Haematologica Atlas on Hematologic Cytology*. Ferrata-Storti Foundation, Pavia, pp. 237–247.

Sun XH, Wang ZY, Yang HY, Cao LJ, Su J, Yu ZQ *et al.* (2013) Clinical, pathological, and genetic analysis of ten patients with MYH9-related disease. *Acta Haematol*, **129**, 106–113.

---

96 Persistent polyclonal B-cell lymphocytosis

Persistent polyclonal B-cell lymphocytosis:

1) Can evolve into chronic lymphocytic leukaemia
2) Can have acquired chromosomal abnormalities
3) Can involve the bone marrow
4) Characteristically occurs in elderly male cigarette smokers
5) Shows an increase of polyclonal IgM

Correct answers 2, 3, 5

Persistent polyclonal B-cell lymphocytosis typically occurs in young and middle-aged female cigarette smokers (Callet-Bauchu *et al.* 2000, Feugier *et al.* 2004, del Giudice *et al.* 2009, Cornet *et al.* 2016). The second patient described in this theme was a 45-year-old female smoker who subsequently died of lung cancer some 7 years later. There is an association with HLA-DR7. Familial cases have been reported. Clinical features sometimes include lymphadenopathy and splenomegaly and there can be interstitial and intrasinusoidal bone marrow infiltration. The immunophenotype is that of a CD27+, IgD+, IgM+ memory B cell. There is no relationship to CLL. This is a curious condition since, although the cells are polyclonal, there can be oligoclonal *BCL2*/IGH rearrangements and not only can there be an acquired cytogenetic abnormality but the same abnormality can be present in both kappa-expressing and lambda-expressing B cells. These abnormalities can include iso(3)(q), dup(3)(q26q29) and trisomy 3. The blood film shows pleomorphic lymphocytes with lobulated, binucleated and occasionally trinucleated cells. These features are very distinctive, since binucleated lymphocytes are very uncommon in any other circumstance, and permit the diagnosis to be predicted.

References

Callet-Bauchu E, Gazzo S, Poncet C, Pages J, Morel D, Alliot C *et al.* (2000) Distinct chromosome 3 abnormalities in persistent polyclonal B-cell lymphocytosis. *Genes Chromosomes Cancer*, **26**, 221–228.

Cornet E, Mossafa H, Courel K, Lesesve J-F and Troussard X (2016) Persistent polyclonal binucleated B-cell lymphocytosis and MECOM gene amplification. *BMC Res Notes*, **9**, 138.

Del Giudice I, Pileri SA, Rossi M, Sabattini E, Campidelli C, Della Starza I *et al.* (2009) Histopathological and molecular features of persistent polyclonal B-cell lymphocytosis (PPBL) with progressive splenomegaly. *Br J Haematol*, **144**, 726–731.

Feugier P, De March AK, Lesesve JF, Monhoven N, Dorvaux V, Braun F *et al.* (2004) Intravascular bone marrow accumulation in persistent polyclonal lymphocytosis: a misleading feature for B-cell neoplasm. *Mod Pathol*, **17**, 1087–1096.

---

97 Acute myeloid leukaemia with t(6;9)(p23;q34.1)

Acute myeloid leukaemia with t(6;9)(p23;q34.1):

1) Can be therapy-related
2) Can occur *de novo* or follow MDS
3) Generally has a good prognosis
4) Often has *FLT3*-ITD
5) Often shows basophilic differentiation

Correct answers 1, 2, 4, 5

Acute myeloid leukaemia with t(6;9)(p23;q34.1) resulting in *DEK-NUP214* is a rare subtype of AML, accounting for only around 1% of cases, which carries a poor prognosis. It is associated with multilineage dysplasia and often shows basophilic as well as neutrophilic differentiation. *FLT3*-ITD is often present. A high white cell count at diagnosis is an additional adverse feature. In the WHO classification, therapy-related cases are categorised as a therapy-related myeloid neoplasm. However, cases following MDS or having myelodysplasia-related changes are assigned to the category of AML with recurrent genetic abnormality rather than AML with myelodysplasia-related changes.

On recognition of this entity it is important to realise that allogeneic stem cell transplantation is necessary and that this should be planned at an early stage but also that remission status is key to a successful outcome (Diaz-Beyá *et al.* 2020). This patient's clinical course illustrates the importance of the integration of morphological, cytogenetic and molecular data in planning treatment when standard chemotherapy-based approaches have failed. Post-transplant, the patient remains well and in remission and on the basis of recent approvals will continue gilteritinib maintenance therapy for a period of 2 years.

Reference

Diaz-Beyá M, Labopin M, Maertens J, Alijurf M, Passweg J, Dietrich B *et al.*; Acute Leukaemia Working Party (ALWP) of the European Society for Blood and Marrow Transplantation (EBMT) (2020) Allogeneic stem cell transplantation in AML with t(6;9)(p23;q34); *DEK-NUP214* shows a favourable outcome when performed in first complete remission. *Br J Haematol*, **189**, 920–925.

98	B-cell prolymphocytic leukaemia

B-cell prolymphocytic leukaemia (B-PLL):

1) Can evolve from chronic lymphocytic leukaemia
2) If associated with t(8;14)(q24;q32), is likely to actually be Burkitt lymphoma
3) If associated with t(11;14)(q13;q32), is likely to actually be mantle cell lymphoma
4) Shows nuclear expression of cyclin D1
5) Usually shows weak or absent CD200 expression

Correct answers 3, 5

B-prolymphocytic leukaemia is a rare mature B-cell lymphoproliferative disorder characterised by a leukaemic presentation with marked splenomegaly. Significant lymphadenopathy is rarely present. B-PLL has no relationship to chronic lymphocytic leukaemia, although smaller numbers of prolymphocytes can be present in CLL. CD200, which is expressed in CLL, is usually weak or negative. Cases with t(11;14)(q13;q32), previously diagnosed as B-PLL, are now considered to be mantle cell lymphoma; the lack of expression of cyclin D1 and SOX11 in B-PLL helps to make the distinction when there is cytological similarity. Unexpectedly, t(8;14)(q24;q32), bringing *MYC* into proximity to the IGH locus, is found in B-PLL as well as in Burkitt lymphoma and does not preclude a diagnosis of B-PLL (Chapiro *et al.* 2019). There is often deletion of the short arm of chromosome 17p and this, with the consequent loss of one allele of *TP53*, largely explains the refractory nature of this disease to chemotherapy. The prognosis is worse if there is *MYC* translocation as well as loss of *TP53* (Chapiro *et al.* 2019).

Reference

Chapiro E, Pramil E, Diop M, Roos-Weil D, Dillard C, Gabillaud C *et al.* (2019) Genetic characterization of B-cell prolymphocytic leukemia: a prognostic model involving *MYC* and *TP53*. *Blood*, **134**, 1821–1831.

99 Various red cell enzyme disorders

Basophilic stippling:

1) Is characteristic of heavy metal poisoning
2) Is often seen in β thalassaemia heterozygosity
3) Leads to a positive Perls stain
4) Represents aggregates of ribosomes
5) Represents ectopically sited DNA

Correct answers 1, 2, 4

Basophilic stippling results from aggregation of ribosomes. It is a common non-specific finding but, when prominent, should lead to suspicion of lead poisoning or deficiency of pyrimidine 5′ nucleotidase, an enzyme responsible for RNA degradation. Toxicity of other heavy metals – arsenic, bismuth, zinc, silver and mercury – can also be responsible.

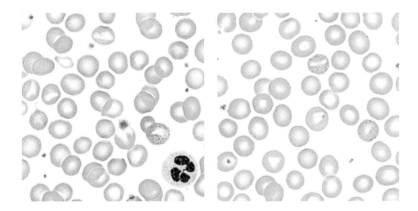

The images above (×100 objective) are from a 10-year-old autistic boy presenting with a chronic non-haemolytic anaemia (Hb 100 g/l, MCV 70 fl), irritability and constipation. Haematinic assays were normal and he had no clinical or laboratory features of systemic infective or inflammatory disease. His blood film showed numerous red cells with basophilic stippling. This prompted a serum lead assay which confirmed a diagnosis of lead poisoning.

Lead toxicity can have many important systemic consequences. In haematology practice it generates an acquired red cell enzymopathy as it binds to sulphhydryl groups on a number of important enzymes but particularly affects the activity in the enzymes involved in haem biosynthesis, generating elevated levels of zinc protoporphyrin. Lead poisoning can be an elusive diagnosis as the symptoms tend to be variable, vague and non-specific; the haematological component and the characteristic microcytic/normocytic anaemia with a film showing basophilic stippling can be a useful diagnostic pointer; haemolytic anaemia can also occur. As lead was traditionally added to paint to improve the intensity and durability of colour (particularly yellow) this can potentially be a source of toxicity. It is suspected that some classical artists, Caravaggio included, might have been afflicted by lead toxicity from their constant exposure to lead-based paints, particularly when using their lips to create a 'point' on the brush. In the modern age one should also be aware that lead is sometimes contained in alternative medications, for example in traditional Tibetan and Indian medicine (Saper *et al.* 2008). Lead poisoning has also resulted from lead added to illegal opium to make it heavier (Helmich and Lock 2018).

References

Helmich F and Lock G (2018) Burton's line from chronic lead intoxication. *N Engl J Med*, **379**, e35.

Saper RB, Phillips RS, Sehgal A, Khouri N, Davis RB, Paquin J *et al.* (2008) Lead, mercury, and arsenic in US- and Indian-manufactured ayurvedic medicines sold via the Internet. *JAMA*, **300**, 915–923.

---

100   Sea-blue histiocytosis in multiple myeloma

Sea-blue histiocytes in the bone marrow can be a feature of:

1) Autoimmune thrombocytopenia
2) Chronic myeloid leukaemia
3) Gaucher disease
4) Niemann–Pick disease
5) Sickle cell anaemia

Correct answers 1, 2, 4, 5

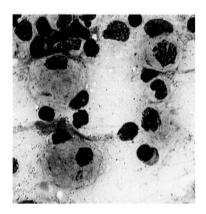

Sea-blue histiocytes (above image ×100 objective) are bone marrow macrophages that acquire this striking cytoplasmic colour on Romanowsky staining as a result of accumulation of ceroid, also known as lipofuscin. This can be the result of an inherited abnormality, resulting from mutation in the apolipoprotein E gene or as a feature of Fabry syndrome or Hermansky–Pudlak syndrome. Sea-blue histiocytes occur in Niemann–Pick disease, in addition to foamy macrophages, but are not a feature of Gaucher disease. More often they result from ingestion of cellular material in a primary bone marrow disorder or with a disturbance of lipid metabolism. They have typically been described in myeloproliferative neoplasms (chronic myeloid leukaemia in particular), myelodysplastic syndromes, lymphoma, autoimmune thrombocytopenia, sickle cell anaemia, multiple myeloma, in lipid disorders and following parenteral feeding with lipid emulsions. Since the inherited causes are rare, the observation of sea-blue histiocytes should alert the morphologist to the likely presence of a primary haematological disorder.

101   Enteropathy-associated T-cell lymphoma

Haematological abnormalities in coeliac disease can result from:

1) Copper deficiency
2) Folic acid deficiency
3) Hyposplenism
4) Refractory iron deficiency anaemia
5) Vitamin B12 deficiency

Correct answers 1, 2, 3, 4, 5

All of these are recognised complications of coeliac disease that produce haematological abnormalities. Those most often seen are hyposplenism (as exemplified by this patient), refractory iron deficiency anaemia and folic acid deficiency. In addition, vitamin K deficiency can lead to haemorrhagic manifestations.

Index

Page numbers in *italics* denote figures; those in **bold** denote a table

Haematology: From the Image to the Diagnosis, First Edition. Mike Leach and Barbara J. Bain.
© 2022 John Wiley & Sons Ltd. Published 2022 by John Wiley & Sons Ltd.